T0293724

Stroke: Pathophysiology, Diagnosis and Management

Stroke: Pathophysiology, Diagnosis and Management

Editor: Robin Deaver

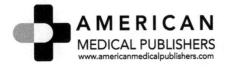

AMERICAN
MEDICAL PUBLISHERS
www.americanmedicalpublishers.com

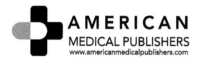

Cataloging-in-Publication Data

Stroke : pathophysiology, diagnosis and management / edited by Robin Deaver.
    p. cm.
Includes bibliographical references and index.
ISBN 978-1-63927-812-1
1. Cerebrovascular disease. 2. Cerebrovascular disease--Pathophysiology. 3. Cerebrovascular disease--Diagnosis.
4. Cerebrovascular disease--Treatment. 5. Brain--Diseases. 6. Neglect (Neurology). I. Deaver, Robin.
RC388.5 .S873 2023
616.81--dc23

American Medical Publishers,
41 Flatbush Avenue,
1st Floor, New York,
NY 11217, USA

ISBN 978-1-63927-812-1 (Hardback)

Contents

Permissions

List of Contributors

Index

Preface

A stroke refers to a medical condition in which there is insufficient blood flow to the brain that leads to cell death. There are two types of stroke, namely, hemorrhagic and ischemic. Hemorrhagic stroke is caused by bleeding, whereas ischemic stroke is caused by a lack of blood flow. High blood pressure is the most important risk factor of stroke. Modifiable and non-modifiable risk factors for stroke are influenced by genetics. The genetic risk is proportional to an individual's gender, age and race. A variety of genetic mechanisms can improve the risk of stroke. Doppler ultrasound, a neurological assessment like NIHSS, arteriography, and MRI scans or CT scans are used to diagnose strokes. If an ischemic stroke is identified within first three to four hours, it can be treated with a medication which can break down the clot. However, surgery is helpful in the case of some hemorrhagic strokes. This book is compiled in such a manner, that it will provide in-depth knowledge about the pathophysiology, diagnosis and management of strokes. It aims to shed light on some of the unexplored aspects of this medical condition. Those in search of information to further their knowledge will be greatly assisted by this book.

This book unites the global concepts and researches in an organized manner for a comprehensive understanding of the subject. It is a ripe text for all researchers, students, scientists or anyone else who is interested in acquiring a better knowledge of this dynamic field.

I extend my sincere thanks to the contributors for such eloquent research chapters. Finally, I thank my family for being a source of support and help.

Editor

Effectiveness of Platelet Function Analysis-Guided Aspirin and/or Clopidogrel Therapy in Preventing Secondary Stroke

Ann-Rong Yan [1], Mark Naunton [1], Gregory M. Peterson [1,2], Israel Fernandez-Cadenas [3] and Reza Mortazavi [1,4,*]

[1] School of Health Sciences, Faculty of Health, University of Canberra, Canberra 2617, Australia; Ann-Rong.Yan@canberra.edu.au (A.-R.Y.); Mark.Naunton@canberra.edu.au (M.N.); g.peterson@utas.edu.au (G.M.P.)
[2] School of Pharmacy and Pharmacology, University of Tasmania, Hobart 7000, Australia
[3] Stroke Pharmacogenomics and Genetics Group, Neurovascular Research Laboratory, Hospital de Sant Pau, 08041 Barcelona, Spain; israel.fernandez@vhir.org
[4] Prehab Activity Cancer Exercise Survivorship Research Group, Faculty of Health, University of Canberra, Canberra 2617, Australia
* Correspondence: reza.mortazavi@canberra.edu.au;

Abstract: Background: Antiplatelet medications such as aspirin and clopidogrel are used following thrombotic stroke or transient ischemic attack (TIA) to prevent a recurrent stroke. However, the antiplatelet treatments fail frequently, and patients experience recurrent stroke. One approach to lower the rates of recurrence may be the individualized antiplatelet therapies (antiplatelet therapy modification (ATM)) based on the results of platelet function analysis (PFA). This review was undertaken to gather and analyze the evidence about the effectiveness of such approaches. Methods: We searched Medline, CINAHL, Embase, Web of Science, and Cochrane databases up to 7 January 2020. Results: Two observational studies involving 1136 patients were included. The overall effects of PFA-based ATM on recurrent strokes (odds ratio (OR) 1.05; 95% confidence interval (CI) 0.69 to 1.58), any bleeding risk (OR 1.39; 95% CI 0.92 to 2.10) or death hazard from any cause (OR 1.19; 95% CI 0.62 to 2.29) were not significantly different from the standard antiplatelet therapy without ATM. Conclusions: The two studies showed opposite effects of PFA-guided ATM on the recurrent strokes in aspirin non-responders, leading to an insignificant difference in the subgroup meta-analysis (OR 1.59; 95% CI 0.07 to 33.77), while the rates of any bleeding events (OR 1.04; 95% CI 0.49 to 2.17) or death from any cause (OR 1.17; 95% CI 0.41 to 3.35) were not significantly different between aspirin non-responders with ATM and those without ATM. There is a need for large, randomized controlled trials which account for potential confounders such as ischemic stroke subtypes, technical variations in the testing protocols, patient adherence to therapy and pharmacogenetic differences.

Keywords: antiplatelet; aspirin; clopidogrel; ischemic stroke; TIA; platelet function analysis; antiplatelet therapy modification; secondary stroke prevention; high on-treatment platelet reactivity

1. Introduction

Recurrent stroke is a major concern in patients with an initial stroke or transient ischemic attack (TIA) [1–3]. On average, the cumulative rate of recurrent ischemic stroke/TIA is 5.4% at one year,

11.3% at five years [4] and as high as 43% within 10 years from an initial event [2,5]. In terms of increased chances of the short-term occurrence of stroke after a TIA event, there are differences in the literature. For example, a Norwegian prospective cohort study reported a 0.9% risk of having stroke within 7 days of a TIA [6]. On the other hand, in a population-based study in the UK, the reported risk for this time point was much higher (8.6%) [7]. Regardless of the magnitude of the reported risks, the risk is real, and recurrent events are a continuing challenge for patients and healthcare systems alike worldwide [2,8]. Therefore, there is an urgent need for effective strategies to prevent stroke recurrence both in the short- and long term.

Platelets have a key role in the development of atherothrombosis and thrombotic events such as ischemic stroke [9–11]. Antiplatelet medications reduce the absolute risk of thrombotic vascular events by 2% per annum, although they concomitantly increase the risk of major extracranial hemorrhage by 0.1% to 0.3% per annum [2]. Current clinical guidelines, for example the living Clinical Guidelines For Stroke Management, published by the Stroke Foundation (Australia), strongly recommend long-term antiplatelet treatment for all patients with ischemic stroke or TIA who are not receiving prophylactic anticoagulants [5]. However, antiplatelet treatments may be ineffective due to various reasons, such as poor patient adherence [12] or individual variations in the genes related to the pharmacokinetics or pharmacodynamics of antiplatelet drugs, which render these drugs non-effective or less effective in the body [13].

Aspirin (acetylsalicylic acid) irreversibly inhibits the bone marrow and blood megakaryocytes and platelets by acetylating the 529th amino acid of the enzyme cyclooxygenase 1 (COX-1), thereby blocking COX-1 from producing prostaglandin G_2/H_2, which is an essential substrate for thromboxane A2 (TXA_2) synthesis [12]. Aspirin ineffectiveness (or resistance) can be attributed to a number of reasons including but not limited to the patient non-adherence, a blocked binding site on COX-1 due to interference by other drugs such as nonsteroidal anti-inflammatory drugs (NSAIDs), common variations (polymorphisms) of the COX-1 gene, non-platelet pathways for TXA_2 production (e.g., biosynthesis by the monocyte/macrophage COX-2), non-thromboxane-dependent platelet activation (e.g., adenosine diphosphate (ADP)—dependent platelet activation), or an over-production of platelets by the bone marrow in response to stress (e.g., inflammation or infection) [14,15].

Clopidogrel is a pro-drug (inactive), which, following oral administration and absorption into the bloodstream, is activated in a two-step metabolic process by hepatic cytochrome P450 enzymes. The active thiol metabolite inhibits ADP-induced platelet activation by binding to the P2Y12 receptors on the platelet surface, thereby preventing the binding of ADP molecules (as platelet activators) to their normal receptors [15–17]. Common causes of clopidogrel resistance include patient non-adherence, inadequate dose or problems with intestinal absorption, inhibition of the cytochrome P (CYP) isoenzymes due to drug interactions (for example, inhibition of CYP2C19 by some proton pump inhibitors), increased platelet production and polymorphisms of CYP450 genes [15,17].

Antiplatelet resistance is commonly referred to as high on-treatment platelet reactivity (HTPR) or platelet non-responsiveness [18]. The overall prevalence of HTPR in ischemic stroke or TIA patients is reported to be 20–28% and 22–32% for aspirin and clopidogrel users respectively, with an estimated range of 5–10% resistance to both drugs in patients taking them simultaneously [19]. Numerous studies have reported associations between HTPR and adverse clinical outcomes. For example, Sabra et al. reported higher rates of HTPR in patients with acute ischemic stroke (AIS) than in healthy volunteers [20], while others highlighted similar differences in patients with recurrent stroke compared with those without a stroke recurrence [21,22]. Other studies have revealed an association between aspirin-HTPR in the initial stages of AIS with stroke severity and infarct volume [23–25], as well as the inflammation status [26]. HTPR could predict 72 h and 10-day early neurological deterioration [27,28], and 1-week early recurrent stroke lesions following the initial ischemic event [29]. These findings are suggestive of a higher risk of stroke recurrence in patients with HTPR. This view is supported by other studies [27,28,30–32].

Given the importance of effective antiplatelet treatments in the prevention of recurrent thrombotic events, there has been a long-lasting interest in the development of laboratory tests for assessing platelet function during antiplatelet treatment. Platelet function analysis (PFA) was initially introduced in the early 1960s by the late Professor G. V. R. Born of King's College, London, based on the aggregation-related changes in the quantity of light transmission from platelet-rich plasma following the addition of ADP as a platelet activator [33]. Since then, there have been major advances in the technologies and methods used. These assays may be used to assess platelets for one or more of their functions, including adhesion, secretion and aggregation. In terms of clinical applications, currently, PFA assays are mainly used in a number of situations such as the assessment of blood coagulability in hospitalized patients before surgery, diagnosis of congenital or acquired platelet dysfunction and monitoring antiplatelet treatment [34].

A sensitive and precise PFA for monitoring antiplatelet treatments would allow clinicians to adjust the drug type or dose (e.g., increase dose, decrease dose, use dual antiplatelet agents or switch to a different drug) to improve the therapeutic outcomes (in this case, decreasing the rate of stroke recurrence). Some researchers are cautiously optimistic about the potential usefulness of standardized PFAs in the development of tailored antiplatelet treatments in patients with cerebrovascular or cardiovascular disease [35,36], while others believe that PFA-guided treatment in stroke patients is currently impractical because of the lack of consensus on the definition of HTPR [13,37], or the lack of a good correlation between PFA results and clinical outcomes [38]. Given these divergent views, the aim of this systematic review was to examine the published evidence for the effectiveness of PFA-based antiplatelet therapy modification (ATM) in patients with ischemic stroke or TIA for the prevention of a recurrent stroke. To the best of our knowledge, this is the first systematic review and meta-analysis undertaken on this topic.

2. Materials and Methods

2.1. Inclusion and Exclusion Criteria

The study's inclusion and exclusion criteria are listed in Box 1.

Box 1. The study's inclusion and exclusion criteria.

Inclusion criteria:

(1) Full text peer-reviewed journal articles
(2) Clinical trials and observational studies
(3) Published in English, Chinese or Persian (Farsi) languages
(4) Published from inception to 7 January 2020
(5) Adults with ischemic stroke or transient ischemic attack
(6) Patients receiving aspirin and/or clopidogrel were followed up for clinical outcomes for at least 3 months
(7) Platelet function analysis (PFA) results were used for making decisions on the choice of antiplatelet drugs or doses

Exclusion criteria:

(1) Not a clinical study (e.g., reviews)
(2) Patients under 18 years of age
(3) Patients with primary diagnosis of coronary or peripheral artery disease
(4) Aspirin or clopidogrel were not administered
(5) Patients were receiving anticoagulants
(6) No PFA-guided antiplatelet drug selection or dose adjustment
(7) Clinical outcomes were not studied
(8) Full text unavailable
(9) Not published in English, Chinese or Persian (Farsi) languages

---

2.2. Participants

Patients with a preliminary diagnosis of ischemic stroke or minor stroke (TIA) who underwent aspirin or clopidogrel therapy following the initial diagnosis were included.

2.3. Types of Interventions

Types of interventions included in the review were PFA-guided modifications in antiplatelet therapies (including increasing the drug dose, adding another antiplatelet drug and switching to another antiplatelet agent), compared to standard antiplatelet therapies based on the current clinical guidelines [3,5], which do not recommend the use of PFA for therapeutic decision making.

2.4. Types of Outcome Measures

Primary outcomes were recurrence of stroke or TIA, and secondary outcomes were death and/or bleeding incidences.

2.5. Search Methods

The systematic review was registered on the International Prospective Register of Systematic Reviews (PROSPERO) (registration ID: CRD42019126946; https://www.crd.york.ac.uk/prospero/display_record.php?ID=CRD42019126946). Full-text peer-reviewed journal articles were searched through five online databases (Embase (Scopus), Cochrane Library, Medline, CINAHL and Web of Science) for articles published in English, Chinese or Persian languages from inception of the databases to 7 January 2020. Different combinations of the following search terms were used: aspirin, clopidogrel, antiplatelet, stroke, cerebrovascular disease, transient ischemic attack, TIA, large-artery atherosclerosis, LAA, platelet function analysis, platelet aggregation, PFA-100, PFA-200, VerifyNow, Multiplate, aggregometry, aspirin resistance, platelet reactivity, clopidogrel resistance, high on-treatment platelet reactivity, HTPR, platelet residual activity, platelet hyperactivity, aspirin non-responder, and clopidogrel non-responder.

2.6. Quality Assessment and Publication Bias

The included observational studies were assessed using the Newcastle-Ottawa Scale (NOS) [39]. For cohort studies, NOS includes the following domains: (1) selection of the exposed cohort and the non-exposed cohort with ascertainment of exposure and demonstration that the outcome of interest was not present at the start of the study, (2) comparability of cohorts on the basis of the design or analysis and (3) assessment of outcome, and adequate follow-up time and rate [39].

2.7. Data Extraction

The following data were extracted: authors; year of publication; sample size; patient diagnosis and demographics; antiplatelet regimen including medication, dosage, duration and any alterations; platelet function test values and cut-off values; therapeutic window of platelet reactivity for antiplatelet regimen adjustment; and prevalence or relative risk or odds risk of secondary stroke.

2.8. Data Analysis

Review Manager 5 software (Copenhagen: The Nordic Cochrane Centre.; version 5.4, The Cochrane Collaboration, London, UK) was employed in all analytic processes. Odds ratios (OR) with 95% confidence intervals (95% CI) of recurrent ischemic stroke were generated to determine the pooled effect of modification in antiplatelet therapy. Heterogeneity was explored by using the chi-square test, with a p-value of < 0.10 indicating significant heterogeneity. Inconsistency across studies was then quantified with the I^2 statistic test, with an I^2 value between 50% and 75% indicating moderate heterogeneity, and a value of $>75\%$ indicating high heterogeneity. Fixed effects were carried out with low levels of clinical or statistical heterogeneity, and random effects were used when the heterogeneity was above 50%.

We analyzed the overall effects of modification in antiplatelet therapy compared to aspirin and/or clopidogrel treatments without adjustment, and the effects of modification in antiplatelet therapy in aspirin non-responders [40,41]. The data for clopidogrel non-responders were not included in the meta-analysis, because they were reported only in one study [40].

3. Results

3.1. Study Selection

Figure 1 depicts the search process for this study using the Preferred Reporting Items for Systematic Reviews and Meta-Analyses (PRISMA) 2009 Flow Diagram. We were able to find only two observational studies which met our inclusion criteria [40,41].

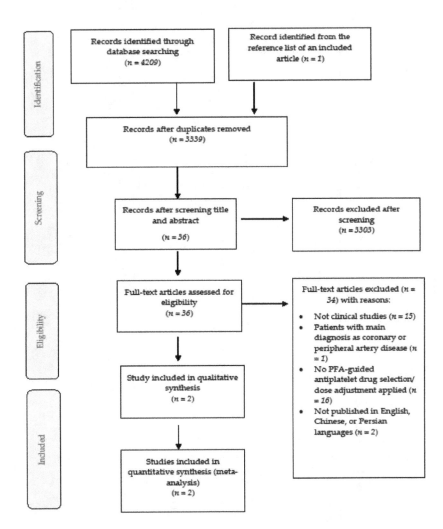

Figure 1. The processes of the study based on the Preferred Reporting Items for Systematic Reviews and Meta-Analyses (PRISMA) 2009 Flow Diagram.

3.2. Characteristics of the Studies

One of the included studies were undertaken in a medical center in the US [40] and the other study in three centers in China [41]. Altogether, these two studies examined 1136 participants who were on antiplatelet therapy after a diagnosis of ischemic stroke or TIA. Depta et al. [40] conducted the comparison in mixed aspirin and/or clopidogrel users, while the study by Yi et al. [41] included patients with aspirin monotherapy before platelet function testing. The accumulated rate of recurrent stroke and treatment side effects was observed within a mean follow-up period of 4.6 ± 1.1 years and 4.8 ± 1.7 years, respectively. The study designs and the characteristics of the participants, interventions and outcome measures are presented in Tables 1 and 2.

Table 1. The study designs and methods of the included studies.

Study	Patient and Sample Size			Intervention	Comparison	Main Outcomes	Follow-Up Time (Mean ± SD)
	Overall	Subgroup 1	Subgroup 2				
Depta et al. [40]	ischemic stroke or TIA (n = 324)	aspirin non-responders * (n = 128)	clopidogrel non-responders # (n = 54)	ATM [a]	aspirin and/or clopidogrel treatment	• recurrence of ischemic stroke • bleeding • death	4.6 ± 1.1 years
Yi et al. [41]	first-ever ischemic stroke with two subtypes of stroke: atherothrombotic or small artery disease (n = 812)	aspirin non-responders * (n = 223)	not studied	ATM [b]	aspirin monotherapy	• recurrence of ischemic stroke • bleeding • death	4.8 ± 1.7 years

SD: standard deviation, ATM: antiplatelet modification, TIA: transient ischemic attack. * ≥20% aggregation with 0.5% mg/mL arachidonic acid (AA), or ≥70% aggregation with 10 μM adenosine diphosphate (ADP), or on-aspirin onset of ischemic stroke or TIA. # ≥70% aggregation with 10 μM ADP. [a] Seven types of modification: added or increased aspirin, added aspirin, added aspirin/clopidogrel, added or increased clopidogrel, added clopidogrel, increased or added both aspirin and clopidogrel, changed from aspirin to clopidogrel. [b] Four kinds of modification: changed from aspirin to clopidogrel, changed from aspirin to cilostazol, increased aspirin, added clopidogrel to aspirin.

Table 2. Characteristics and outcomes of the included studies.

Study	Intervention and Patient Characteristics Mean ± SD	Recurrent Ischemic Stroke	p-Value	Bleeding	p-Value	Death	p-Value
				Main Outcomes			
Depta et al. [40]	With ATM [a] age: 71.4 ± 11.9 years aggregation with AA, %: 26.7 ± 19.7 aggregation with ADP, %: 56.2 ± 22.9	6/73 (8%)	0.23	14/73 (19%)	0.04	6/73 (8%)	0.60
	Without ATM [a] age: 65.6 ± 13.5 years aggregation with AA, %: 19.1 ± 14.0 aggregation with ADP, %: 46.5 ± 23.5	11/251 (4%)		26/251 (10)		16/251 (6%)	
Yi et al. [41]	With ATM [b] age: 71.8 ± 11.6 years aggregation with AA, %: 26.8 ± 10.2 aggregation with ADP, %: 58.4 ± 18.6	29/204 (14.2%)	0.82	23/204 (11.3%)	0.61	7/204 (3.4%)	0.84
	Without ATM [b] age: 67.1 ± 13.6 years * aggregation with AA, %: 20.1 ± 8.7 * aggregation with ADP, %: 47.6 ± 16.4	91/608 (15.0%)		60/608 (9.9%)		19/608 (3.1%)	

Study	Subgroup: Aspirin Non-Responders *,a	Recurrent Ischemic Stroke	p-Value	Bleeding	p-Value	Death	p-Value
				Main Outcomes			
Depta et al. [40]	With ATM [a] Patient characteristics not stated	4/42 (10%)	0.04	5/42 (12%)	0.89	4/42 (10%)	0.44
	Without ATM [a] Patient characteristics not stated	1/86 (1%)		11/86 (13%)		4/86 (5%)	
Yi et al. [41]	With ATM [b] Patient characteristics not different significantly	18/154 (11.7%)	0.008	15/154 (9.7%)	0.81	4/154 (2.6%)	0.67
	Without ATM [b] Patient characteristics not different significantly	17/69 (24.6%)		6/69 (8.7%)		3/69 (4.3%)	

SD: standard deviation, ATM: antiplatelet modification, AA: arachidonic acid, ADP: adenosine diphosphate. * Aspirin non-responsiveness was defined as ≥20% aggregation with 0.5% mg/mL AA, or ≥70% aggregation with 10 μM ADP, or on-aspirin onset of ischemic stroke or TIA. [a] Seven types of modification: added or increased aspirin, added aspirin, added aspirin/clopidogrel, added or increased clopidogrel, added both aspirin and clopidogrel, increased or added both aspirin and clopidogrel, changed from aspirin to clopidogrel. [b] Four kinds of modification: changed from aspirin to clopidogrel, changed from aspirin to cilostazol, increased aspirin, added clopidogrel to aspirin.

3.3. Comparisons

In both studies, the participants were originally prescribed an antiplatelet for the prevention of recurrent thrombotic events, and antiplatelet therapy modification was defined as any changes in antiplatelet regimen within 24 h after platelet function testing. However, the two studies varied in original antiplatelet therapy and the specific modification in antiplatelet regimens. Yi et al. [41] studied aspirin monotherapy and four types of modification: (1) changed from aspirin to clopidogrel, (2) changed from aspirin to cilostazol, (3) increased aspirin doses and (4) added clopidogrel to aspirin. Depta et al. [40] studied aspirin and/or clopidogrel treatment and seven types of modification: (1) added or increased aspirin doses, (2) added aspirin, (3) added aspirin/dipyridamole, (4) added or increased clopidogrel, (5) added clopidogrel, (6) increased or added both aspirin or clopidogrel, and (7) changed from aspirin to clopidogrel. The comparison of the rates of recurrent stroke was conducted in overall patients and subgroups (i.e., aspirin non-responders and/or clopidogrel non-responders) between those with antiplatelet modification (ATM) and without ATM.

3.4. Outcomes

Both studies recorded ischemic events (ischemic stroke, transient ischemic attack and myocardial infarction), any bleeding events and deaths from any cause.

3.5. Quality

The studies had similar methodologies, but there were some improvements in the study by Yi et al. [41]. Although the non-exposure cohort (without ATM) were drawn from the same register as the exposed cohort (with ATM), potential selection bias, caused by unknown clinical factors that may affect physicians' decisions regarding platelet function test results and antiplatelet regimens, existed in both studies. For exclusion of cases in which the study outcome (i.e., recurrent stroke) had already occurred at the start of the study, Yi et al. [41] included only the first-ever ischemic stroke patients, while Depta et al. [40] did not.

In terms of comparability, both studies conducted adjustments for propensity scores, which included age, male, inpatient and risk factors for stroke, such as smoking status, diabetes, hypertension, prior cardiovascular disease and surgical treatment, as well as history of medications like antiplatelet, antihypertensive and hypoglycemic agents. However, adherence to the antiplatelet therapy was not assessed in either of the studies. The diagnosis of ischemic stroke subtypes was undertaken only in the study by Yi et al. [41]. Neither of the studies described the subjects lost to follow-up in any detail.

3.6. The Overall Effects of Modified Antiplatelet Therapy

The meta-analysis of the incidence rates of recurrent ischemic stroke in ischemic stroke or TIA patients with ATM versus those without ATM, using a fixed effects model because of low heterogeneity, indicated an overall effect size of 0.22 without statistical significance (OR 1.05; 95% CI 0.69 to 1.58) (Figure 2).

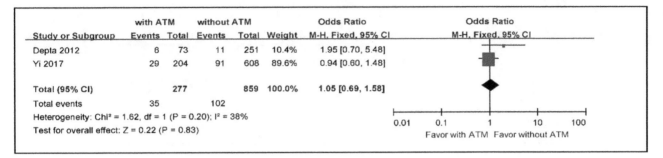

Figure 2. The meta-analysis of the incidence rate of recurrent ischemic stroke in ischemic stroke or TIA patients with ATM versus those without ATM (*n* = 1136). TIA: transient ischemic attack, ATM: antiplatelet therapy modification.

The meta-analysis of the incidence rate of any bleeding in ischemic stroke or TIA patients with ATM versus those without ATM, using a fixed effects model because of low heterogeneity, indicated an overall effect size of 1.58 without statistical significance (OR 1.39; 95% CI 0.92 to 2.10) (Figure 3).

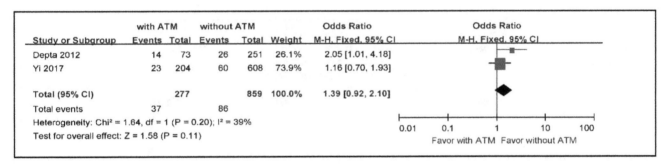

Figure 3. The meta-analysis of the incidence rate of bleeding in ischemic stroke or TIA patients with ATM versus those without ATM (*n* = 1136). TIA: transient ischemic attack, ATM: antiplatelet therapy modification.

The meta-analysis of the incidence of death from any cause in ischemic stroke or TIA patients with ATM versus those without ATM, using a fixed effects model because of low heterogeneity, indicated an overall effect size of 0.52 without statistical significance (OR 1.19; 95% CI 0.62 to 2.29) (Figure 4).

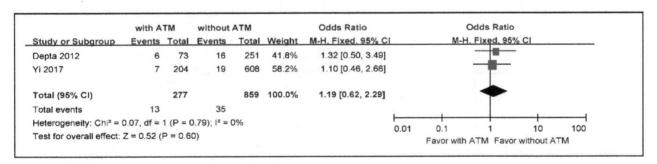

Figure 4. The meta-analysis of the incidence rate of death in ischemic stroke or TIA patients with ATM versus those without ATM (*n* = 1136). TIA: transient ischemic attack, ATM: antiplatelet therapy modification.

3.7. Effect of Modified Antiplatelet Therapy in Aspirin Non-Responders

The subgroup meta-analysis of the incidence rate of recurrent ischemic stroke in ischemic stroke or TIA aspirin non-responders with ATM versus those without ATM, using a random effects model because of high heterogeneity, indicated an effect size of 0.30 without statistical significance (OR 1.59; 95% CI 0.07 to 33.77) (Figure 5).

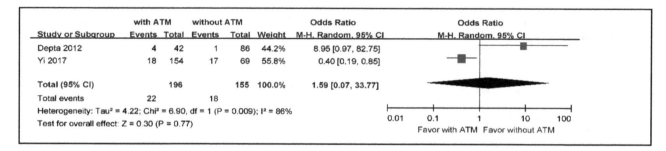

Figure 5. The meta-analysis of the incidence rate of recurrent ischemic stroke in ischemic stroke or TIA aspirin non-responders with ATM versus those without ATM (*n* = 351). TIA: transient ischemic attack, ATM: antiplatelet therapy modification.

The subgroup meta-analysis of the incidence rate of any bleeding in ischemic stroke or TIA aspirin non-responders with ATM versus those without ATM, using a fixed effects model because of low heterogeneity, indicated an effect size of 0.09 without statistical significance (OR 1.04; 95% CI 0.49 to 2.17) (Figure 6).

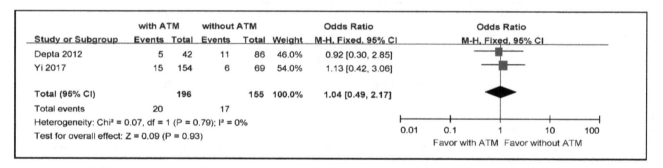

Figure 6. The meta-analysis of the incidence rate of bleeding in ischemic stroke or TIA aspirin non-responders with ATM versus those without ATM (*n* = 351). TIA: transient ischemic attack, ATM: antiplatelet therapy modification.

The subgroup meta-analysis of the incidence rate of death from any cause in ischemic stroke or TIA aspirin non-responders with ATM versus those without ATM, using a fixed effects model because of low heterogeneity, indicated an effect size of 0.29 without statistical significance (OR 1.17; 95% CI 0.41 to 3.35) (Figure 7).

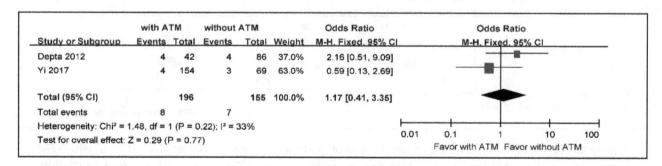

Figure 7. The meta-analysis of the incidence rate of death in ischemic stroke or TIA aspirin non-responders with ATM versus those without ATM (*n* = 351). TIA: transient ischemic attack, ATM: antiplatelet therapy modification.

4. Discussion

The analyses of the pooled data indicated that, compared with standard antiplatelet therapy (i.e., without ATM), the overall effects of PFA-guided ATM on recurrent strokes, any bleeding risk or death hazard were not statistically significant, although the group with ATM had a significantly higher residual platelet reactivity than the group without ATM. Higher residual platelet reactivity has been known as an independent risk factor for recurrent stroke in patients with ischemic stroke or transient ischemic attack [19], but ATM was successful in keeping the rate of recurrent ischemic stroke for ischemic stroke or TIA patients with higher residual platelet reactivity down to the same value as for the antiplatelet responders.

Modification in antiplatelet therapy was associated with an increased risk for any bleeding event in the study by Depta et al. [40] (19% vs. 10%, $p = 0.04$), while there was no significant change in the rate for any bleeding event after antiplatelet therapy modification in the study by Yi et al. [41] (11.3% vs. 9.9%, $p = 0.61$). Moreover, the effects of PFA-guided ATM on the risk of recurrent ischemic stroke in the subgroup of aspirin non-responders were opposite, leading to a result without statistical significance in the meta-analysis. In one study (Yi et al. [41]), it was reported that the antiplatelet therapy modification significantly lowered the recurrence rate of ischemic stroke (11.7% vs. 24.6%, $p = 0.02$), whereas the other study (Depta et al. [40]) reported an increase in the recurrence rate of ischemic stroke by antiplatelet therapy modification with borderline significance (10% vs. 1%, $p = 0.04$).

To be able to justify these kinds of inconsistencies between the two studies, they should be looked at from different perspectives. Firstly, the predictive value of HTPR for clinical outcomes may be complicated because of multiple etiologies [42], as the roles of the platelet reactivity may be different in different vascular diseases (cardiovascular versus cerebrovascular) [43], or even different subtypes of ischemic stroke [44–46]. Between the two included studies in this systematic review, this is only the study by Yi et al. [41] which identifies the stroke subtypes in the patients. The study sample was more homogeneous in the study by Yi et al. [41], as only two subtypes were included (i.e., the atherothrombotic and small artery disease). Although small artery disease could be thrombotic or embolic, cerebral embolism was excluded in this study.

Additionally, the prevalence of aspirin non-response in the study by Depta et al. [40] was much higher than in the study by Yi et al. [41] (43% vs. 27.5%), while both studies adopted the same technology (optical platelet aggregometry) for platelet function analysis. The latter included patients with first-time stroke only, while the former did not clarify this. Hence, the study by Depta et al. [40] may have enrolled patients with recurrent stroke, and it is known that patients with prior stroke or TIA have an increased risk for recurrent stroke [47].

Regardless of the above inconsistencies, both studies had limitations in controlling the potential confounders, which should be taken into consideration in future studies. Firstly, neither of the studies did report the patient adherence to antiplatelet treatment, which could be a confounder in assessing the efficacy of antiplatelet agents, and in evaluating the effect of true HTPR compared to pseudo HTPR (due to non-compliance). This is probably a common issue in antiplatelet treatments, as Dawson et al. [48] reported a 60% patient non-adherence rate following the urinary measurement of aspirin metabolites. In addition, the reported drop of nearly 50% in the HTPR rates in two studies of stroke patients following the supervised administration of aspirin indicates the role of patients' non-compliance in influencing HTPR results [49,50].

Secondly, the proportion of patients undergoing platelet function re-testing after antiplatelet therapy modification was quite low in both studies. Not only the platelet function re-testing can be used for assessing the effectiveness of the modified antiplatelet therapies [51], but also it can help detect a sustained HTPR as a risk factor for recurrent stroke. Accounting for the dynamic feature of HTPR may be essential for optimizing the protocols for platelet function analyses and establishing specific criteria for the frequency of retesting and the choice of antiplatelet therapy modification [13,52]. Although the included studies involved the same method of laboratory testing, it is necessary to understand that the laboratory identification of HTPR depends on assay-specific factors such as the exact method, the device, and the cut-off values used [13]. As a result, more research should be done to rectify these technical issues so that PFA can be used consistently in different clinical practices.

Thirdly, although HTPR can be, in some cases, improved by either increasing the antiplatelet dose [20,43,53] or adding another type of platelet inhibitor [54], the pharmacological response to an antiplatelet therapy (i.e., clinical responsiveness) may not be exactly the same phenomenon that is measured through laboratory testing. In other word, the concepts of clinical resistance and laboratory-measured resistance may be quite different [55].

As our study limitation, we could not find any randomized controlled clinical trials or prospective cohort studies to meet our inclusion criteria, so we had to include only two retrospective cohort studies with relatively small sample sizes. This affects the power of our meta-analysis and the generalizability of the results. However, as mentioned in the discussions above, due to the scarcity of clinical studies in this area, and given the serious consequences of recurrent stroke, there is a strong need for more research in this area to find ways to improve the effectiveness of antiplatelet treatments in stroke patients.

5. Conclusions

Given the small number of participants in the included studies and the lack of randomized clinical trials in this area, it is not certain whether a PFA-guided antiplatelet therapy would be successful in improving patient outcomes by decreasing the rates of secondary stroke while minimizing the risk of bleeding. Thus, well-designed randomized controlled trials are needed to obtain stronger evidence to address the research question.

Author Contributions: Two of the authors, A.-R.Y. and R.M., independently screened the preliminary search results for titles and abstracts using the inclusion and exclusion criteria and read the full text of relevant articles. The reference lists of the relevant papers were manually searched by A.-R.Y. Discrepancies between search results were resolved by discussion. All authors participated in the critical analysis of the manuscript, as well as its conceptual development. All authors have read and agreed to the published version of the manuscript.

References

1. Australian Institute of Health and Welfare. *Stroke and Its Management in Australia: An Update*; Australian Institute of Health and Welfare: Canberra, Australia, 2013.
2. Esenwa, C.; Gutierrez, J. Secondary stroke prevention: Challenges and solutions. *Vasc. Health Risk Manag.* **2015**, *11*, 437–450. [PubMed]
3. Kernan, W.N.; Ovbiagele, B.; Black, H.R.; Bravata, D.M.; Chimowitz, M.I.; Ezekowitz, M.D.; Fang, M.C.; Fisher, M.; Furie, K.L.; Heck, D.V.; et al. Guidelines for the prevention of stroke in patients with stroke and transient ischemic attack: A guideline for healthcare professionals from the American Heart Association/American Stroke Association. *Stroke* **2014**, *45*, 2160–2236. [CrossRef] [PubMed]
4. Khanevski, A.N.; Bjerkreim, A.T.; Novotny, V.; Naess, H.; Thomassen, L.; Logallo, N.; Kvistad, C.E. Recurrent ischemic stroke: Incidence, predictors, and impact on mortality. *Acta Neurol. Scand.* **2019**, *140*, 3–8. [CrossRef] [PubMed]
5. Stroke Foundation. Clinical Guidelines for Stroke Management 2017. Available online: https://informme.org.au/Guidelines/Clinical-Guidelines-for-Stroke-Management-2017 (accessed on 12 April 2020).
6. Ildstad, F.; Ellekjær, H.; Wethal, T.; Lydersen, S.; Sund, J.K.; Fjærtoft, H.; Schüler, S.; Horn, J.W.; Bråthen, G.; Midtsæther, A.G.; et al. Stroke risk after transient ischemic attack in a Norwegian prospective cohort. *BMC Neurol.* **2019**, *19*, 2. [CrossRef]
7. Lovett, J.K.; Dennis, M.S.; Sandercock, P.A.G.; Bamford, J.; Warlow, C.P.; Rothwell, P.M. Very Early Risk of Stroke After a First Transient Ischemic Attack. *Stroke* **2003**, *34*, e138–e140. [CrossRef]
8. Moretti, A.; Ferrari, F.; Villa, R.F. Pharmacological therapy of acute ischaemic stroke: Achievements and problems. *Pharmacol. Ther.* **2015**, *153*, 79–89. [CrossRef]
9. Spronk, H.M.H.; Padró, T.; Siland, J.E.; Prochaska, J.H.; Winters, J.; van der Wal, A.C.; Posthuma, J.J.; Lowe, G.; D'Alessandro, E.; Wenzel, P.; et al. Atherothrombosis and thromboembolism: Position paper from the second maastricht consensus conference on thrombosis. *Thromb. Haemost.* **2018**, *118*, 229–250. [CrossRef]
10. Kannan, M.; Ahmad, F.; Saxena, R. Platelet activation markers in evaluation of thrombotic risk factors in various clinical settings. *Blood Rev.* **2019**, *37*, 100583. [CrossRef]

11. Paniccia, R.P.R.; Liotta, A.A.; Abbate, R. Platelet function tests: A comparative review. *Vasc. Health Risk Manag.* **2015**, *11*, 133–148. [CrossRef]

12. Michelson, A.D.; Bhatt, D.L. How i use laboratory monitoring of antiplatelet therapy. *Blood* **2017**, *130*, m713–m721. [CrossRef]

13. Lim, S.T.; Coughlan, C.A.; Murphy, S.J.X.; Fernandez-Cadenas, I.; Montaner, J.; Thijs, V.; Marquardt, L.; McCabe, D.J. Platelet function testing in transient ischaemic attack and ischaemic stroke: A comprehensive systematic review of the literature. *Platelets* **2015**, *26*, 402–412. [CrossRef]

14. Hankey, G.J.; Eikelboom, J.W. Aspirin resistance. *Lancet* **2006**, *367*, 606–617. [CrossRef]

15. Marginean, A.; Banescu, C.; Scridon, A.; Dobreanu, M. Anti-platelet Therapy Resistance—Concept, Mechanisms and Platelet Function Tests in Intensive Care Facilities. *J. Crit. Care Med.* **2016**, *2*, 6–15. [CrossRef]

16. Ford, N.F. The Metabolism of Clopidogrel: CYP2C19 Is a Minor Pathway. *J. Clin. Pharmacol.* **2016**, *56*, 1474–1483. [CrossRef]

17. Gurbel, P.A.; Tantry, U.S. Drug Insight: Clopidogrel nonresponsiveness. *Nat. Clin. Pract. Cardiovasc. Med.* **2006**, *3*, 387–395. [CrossRef]

18. Topcuoglu, M.A.; Arsava, E.M.; Ay, H. Antiplatelet resistance in stroke. *Expert Rev. Neurother.* **2011**, *11*, 251–263. [CrossRef]

19. Fiolaki, A.; Katsanos, A.H.; Kyritsis, A.P.; Papadaki, S.; Kosmidou, M.; Moschonas, I.C.; Tselepis, A.D.; Giannopoulos, S. High on treatment platelet reactivity to aspirin and clopidogrel in ischemic stroke: A systematic review and meta-analysis. *J. Neurol. Sci.* **2017**, *376*, 112–116. [CrossRef]

20. Sabra, A.; Stanford, S.N.; Storton, S.; Lawrence, M.; D'Silva, L.; Morris, R.H.K.; Evans, V.; Wani, M.; Potter, J.F.; Evans, P.A. Assessment of platelet function in patients with stroke using multiple electrode platelet aggregometry: A prospective observational study. *BMC Neurol.* **2016**, *16*, 254–261. [CrossRef]

21. Grundmann, K.; Jaschonek, K.; Kleine, B.; Dichgans, J.; Topka, H. Aspirin non-responder status in patients with recurrent cerebral ischemic attacks. *J. Neurol.* **2003**, *250*, 63–66. [CrossRef]

22. Gengo, F.M.; Rainka, M.; Robson, M.; Gengo, M.E.; Forrest, A.; Hourihane, M.; Bates, V. Prevalence of platelet nonresponsiveness to aspirin in patients treated for secondary stroke prophylaxis and in patients with recurrent ischemic events. *J. Clin. Pharmacol.* **2008**, *48*, 335–343. [CrossRef] [PubMed]

23. Oh, M.S.; Yu, K.H.; Lee, J.H.; Jung, S.; Kim, C.; Jang, M.U.; Lee, J.; Lee, B.C. Aspirin resistance is associated with increased stroke severity and infarct volume. *Neurology* **2016**, *86*, 1808–1817. [CrossRef] [PubMed]

24. Zheng, A.S.Y.; Churilov, L.; Colley, R.E.; Goh, C.; Davis, S.M.; Yan, B. Association of Aspirin Resistance with Increased Stroke Severity and Infarct Size. *JAMA Neurol.* **2013**, *70*, 208–213. [CrossRef] [PubMed]

25. Ozben, S.; Ozben, B.; Tanrikulu, A.M.; Ozer, F.; Ozben, T. Aspirin resistance in patients with acute ischemic stroke. *J. Neurol.* **2011**, *258*, 1979–1986. [CrossRef] [PubMed]

26. Coignion, C.; Poli, M.; Sagnier, S.; Freyburger, G.; Renou, P.; Debruxelles, S.; Rouanet, F.; Sibon, I. Interest of Antiplatelet Drug Testing after an Acute Ischemic Stroke. *Eur. Neurol.* **2015**, *74*, 135–139. [CrossRef]

27. Yi, X.; Wang, C.; Liu, P.; Fu, C.; Lin, J.; Chen, Y. Antiplatelet drug resistance is associated with early neurological deterioration in acute minor ischemic stroke in the Chinese population. *J. Neurol.* **2016**, *263*, 1612–1619. [CrossRef]

28. Yi, X.; Lin, J.; Zhou, Q.; Wu, L.; Cheng, W.; Wang, C. Clopidogrel Resistance Increases Rate of Recurrent Stroke and Other Vascular Events in Chinese Population. *J. Stroke Cerebrovasc. Dis.* **2016**, *25*, 1222–1228. [CrossRef]

29. Jeon, S.B.; Song, H.S.; Kim, B.J.; Kim, H.J.; Kang, D.W.; Kim, J.S.; Kwon, S.U. Biochemical Aspirin Resistance and Recurrent Lesions in Patients with Acute Ischemic Stroke. *Eur. Neurol.* **2010**, *64*, 51–57. [CrossRef]

30. Wang, C.W.; Su, L.L.; Hua, Q.J.; He, Y.; Fan, Y.N.; Xi, T.T.; Yuan, B.; Liu, Y.X.; Ji, S.B. Aspirin resistance predicts unfavorable functional outcome in acute ischemic stroke patients. *Brain Res. Bull.* **2018**, *142*, 176–182. [CrossRef]

31. Rao, Z.; Zheng, H.; Wang, F.; Wang, A.; Liu, L.; Dong, K.; Zhao, X.; Cao, Y.; Wang, Y. High On-Treatment Platelet Reactivity to Adenosine Diphosphate Predicts Ischemic Events of Minor Stroke and Transient Ischemic Attack. *J. Stroke Cerebrovasc. Dis.* **2017**, *26*, 2074–2081. [CrossRef]

32. Rao, Z.; Zheng, H.; Wang, F.; Wang, A.; Liu, L.; Dong, K.; Zhao, X.; Wang, Y. The association between high on-treatment platelet reactivity and early recurrence of ischemic events after minor stroke or TIA. *Neurol. Res.* **2017**, *39*, 719–726. [CrossRef]

33. Born, G.V.R. Aggregation of Blood Platelets by Adenosine Diphosphate and its Reversal. *Nature* **1962**, *194*, 927–929. [CrossRef] [PubMed]

34. Harrison, P. Platelet function analysis. *Blood Rev.* **2005**, *19*, 111–123. [CrossRef] [PubMed]

35. Bonello, L.; Camoin-Jau, L.; Arques, S.; Boyer, C.; Panagides, D.; Wittenberg, O.; Simeoni, M.C.; Barragan, P.; Dignat-George, F.; Paganelli, F. Adjusted clopidogrel loading doses according to vasodilator-stimulated phosphoprotein phosphorylation index decrease rate of major adverse cardiovascular events in patients with clopidogrel resistance: A multicenter randomized prospective study. *J. Am. Coll. Cardiol.* **2008**, *51*, 1404–1411. [CrossRef] [PubMed]

36. Le Quellec, S.B.J.; Negrier, C.; Dargaud, Y. Comparison of current platelet functional tests for the assessment of aspirin and clopidogrel response. A review of the literature. *Thromb. Haemost.* **2016**, *116*, 638–650. [PubMed]

37. Eikelboom, J.W.; Emery, J.; Hankey, G.J. The use of platelet function assays may help to determine appropriate antiplatelet treatment options in a patient with recurrent stroke on baby aspirin: Against. *Stroke* **2010**, *41*, 2398–2399. [CrossRef]

38. Dahlen, J.R.; Price, M.J.; Parise, H.; Gurbel, P.A. Evaluating the clinical usefulness of platelet function testing: Considerations for the proper application and interpretation of performance measures. *Thromb. Haemost.* **2013**, *109*, 808–816.

39. Wells, G.A.; Shea, B.; O'Connell, D.; Peterson, J.; Welch, V.; Losos, M.; Tugwell, P. The Newcastle-Ottawa Scale (NOS) for Assessing the Quality of Nonrandomised Studies in Meta-Analyses. 2020. Available online: http://www.ohri.ca/programs/clinical_epidemiology/oxford.asp (accessed on 12 April 2020).

40. Depta, J.P.; Fowler, J.; Novak, E.; Katzan, I.; Bakdash, S.; Kottke-Marchant, K.; Bhatt, D.L. Clinical Outcomes Using a Platelet Function-Guided Approach for Secondary Prevention in Patients With Ischemic Stroke or Transient Ischemic Attack. *Stroke* **2012**, *43*, 2376–2381. [CrossRef]

41. Yi, X.; Lin, J.; Wang, C.; Huang, R.; Han, Z.; Li, J. Platelet function-guided modification in antiplatelet therapy after acute ischemic stroke is associated with clinical outcomes in patients with aspirin nonresponse. *Oncotarget* **2017**, *8*, 106258. [CrossRef]

42. Agayeva, N.; Gungor, L.; Topcuoglu, M.A.; Arsava, E.M. Pathophysiologic, Rather than Laboratory-defined Resistance Drives Aspirin Failure in Ischemic Stroke. *J Stroke Cereb. Dis.* **2015**, *24*, 745–750. [CrossRef]

43. Meves, S.H.; Hummel, T.; Endres, H.G.; Mayboeck, N.; Kaiser, A.F.C.; Schroeder, K.D.; Rüdiger, K.; Overbeck, U.; Mumme, A.; Mügge, A.; et al. Effectiveness of antiplatelet therapy in atherosclerotic disease: Comparing the ASA low-response prevalence in CVD, CAD and PAD. *J. Thromb. Thrombolysis* **2014**, *37*, 190–201. [CrossRef]

44. Adams, H.P., Jr.; Bendixen, B.H.; Kappelle, L.J.; Biller, J.; Love, B.B.; Gordon, D.L.; Marsh, E.E., 3rd. Classification of subtype of acute ischemic stroke. Definitions for use in a multicenter clinical trial. TOAST. Trial of Org 10172 in Acute Stroke Treatment. *Stroke* **1993**, *24*, 35–41. [CrossRef] [PubMed]

45. Tuttolomondo, A.; Pecoraro, R.; di Raimondo, D.; Arnao, V.; Clemente, G.; Della Corte, V.; Carlo, M.; Irene, S.; Giuseppe, L.; Antonio, P. Stroke subtypes and their possible implication in stroke prevention drug strategies. *Curr. Vasc. Pharmacol.* **2013**, *11*, 824–837. [CrossRef] [PubMed]

46. Cha, J.K.; Park, H.S.; Nah, H.W.; Kim, D.H.; Kang, M.J.; Choi, J.H.; Huh, J.T.; Suh, H.K. High residual platelet reactivity (HRPR) for adenosine diphosphate (ADP) stimuli is a determinant factor for long-term outcomes in acute ischemic stroke with anti-platelet agents: The meaning of HRPR after ADP might be more prominent in large atherosclerotic infarction than other subtypes of AIS. *J. Thromb. Thrombolysis* **2016**, *42*, 107–117. [PubMed]

47. Bernstein, P.L.; Jacobson, B.F.; Connor, M.D.; Becker, P.J. Aspirin resistance in South African Caucasian patients with thrombotic cerebrovascular events. *J. Neurol. Sci.* **2009**, *277*, 80–82. [CrossRef]

48. Dawson, J.; Quinn, T.; Rafferty, M.; Higgins, P.; Ray, G.; Lees, K.R.; Walters, M.R. Aspirin Resistance and Compliance with Therapy. *Cardiovasc. Ther.* **2011**, *29*, 301–307. [CrossRef]

49. Halawani, S.H.M.; Williams, D.J.P.; Webster, J.; Greaves, M.; Ford, I. Aspirin failure in patients presenting with acute cerebrovascular ischaemia. *Thromb. Haemost.* **2011**, *106*, 240–247. [CrossRef]

50. El-Mitwalli, A.; Azzam, H.; Abu-Hegazy, M.; Gomaa, M.; Wasel, Y. Clinical and biochemical aspirin resistance in patients with recurrent cerebral ischemia. *Clin. Neurol. Neurosurg.* **2013**, *115*, 944–947. [CrossRef]

51. Berrouschot, J.; Schwetlick, B.; von Twickel, G.; Fischer, C.; Uhlemann, H.; Siegemund, T.; Siegemund, A.; Roessler, A. Aspirin resistance in secondary stroke prevention. *Acta Neurol. Scand.* **2006**, *113*, 31–35. [CrossRef]

52. Kim, J.T.; Choi, K.H.; Park, M.S.; Lee, J.S.; Saver, J.L.; Cho, K.H. Clinical significance of acute and serial platelet function testing in acute ischemic stroke. *J. Am. Heart Assoc.* **2018**, *7*, e008313. [CrossRef]

53. Uchiyama, S.; Nakamura, T.; Yamazaki, M.; Kimura, Y.; Iwata, M. New modalities and aspects of antiplatelet therapy for stroke prevention. *Cerebrovasc. Dis.* **2006**, *21* (Suppl. 1), 7–16. [CrossRef]

54.　Lee, J.H.; Cha, J.K.; Lee, S.J.; Ha, S.W.; Kwon, S.U. Addition of cilostazol reduces biological aspirin resistance in aspirin users with ischaemic stroke: A double-blind randomized clinical trial. *Eur. J. Neurol.* **2010**, *17*, 434–442. [CrossRef] [PubMed]

55.　Sambu, N.; Radhakrishnan, A.; Englyst, N.; Weir, N.; Curzen, N. "Aspirin Resistance" in Ischemic Stroke: Insights Using Short Thrombelastography. *J. Stroke Cerebrovasc. Dis.* **2013**, *22*, 1412–1419. [CrossRef] [PubMed]

The Role of Resolvins: EPA and DHA Derivatives Can Be Useful in the Prevention and Treatment of Ischemic Stroke

Nikola Tułowiecka [1], Dariusz Kotlęga [2,3]⓪, Piotr Prowans [4] and Małgorzata Szczuko [1,*]⓪

[1] Department of Human Nutrition and Metabolomics, Pomeranian Medical University in Szczecin, 71-460 Szczecin, Poland; ntulowiecka97@gmail.com

[2] Department of Neurology, Pomeranian Medical University in Szczecin, 71-252 Szczecin, Poland; dkotlega@uz.zgora.pl

[3] Department of Applied and Clinical Physiology, Collegium Medicum University of Zielona Gora, 65-417 Zielona Gora, Poland

[4] Clinic of Plastic, Endocrine and General Surgery, Pomeranian Medical University in Szczecin, 72-009 Police, Poland; Pprowans@wp.pl

* Correspondence: malgorzata.szczuko@pum.edu.pl;

Abstract: Introduction: Most ischemic strokes develop as a result of atherosclerosis, in which inflammation plays a key role. The synthesis cascade of proinflammatory mediators participates in the process induced in the vascular endothelium and platelets. Resolvins are anti-inflammatory mediators originating from eicosapentaenoic acid (EPA) and docosahexaenoic acid (DHA), which may improve the prognosis related to atherosclerosis by inhibiting the production of proinflammatory cytokines, limiting neutrophil migration, or positively influencing phagocytosis. Although clinical trials with resolvin in humans after stroke have not been realized, they may soon find application. Aim: The aim of the study was to review the available literature on the scope of the possibilities of the prevention and treatment of stroke with the use of resolvins, EPA and DHA derivatives. Materials and methods: The review features articles published until 31 January 2020. The search for adequate literature was conducted using the keywords: stroke and resolvins. Over 150 articles were found. Studies not written in English, letters to the editor, conference abstracts, and duplicate information were excluded. Results: In several studies using the animal model, the supplementation of resolvin D2 decreased brain damage caused by myocardial infarction, and it reversed the neurological dysfunction of the brain. A decrease in the concentration of proinflammatory cytokines, such as TNF-α, Il-6, and Il-1β, was also observed, as well as a decrease in the scope of brain damage. In the context of stroke in animals, the treatment with resolvin D2 (RvD2) (injection) has a better effect than supplementation with DHA. Conclusions: Resolvins are characterised by strong anti-inflammatory properties. Resolvins improve prognosis and decrease the risk of developing cardiovascular disease, consequently lowering the risk of stroke, and may find application in the treatment of stroke.

Keywords: resolvin; maresin; DHA; EPA; cardiovascular disease; stroke

---

1. Introduction

Ischemic stroke is currently the most frequent cause of disability in adults and one of the most common causes of death in the USA [1]. Despite the fact that the mortality rate resulting from strokes has decreased in the recent decade in the USA, it still constitutes a large percentage of the population [1]. In the case of European countries at the beginning of the 21st Century, the rate of cases was between 95 and 290 per 100,000 people a year (the data are from 2000–2010 and were extracted from the Register of

Strokes or Stroke Reports), so it is in the range of 0.29%. A higher prevalence of this illness was observed in Eastern Europe, less in the south [2]. The geographical differences associated with the prevalence of strokes may be related to environmental conditions, diet type, genetic factors, lower income, and thus, limited access to and the lower quality of the healthcare system [2]. The prevalence increases with age, especially after the age of 80, and the stroke incidence is more frequent in men than women over 60 years of age, as is also confirmed by European studies [1,2]. Fatigue, cognitive impairment, and lower quality of daily life can be present even after a minor stroke [3]. Continued and complex posthospitalization care, including treatment for depression and increased social support, covers the vast financial resources of healthcare [4]. Moreover, the perceived impact of stroke becomes more prominent with time, even for persons with mild-to-moderate stroke [5]. There are two main types of stroke leading to focal neurological deficit: ischemic and haemorrhagic stroke, which constitute 80–85% and 10–15% of all strokes, respectively. The standard treatment of ischemic stroke is to administer thrombolytic drugs to the patient or mechanical thrombectomy, while the haemorrhagic stroke methods are limited [6,7]. Current studies show that the level of DHA derivatives significantly decreases in the early post-stroke stage (up to seven days) compared to the control group. It is also related to the decrease of its precursor, DHA. Moreover, EPA was also lowered, but not resolvin E1 (RvE1) [8]. The same authors found that there was a relationship between the severity of depressive symptoms in stroke patients and the level of eicosanoids and free fatty acid (measured seven days after the incident and six months later). Patients with lower levels of DHA and its derivative (RvD1) had worse results by the Beck Depression Inventory-II [9]. The aim of this study is to overview the risk factors associated with stroke, the role of inflammation in stroke and the effects of EPA and DHA derivatives on the aspects of stroke pathomechanisms. We also discuss the potential beneficial effects of resolvins in the prevention and treatment of stroke taking into consideration the pre-stroke period and the acute phase of stroke. As clinical trials have not been conducted in humans, the last of the goals will be the discussion of the examples of experimental treatment in the animal models.

2. The Risk Factors for Developing Stroke

The risk factors of stroke development are associated both with some diseases, such as hypertension, dyslipidemia, obesity, and diabetes, as well as lifestyle (not enough physical activity, bad diet, smoking tobacco, and the overuse of alcohol) [10]. The modifiable factors listed above are responsible for as much as 90% of the possibility of developing stroke, whereas the remaining 10% are non-modifiable factors [11]. The latter include age, male gender, race and ethnicity, positive family history, socioeconomic status, and genetic factors (e.g., gene mutations of coagulation factors, proteins involved in lipid or homocysteine metabolism) [12].

One of the most important interventions that can prevent ischemic stroke is the treatment of hypertension. Hypertension is defined as systolic blood pressure ≥ 140 mm Hg or diastolic blood pressure ≥ 90 mm Hg. The occurrence of hypertension in stroke patients is more than 70% [13]. The effectiveness of treatment in the prevention of this illness has been confirmed more than once in randomised clinical studies: the risk of another stroke decreased by about 30% [13]. Studies also show a positive influence of the treatment of lipid disorders in patients after ischemic stroke, particularly when accompanied by an excessive level of LDL-C and an insufficient level of HDL in the blood serum of these patients. Treatment with statins decreased the risk of a subsequent ischemic stroke by 3.5–18% [11,14]. In patients after stroke, there are often problems with glucose metabolism disruptions: type 2 diabetes or impaired fasting glycemia (glucose levels: 100–125 mg/dL) were observed in about 70% of patients with ischemic stroke [13]. In persons suffering from diabetes, there is a risk of not only subsequent strokes, but also of the first ischemic stroke [15]. Obesity is another frequent disorder in stroke patients (44% of patients). In obese patients, most frequently, there are several connected risk factors related to stroke, including the abovementioned type 2 diabetes, hypertension, and dyslipidemia. Numerous studies indicate that obesity is associated with increased mortality, especially in young, post-stroke patients [16]. On the basis of the BMI analysis of stroke patients, it has been established that obese and overweight patients (BMI $\geq$ 25 kg/m^2) are characterised by much lower mortality in comparison to patients with correct BMI (<25 kg/m^2). This is why it is suggested that BMI (the interpretation of <25/ kg/m^2 considered as correct) is not an accurate indicator of the presence of obesity, particularly in elderly people. The study also did not take into account the distribution of adipose tissue, which is also an important factor determining the mortality in stroke [17–20]. In summary, modifiable risk factors of stroke pose the greatest risk of stroke and complications associated with this disease. The modifiable risk factors of stroke affect the inflammatory system leading to multidirectional, inflammatory changes and the development of atherosclerosis [21].

3. Inflammation in Stroke

Inflammation constitutes the significant pathogenetical factor of ischemic stroke because it is associated with the development of atherosclerosis. During a stroke, the death of neurons progresses very rapidly, from a few minutes to up to a few hours. This is caused by energy deficit, the lack of ion balance, the ineffectiveness of mitochondria, and the activation of intracellular lipases, proteases, and ribonucleases, which cause a rapid breakdown of the structural elements of cells and their integrity [21,22]. Immunological response begins locally in the vessel and, in the case of ischemic stroke, in ischemic brain cells. The inflammation cascade is activated immediately after the obstruction of blood vessels. Vascular stasis causes stress in the vascular endothelium and activates platelets. The distribution of P-selectin takes place on the cell surface, which is key for the deceleration of circulating leukocytes [21]. P-selectin binds with leukocytes, further increasing ischemic damage. Other adhesive molecules, such as E-selectin, intercellular adhesion molecule-1, and the vascular cell adhesion molecule-1, play a key role in the coordination, recruitment, adhesion, and migration of leukocytes in blood [23]. The basis of inflammation in ischemic stroke is the adhesion of neutrophils to endothelium cells and the cascades of blood coagulation, additionally stimulating inflammation signals. Thrombin induces the expression of adhesive molecules on endothelial cells and activates the C3 and C5 constituents of the complement system, and it may disrupt the function of the endothelial barrier. It forms a strong anticoagulation and anti-inflammatory complex, and it leads to the activation of monocytes and the complement system [21–24]. Inflammation mediators are spread throughout the entire body, leading to a systemic inflammatory response and, later, immunosuppression aiming at the suppression of a potentially damaging proinflammatory environment [24]. In experimental stroke, the systemic inflammatory response signal is characterised by an increased level of cytokines in the serum (interleukin-6, interferon-γ, CXC-chemokine ligand) and the increased production of inflammatory mediators in immune cells (TNF, IL-6, IL-2, CXC-chemokine ligand 12) within a few hours of ischemia [22–24]. Most of these parameters return to initial output levels within 24 h after stroke. The level of IL-6 in the serum is positively correlated with the exacerbation of stroke [25]. Ischemic stroke is associated with the presence of a strong inflammatory response in which arachidonic acid (AA) also plays a key role. Derivatives are synthesised by using three pathways, 5LOX, 15LOX, and COX1, 2 together with prostaglandins. It seems that 12LOX plays only a minor, insignificant role in this process [26–28].

Omega-3 PUFAs represent the precursors of lipid mediators, including resolvins, maresins, and protectins, which are collectively termed "specialized pro-resolving mediators" (SPMs) [29]. EPA and DHA can be incorporated into platelet phospholipid membranes at the expense of AA, and thus can decrease the synthesis of AA-derived metabolites and reduce the platelet aggregation [30]. The paths leading to the synthesis of EPA derivatives, DHA in particular, are also amplified as a result of the increased use of resolvins. There is growing evidence pointing to different mechanisms in the pathogenesis of stroke, but its progression depends on the intensity of the inflammation. Therefore, resolvins may improve the prognosis in numerous illnesses, including atherosclerosis, which is the main cause of stroke. The atherosclerotic plaque is characterised by a high presence of oxidised lipids and low-density lipoproteins, as well as the accumulation of monocytes and neutrophils [31]. Due to the dominating role of the inflammatory process in the pathogenesis of ischemic stroke, we concentrate in our work on the analysis of the role of resolvins in this type of stroke.

4. Resolvins: Synthesis

Excessive or uncontrolled inflammatory processes in the body contribute to the development of many illnesses that influence numerous cells and mediators. In recent years, there have been intensive studies regarding the identification of proinflammatory mediators originating from the enzymatic oxidation of polyunsaturated omega-3 acids: eicosapentaenoic acid (EPA) and docosahexaenoic acid (DHA) [32]. n-3 α-linolenic acid (ALA) is an important constituent of the cell membrane and is transformed into EPA with an efficiency of about 8%, whereas DHA is transformed with an efficiency of about 0.5%. The human ability to enzymatically convert ALA into DHA or EPA is limited, so they should be supplemented with diet [33]. The main source of DHA in diet are sea fish and seafood, out of which wild fish (sea fish) contain more omega-3 acids than farmed fish due to the fact that most of them feed on phytoplankton and zooplankton, which are rich in these fatty acids [33,34]. Most plant seeds and oils, e.g., rapeseed, soy, corn, and sunflower, are mainly a source of omega-6 acids, with a small amount of omega-3. The exceptions are the seeds of chia, flax, and hemp, which are rich in omega-3 acids, and they should be used for diet supplementation [33,35]. Studies show that EPA and DHA can have a positive influence on the resolution of atherosclerotic inflammation by reducing the synthesis of proinflammatory lipid mediators [30]. One such mediator is resolvins, which are synthesized with the involvement of cyclooxygenase pathways (COX) and lipoxygenase pathways (LOX) [32]. EPA serves as a substrate for the creation of resolvins E, whereas resolvins D are formed from DHA [36].

Acetylsalicylic acid (ASA), known as aspirin, acetylates cyclooxygenase-2 (COX-2) and enables the biosynthesis of precursors for anti-inflammatory mediators. Experimental studies show that, when influenced by ASA, EPA in mice is transformed into completely new products with anti-inflammatory properties. Because DHA has a cardioprotective effect, is abundantly present in the brain and the retina, and has an influence on numerous physiological processes, analyses were conducted to determine whether during inflammation, DHA was used in the treatment of ASA [37]. The analysis revealed that in mice treated with ASA and DHA, new bioactive docosanoids were formed, such as 17R-hydro(peroxy)-docosahexaenoic acid (17R-H (p) DHA), which is then transformed into resolvins D1-D4 thanks to COX-2 [37], as presented in Figure 1.

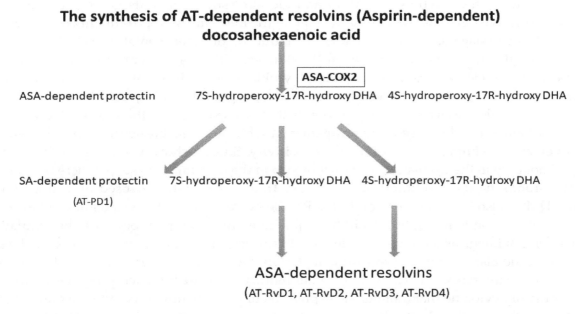

Figure 1. The biosynthesis of resolvins D with the presence of acetylsalicylic acid (ASA) [38,39]. Rv, resolvin.

A similar observation was made in the case of the synthesis of resolvins E. In mice treated with ASA, EPA was transformed into 18R-hydro (peroxy)-eicosapentaenoic acid (18R-H (p) EPA) thanks to the capabilities of the ASA-COX-2 enzyme [39,40]. Subsequently, this acid, in conjunction with 5-LOX, underwent further transformations into resolvins E, as presented in Figure 2.

The synthesis of AT-dependent resolvins (Aspirin-dependent)

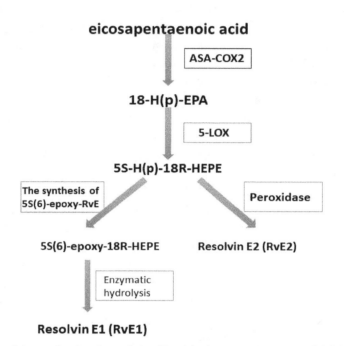

Figure 2. The biosynthesis of resolvins E with the participation of ASA [38,39].

It has been proven that resolvin E1 (RvE1) significantly decreases inflammation and the migration of neutrophils, activating the resolution of inflammation [38]. Moreover, it decreases the release of pro-inflammatory cytokines, mainly interleukins (Il-1, Il-6, Il-12, Il-17, and Il-23). One of the most studied cytokines in the cerebrospinal fluid and blood of stroke patients is the proinflammatory IL-6 [38–40]. However, there is still not many data on the mechanism of pro-inflammatory cytokines' activities in the early stage of stroke (4–6 h after the induction of experimental stroke). It is known that TNF-α, Il-1, and Il-6 increase in amount, even 40–60 times, within 24 h after a stroke [40]. Apart from the decrease in the release of pro-inflammatory cytokines, resolvin E1 also inhibits inflammatory angiogenesis and stimulates phagocytosis through macrophages. The strong anti-inflammatory activity of this resolvin was also observed in an in vivo study that focused, among others, on the kidney damage caused by ischemia, the decrease of inflammation in white adipose tissue (in mice), the reduction of fatty liver, and the improvement of insulin sensitivity. Studies show a strong protective effect of resolvins E not only in the circulatory system, but also in the respiratory system, where they facilitate apoptosis, promoting the resolution of respiratory tract inflammation caused by contact with an allergen [41]. It is also known that resolvin E2 (RvE2) is characterised by weaker anti-inflammatory activity in comparison to RvE1, but it still has a positive impact on phagocytosis, the regulation of the functioning of integrins located on the leukocyte surface, facilitating their migration to the site of inflammation, and also limiting the recruitment of granulocytes. Moreover, it has an influence on the production of the interleukin-10 (Il-10) anti-inflammatory cytokine by macrophages [42]. Il-10 is an anti-inflammatory cytokine that inhibits the expression of pro-inflammatory cytokines and regulates the innate immune response. In studies conducted on rats, Il-10 decreased the scope of ischemic stroke and the damage caused by cerebral artery obstruction [43]. It has also been demonstrated that lower levels of Il-10 are associated with an increased risk of stroke [44].

Resolvins D are created from DHA, and similarly to resolvins E, they have a strong anti-inflammatory effect. They contribute to the decrease in the migration of neutrophils. Furthermore, the activity of resolvin D1 (RvD1) is a mechanism that limits the damage that free radicals cause to tissues during oxygen explosion while the microorganism removal takes place. Resolvin D1 also inhibits the production of the Il-1β pro-inflammatory cytokine [44]. This is an acute-phase pro-inflammatory cytokine that serves as a chemoattractant for neutrophils, natural killer cells (NK), and T-lymphocytes. Most probably, it plays a key role already after the occurrence of stroke, and it may be a marker for the long-term changes after a stroke or brain damage [45]. Studies show that resolvin D4 promotes the synthesis of other D-series resolvins involved in the inhibition of inflammation. Moreover, it decreases the infiltration of neutrophilic granulocytes, and it increases the number of monocytes in the case of blood vessel thrombosis [46].

5. Receptors for Resolvins

So far, four G-protein coupled transmembrane receptors have been identified serving as receptors for resolvins D and E: DRV1/GPR32 (resolvin D1 receptor/G-23 protein coupled receptor), DRV2/GPR18 (resolvin D2 receptor/G-18 protein coupled receptor) for D-series resolvins, ERV1/ChemR23 (resolvin E1 receptor/chemerin receptor 23) and the leukotriene B_4 receptor 1 (BLT1) for E-series resolvins (resolvin E1 and resolvin E2) [47,48]. The latest studies conducted on mice revealed the significant therapeutic role of these receptors in the course of atherosclerosis via the ability to induce the resolution of inflammation in cardiovascular diseases [47]. Resolvins D1 and D3 transmit signals through the DRV1/GPR32 receptor, which is also activated by resolvin D5 and the analogues of D-series resolvins released through aspirin. The receptor undergoes expression in macrophages, increasing phagocytosis. D-series resolvins, through the DRV1/GPR32 receptor, also regulate the functioning of the immune system, preventing the differentiation of T-lymphocytes towards Th1 and Th12, and promoting regulatory cell (Tr) formation [47,48]. It has been proven that the atherosclerotic process features the transformation of vascular smooth muscle cells (SMCs) into a proliferative and migratory phenotype [49]. As a result, SMCs migrate to the site that was altered by atherosclerosis and stabilise the atherosclerotic plaque, forming its main constituent. Therefore, D-series resolvins may have a positive anti-inflammatory influence on blood vessel walls due to the presence of the DRV1/GRP32 receptor also in the vascular endothelium and SMCs [50,51]. Moreover, RvD3 is also associated with the DRV1/GPR32 receptor, which promotes macrophage phagocytosis [52]. Currently, there are no in vivo studies oriented towards the impact of the DRV1/GPR32 receptor on cardiovascular diseases due to the lack of a similar receptor in the studied mice. However, it seems that it can play a significant role in humans [53].

The DRV2/GPR18 receptor was detected in immune cells with various functions. It participates in the development of CD8a lymphocytes in the small intestine. In mice with a decreased amount of this receptor, we observed a smaller number and the migration ability of immune cells [54]. The development of CD8 lymphocytes is significant in the immune therapy of neoplasms, as well as in the treatment of inflammatory bowel diseases and viral infections. The DRV2/GPR18 receptor is also present in skeletal muscles. It has an influence on the resolution of inflammation: studies indicate that resolvin D2, after combining with the DRV2/GPR18 receptor, participates in the recruitment of granulocytes [54]. It has also been proven that DRV2/GPR18 undergoes expression in the heart of mice, particularly in cardiomyocytes. The chronic activation of this receptor leads to a decrease in blood pressure and an improvement of the functioning of the left ventricle in mice [51]. A combination of resolvin E1 and the ERV1/ChemR23 receptor stimulates phagocytosis, contributing to the reduction of inflammation and atherosclerotic processes in the arteries. Studies indicate that RvE1 may indirectly influence the development of cardiovascular diseases also through the change in metabolic factors because increased expression of the ERV1/ChemR23 receptor in fat tissue and a simultaneous decrease in the level of proinflammatory cytokines were observed [51,52]. The BLT1 receptor is expressed on human neutrophils, eosinophils, monocytes, macrophages, mast cells, dendritic cells, and T cells [48]. Both resolvins (RvE1, RvE2) are antagonists of the BLT1 receptor and have counterregulatory effects that lead to the inhibition of neutrophil chemotaxis, calcium mobilization, and NF-kB activation [55,56]. The types of resolvins and their roles are presented in Table 1.

Table 1. Characterization of resolvin subtypes and their receptors.

Omega-3	Resolvin Subtypes	Corresponding Receptors	Localisation	Function
EPA	RvE1	ChemR23 (ERV, CMKLR1)	Chemerin receptor 23 is expressed on NK cells, ILCs, macrophages, dendritic cells, and epithelial cells	stimulation of phagocytosis decrease in the level of proinflammatory cytokines
		BLT1		
	RvE2	BLT1	Leukotriene LTB4 is expressed on human neutrophils, eosinophils, monocytes, macrophages, mast cells, dendritic cells, and T cells	reduction in neutrophil mobilization
DHA-	RvD1	ALX/FPR2	Expression on neutrophils, macrophages, monocytes, macrophages, and T cells	increase of phagocytosis prevention of the differentiation of T-lymphocytes towards Th1 and Th12, promotion of regulatory cell (Tr) formation
		DRV1/GPR32	The G-23 protein coupled receptor is expressed on human neutrophils, lymphocytes, macrophages, and monocytes, as well as vascular tissues	
	RvD2	DRV1/GPR32	The G-18 protein coupled receptor is expressed on human and murine neutrophils, monocytes, and macrophages	development of CD8a lymphocytes in the small intestine migration ability of immune cells recruitment of granulocytes decrease in blood pressure
		DRV2/GPR18		
	RvD3	DRV1/GPR32	The G-23 protein coupled receptor is expressed on human neutrophils, lymphocytes, macrophages, and monocytes, as well as vascular tissues	promotion of macrophage phagocytosis
	RvD4	G protein-coupled receptors: no data		inhibition of metastases and induced T cell responses
	RvD5	DRV1/GPR32	The G-23 protein coupled receptor is expressed on human neutrophils, lymphocytes, macrophages, and monocytes, as well as vascular tissues	expression of macrophages increase of phagocytosis.

6. The Role of Resolvins in Stroke

Though preliminary studies indicate a decrease in the risk of cardiovascular diseases thanks to the introduction of omega-3 acid supplementation, large double-blind studies did not show clear beneficial effects [26]. Omega-3 fatty acids may contribute to the reduction of inflammation both through the reduction of pro-inflammatory factors, as well as through the stimulation of the resolution of inflammation. The potentially protective effect of these acids in cardiovascular diseases, including atherosclerosis and stroke, may refer to their influence on lipid metabolism, thrombosis, and the abovementioned inflammations, which are the risk factors of stroke [26,46].

Dong et al. conducted studies on experimental models: mice with ischemic stroke caused by the obstruction of the middle cerebral artery [57]. RvD2 was supplied to the brain of mice in the form of nanoparticles. The results showed that RvD2 nanoparticles aim precisely at the inflammation of endothelium in the brain. After the supply of RvD2, there was a decrease in the concentration of pro-inflammatory cytokines, such as TNF-α, IL-6, and IL-1β. Furthermore, in mice treated with RvD2, the volume of brain damage after a stroke decreased to 16%, in comparison to 46% in the control group. After the intraperitoneal injection of this resolvin, a decrease of inflammation, a reversal of the formed brain damage, and a reversal of the neurological dysfunction of the brain were observed [57]. The available data points to the benefits of using resolvins in ischemic stroke. The supply of RvD2 also increased the amount of GPR18 protein, which is a receptor for RvD2, particularly in neurons and brain endothelial cells [57,58]. In the animal model of ischemic stroke in rats, the effective dose of RvD2 was 50 µg/kg or 100µg/kg. The beneficial effects were elucidated by the decrease in the volume of the infarcted area of the brain, as well as by the anti-inflammatory properties. The exogenous RvD2 reduces the release of TNF-α and IL6 in the brain, decreases the infarct area, and protects the neurons and endothelial cells of the blood-brain barrier (BBB) from apoptosis and necrosis, maintaining the BBB's integrity [54,59].

Correia et al. proved that preliminary DHA treatment may successfully improve the process of memory recovery in rats with ischemic stroke. In the context of stroke, treatment with RvD2 (administered directly in the form of an injection) had better treatment results [55,60]. The basis for inflammation in ischemic stroke is the adhesion of neutrophils to endothelium cells. Studies show that RvD2 can decrease the interaction between leukocytes: endothelium cells, as well as the production of cytokines. This happens through the induction of the creation of nitrogen oxide in endothelium cells in order to decrease this interaction [57]. Similar results pointing to the reduction of the concentration of pro-inflammatory cytokines by resolvins were achieved by Xu et al. [61]. They determined that RvD1 prevents the lipopolysaccharide-induced (LPS induced) inflammatory response in microglia cells of mice (in vitro). The LPS-activated microglia cells cause a release of pro-inflammatory factors through the interaction of LPS-TLR4 (lipopolysaccharide-Toll-like receptor-4). After the supply of RvD1, the expression of TNF-α and IL-1β was stopped, and the process of forming pro-inflammatory factors in microglia cells did not occur in the studied mice [61]. According to the study of related signaling pathways, RvD1 attenuated LPS-induced microglia NF-κB activation and MAPK phosphorylation and inhibited the transcriptional activity of protein-1 activator [60,61].

In other studies conducted on mice, it was demonstrated that the supply of RvD2 supported the activity of macrophages, contributing to the increase in the stabilisation of atherosclerotic plaque. The treatment with RvD2 and maresin R1 decelerated the progression of atherosclerosis without influencing body mass, the level of lipids in the plasma, and the number of blood cells of the studied mice [62].

Macrophages in blood have the ability to adapt to the changes in their surroundings due to the fact that they react to receptors and signalling particles. It is usually not possible to clearly determine their phenotype because they swiftly adapt to changes in their surroundings. Macrophages with the M1 phenotype dominate in the early inflammation response: pro-inflammatory pathways are activated in cells. On the other hand, macrophages with the M2 phenotype participate in regeneration processes after inflammation, including in atherosclerotic processes [63,64]. Studies confirmed that in mice supplied with RvD2 and MaR1, the phenotype of macrophages changes from pro-inflammatory M1 into M2, the latter playing an important role in maintaining homeostasis against inflammation and atherosclerosis, as well as supporting regenerative processes [65–67].

Additionally, in a study conducted on a mice model of atherosclerosis, it was determined that the supply of resolvin E1 (RvE1) significantly decreases atherosclerotic changes by inhibiting the expression of TNF-α, without changing the amount of macrophages. When supplying RvE1 orally once per day for 16 weeks, there was a decrease in atherosclerotic changes in mice by 35%, and they were classified as mild. Moreover, RvE1 did not have an influence on the level of cholesterol in the plasma [67]. The potential effects of resolvin injections can be expected even faster, because after the intraperitoneal administration of RvD1, its plasma level peaks at one hour, stays constant at three hours, and returns to baseline after 36 h. Such an observation is promising for potential clinical use in humans, as it could be used as an option for treatment in the acute phase of stroke [68].

Similar results were achieved in rabbits with a high-cholesterol diet, in which the supply of RvE1 caused a decrease in atherosclerotic changes in the aorta and a significant decrease in C-reactive protein (CRP), which, as an acute-phase protein, appears in blood during an inflammation, becoming an inflammation marker [69]. The aggregation of platelets and thrombosis are two factors that, similarly to atherosclerosis and inflammation, support the development of stroke. However, in recent studies, it has been demonstrated that resolvins may also prevent the aggregation of platelets and induce the extension of blood vessels [70]. The hypothetical effects of resolvin after stroke are shown in Figure 3.

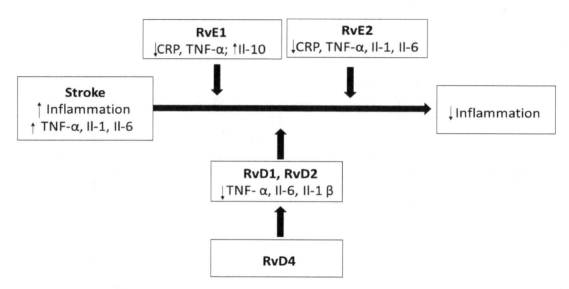

Figure 3. The effect of resolvins on inflammation after a stroke.

Although no studies on the effects of resolvins have been found in humans after stroke, a great deal of research has been done on the effects of omega-3 fatty acids. Yokoyama M. et al. conducted studies on the effect of omega-3 fatty acid supplementation on the prevention of cardiovascular diseases [71]. This randomized placebo-controlled trials proved that EPA supplementation (1.8 g/24 h) may reduce the risk of coronary events by 19% [71]. Similar results were obtained by Bhatt D. et al. in a randomized, placebo-controlled trial (REDUCE-IT) [72]. They studied the effects of EPA supplementation (4 g of icosapent ethyl-EPA ethyl ester/24h) on cardiovascular risk in patients with cardiovascular risk factors. The incidence of cardiovascular incidents and deaths from cardiovascular causes were significantly lower in the group that was supplemented with EPA [72]. The opposite results were presented in the ASCEND and Risk and Prevention trials. The supplementation with EPA and DHA or omega-3 fatty acids in the amount of 1 g per day does not significantly reduce the overall and cardiovascular morbidity of patients with cardiovascular risk factors [73,74].

Clinical studies suggest that omega-3 fatty acids may play a beneficial role in preventing CVD episodes when administered at higher doses. However, more research is needed on resolvins, especially in regard to primary and secondary prevention, as well as in the treatment of the acute phase of stroke in humans.

7. Conclusions

Excessive or uncontrolled inflammatory processes contribute to the development of many illnesses. The significant role of omega-3 acids, out of which resolvins with anti-inflammatory influence are formed, was proven in the treatment of cardiovascular diseases, including stroke. It has been confirmed that resolvins have a positive influence on the resolution of inflammation by synthesizing the anti-inflammatory mediators and inhibiting the synthesis of pro-inflammatory mediators. As a result, resolvins influence the improvement of prognosis in stroke cases, but the studies were mostly carried out on rodents.

The limitation of the use of resolvins in stroke patients is mainly connected with the safety profile; thus, there should be a standard safety protocol of the clinical studies performed. The initial, promising treatment with the use of resolvins in animal models may be limited by the potential disadvantages of such a treatment in humans. Secondary intracerebral haemorrhage is a serious, harmful complication of ischemic stroke itself or the thrombolytic therapy in such patients, especially when, additionally, antiplatelet or anticoagulant treatment is used. Taking into consideration the interaction with the inflammatory system, platelets, adhesion molecules, and BBB stability, the risk of haemorrhagic complications after resolvins' administration should be cautiously analysed.

The future direction for resolvin therapy in humans should start with the analysis of the safety, then the bioavailability and effectiveness need to be established. Rapid bioavailability may give a chance that the beneficial effects of resolvins' administration would be observed in stroke patients directly after the onset. If the safety profile is granted, we suggest testing such treatment in the time-window as fast as possible after the ischemic stroke onset. This seems to be important, because secondary to brain tissue ischemia, the inflammatory, cytotoxic cascade appears and could potentially be inhibited at an early stage by the use of resolvins. The protective effect on the BBB is also of note, as the cytotoxic cascade after stroke disrupts this barrier. Different neuroprotective strategies have been discussed and tested, but this type of treatment is a promising method of neuroprotection and treatment. The prolonged effect of resolvins would also be beneficial by means of reducing the risk of recurrent stroke or malignant brain oedema, which are serious complications of ischemic stroke. We also suggest taking into consideration the interaction of resolvins with other drugs that can affect the inflammatory system. A number of stroke patients are treated with the use of statins or hypotensives that can interact with resolvins within inflammation.

The mechanism of resolvins' activity takes place through phagocytosis, the decrease in the migration of neutrophils, the reduction in the synthesis of pro-inflammatory cytokines, and the strengthening of the resolution of the inflammatory process. However, further studies are necessary to determine the existing mechanisms in humans and to determine the efficiency, pharmacokinetics, and safety profile of the preventive or therapeutical dose of resolvins and the way of administration.

8. Method of Article Search

The review takes into account articles published until 31 January 2020. The literature was searched for in PubMed and Embase databases using the following keywords: resolvin, stroke, and cardiovascular disease. We analysed 153 articles, and 56 of the works were included in the study. Studies not written in English, letters to the editor, conference abstracts, and duplicate information were excluded. Another 18 studies were included by analysing the individual sections of this review. All included studies were screened and discussed by the authors until a general consensus was reached.

Author Contributions: Conceptualization, M.S.; methodology N.T., M.S.; software, N.T., D.K., P.P., M.S.; validation, N.T., D.K., M.S.; formal analysis, N.T., D.K., M.S.; investigation, N.T., D.K., M.S.; writing—original draft preparation, N.T., D.K., M.S.; writing—review and editing, N.T., D.K., P.P., M.S.; visualization, N.T., M.S.; supervision, D.K., M.S.; project administration, M.S.; funding acquisition, P.P., M.S. All authors have read and agreed to the published version of the manuscript.

References

1.   Guzik, A.; Bushnell, C. Stroke epidemiology and risk factor management. *Continuum (Minneap. Min.)* **2017**, *23*, 15–39. [CrossRef] [PubMed]
2.   Bejot, Y.; Bailly, H.; Durier, J.; Giroud, M. Epidemiology of stroke in Europe and trends for the 21st century. *La Presse Med.* **2016**, *45*, e391–e398. [CrossRef] [PubMed]
3.   Ramírez-Moreno, J.M.; Muñoz-Vega, P.; Alberca, S.B.; Peral-Pacheco, D. Health-related quality of life and fatigue after transient ischemic attack and minor stroke. *J. Stroke Cerebrovasc. Dis.* **2019**, *28*, 276–284. [CrossRef] [PubMed]
4.   Dąbrowska-Bender, M.; Milewska, M.; Gołąbek, A.; Duda-Zalewska, A.; Staniszewska, A.J. The impact of ischemic cerebral stroke on the quality of life of patients based on clinical, social, and psychoemotional factors. *Stroke Cerebrovasc. Dis.* **2017**, *26*, 101–107. [CrossRef]

5. Skoglund, E.; Westerlind, E.; Persson, H.C.; Sunnerhagen, K.S. Self-perceived impact of stroke: A longitudinal comparison between one and five years post-stroke. *J. Rehabil. Med.* **2019**, *51*, 660–664. [CrossRef]

6. Davis, C.M.; Fairbanks, S.L.; Alkayed, N.J. Mechanism of the sex difference in endothelial dysfunction after stroke. *Transl. Stroke Res.* **2013**, *4*, 381–389. [CrossRef]

7. Shu, S.; Pei, L.; Lu, Y. Promising targets of cell death signaling of NR2B receptor subunit in stroke pathogenesis. *Regen. Med. Res.* **2014**, *2*, 8. [CrossRef]

8. Szczuko, M.; Kotlęga, D.; Palma, J.; Zembroń-Łacny, A.; Tylutka, A.; Gołąb-Janowska, M.; Drozd, A. Lipoxins, RevD1 and 9, 13 HODE as the most important derivatives after an early incident of ischemic stroke. *Sci. Rep.* **2020**, *10*, 12849. [CrossRef]

9. Kotlega, D.; Zembron-Lacny, A.; Golab-Janowska, M.; Nowacki, P.; Szczuko, M. The association of free fatty acids and eicosanoids with the severity of depressive symptoms in stroke patients. *Int. J. Mol. Sci.* **2020**, *21*, 5220. [CrossRef]

10. Sakakibara, B.; Kim, A.; Eng, J. A systematic review and meta-analysis on self-management for improving risk factor control in stroke patients. *Int. J. Behav. Med.* **2017**, *24*, 42–53. [CrossRef]

11. Kotlęga, D.; Gołąb-Janowska, M.; Meller, A.; Pawlukowska, W.; Nowacki, P. Detection of stroke risk factors over the decade in the polish population of ischemic stroke patients. *Adv. Psychiatry Neurol. Postępy Psychiatrii i Neurologii* **2019**, *28*, 83–87. [CrossRef]

12. Kariasa, I.M.; Nurachmah, E.; Setyowati, S.; Koestoer, R.A. Analysis of participants' characteristics and risk factors for stroke recurrence. *Enferm. Clin.* **2019**, *29*, 286–290. [CrossRef]

13. Kernan, W.; Ovbiagele, B.; Black, H.; Bravata, D.; Chimowitz, M.; Ezekowitz, M.; Fang, M.C.; Fisher, M.; Furie, K.L.; Heck, D.V.; et al. Guidelines for prevention of stroke in patients with stroke and transient ischemic attack: A guideline for healthcare professionals from the American Heart Association/American Stroke Association. *Stroke* **2014**, *45*, 2160–2236. [CrossRef]

14. Kotlęga, D.; Ciećwież, S.; Turowska-Kowalska, J.; Nowacki, P. Pathogenetic justification of statin use in ischaemic stroke prevention according to inflammatory theory in development of atherosclerosis. Advances in Psychiatry and Neurology/Postępy Psychiatrii i Neurologii. *Neurol. Neurochir. Polska* **2012**, *46*, 176–183. [CrossRef] [PubMed]

15. Goldstein, L.B.; Bushnell, C.D.; Adams, R.J.; Appel, L.J.; Braun, L.T.; Chaturvedi, S.; Creager, M.A.; Culebras, A.; Eckel, R.H.; Hart, R.G.; et al. Guidelines for the primary prevention of stroke. *Stroke* **2011**, *42*, 517–584. [CrossRef] [PubMed]

16. Sahlin, C.; Sandberg, O.; Gustafson, Y.; Bucht, G.; Carlberg, B.; Stenlund, H.; Franklin, G.A. Obstructiove sleep apnea is a risk factor for death in patients with stroke: A 10-year follow-up. *Arch. Intern. Med.* **2008**, *168*, 297–301. [CrossRef] [PubMed]

17. Kernan, W.; Inzucchi, S.; Sawan, C.; Macko, R.; Furie, K. Obesity: A stubbornly obvious target prevention. *Stroke* **2013**, *44*, 278–286. [CrossRef]

18. Vemmos, K.; Ntaios, G.; Spengos, K.; Savvari, P.; Vemmou, A.; Pappa, T.; Manios, E.D.; Georgiopoulos, G.; Alevizaki, M. Association between obesity and mortality after acute first-ever stroke. *Stroke* **2011**, *42*, 30–36. [CrossRef]

19. Ovbiagele, B.; Bath, P.M.; Cotton, D.; Vinisko, R.; Diener, H.-C. Obesity and recurrent vascular risk after a recent ischemic stroke. *Stroke* **2011**, *42*, 3397–3402. [CrossRef]

20. Haley, M.J.; Lawrence, C.B. Obesity and stroke: Can we translate from rodents to patients? *Br. J. Pharmacol.* **2016**, *36*, 2007–2021. [CrossRef]

21. Anrather, J.; Iadecola, C. Inflammation and stroke: An overview. *Neurotherapeutics* **2016**, *13*, 661–670. [CrossRef]

22. Jackman, K.; Iadecola, C. Neurovascular regulation in the ischemic brain. *Antioxid. Redox Signal.* **2015**, *22*, 149–160. [CrossRef] [PubMed]

23. Petrovic-Djergovic, D.; Goonewardena, S.N.; Pinsky, D.J. Inflammatory disequilibrium in stroke. *Circ. Res.* **2016**, *119*, 142–158. [CrossRef]

24. Chapman, K.Z.; Dale, V.Q.; Dénes, Á.; Bennett, G.; Rothwell, N.J.; Allan, S.M.; McColl, B.W. A rapid and transient peripheral inflammatory response precedes brain inflammation after experimental stroke. *Br. J. Pharmacol.* **2009**, *29*, 1764–1768. [CrossRef]

25. Kes, V.B.; Simundic, A.-M.; Nikolac, N.; Topic, E.; Demarin, V. Pro-inflammatory and anti-inflammatory cytokines in acute ischemic stroke and their relation to early neurological deficit and stroke outcome. *Clin. Biochem.* **2008**, *41*, 1330–1334. [CrossRef]

26. Zhao, L.; Funk, C.D.; Zhao, L.; Funk, C.D. Lipoxygenase pathways in atherogenesis. *Trends Cardiovasc. Med.* **2004**, *14*, 191–195. [CrossRef]

27. Hampel, J.K.; Brownrigg, L.M.; Vignarajah, D.; Croft, K.D.; Dharmarajan, A.M.; Bentel, J.M.; Puddey, I.B.; Yeap, B.B. Differential modulation of cell cycle, apoptosis and PPARγ2 gene expression by PPARγ agonists ciglitazone and 9-hydroxyoctadecadienoic acid in monocytic cells. *Prostaglandins Leukot. Essent. Fat. Acids* **2006**, *74*, 283–293. [CrossRef]

28. Limor, R.; Sharon, O.; Knoll, E.; Many, A.; Weisinger, G.; Stern, N. Lipoxygenase-derived metabolites are regulators of peroxisome proliferator-activated receptor -2 expression in human vascular smooth muscle cells. *Am. J. Hypertens.* **2008**, *21*, 219–223. [CrossRef]

29. Simonetto, M.; Infante, M.; Sacco, R.L.; Rundek, T.; Della-Morte, D. A novel anti-inflammatory role of omega-3 PUFAs in prevention and treatment of atherosclerosis and vascular cognitive impairment and dementia. *Nutrients* **2019**, *11*, 2279. [CrossRef] [PubMed]

30. Carracedo, M.; Artiach, G.; Arnardottir, H.; Bäck, M. The resolution of inflammation through omega-3 fatty acids in atherosclerosis, intimal hyperplasia, and vascular calcification. *Semin. Immunopathol.* **2019**, *41*, 757–766. [CrossRef]

31. Viola, J.; Lemnitzer, P.; Jansen, Y.; Csaba, G.; Winter, C.; Neideck, C.; Silvestre-Roig, C.; Dittmar, G.; Döring, Y.; Drechsler, M.; et al. Resolving lipid mediatrs maresin 1 and resolvin D2 prevent atheroprogression in mice. *Circ. Res.* **2016**, *119*, 1030–1038. [CrossRef] [PubMed]

32. Bäck, M.; Hansson, G.K. Omega-3 fatty acids, cardiovascular risk, and the resolution of inflammation. *FASEB J.* **2019**, *33*, 1536–1539. [CrossRef] [PubMed]

33. Saini, R.K.; Keum, Y.-S. Omega-3 and omega-6 polyunsaturated fatty acids: Dietary sources, metabolism, and significance—A review. *Life Sci.* **2018**, *203*, 255–267. [CrossRef] [PubMed]

34. Brenna, J.; Salem, N.; Sinclair, A.J.; Cunnane, S.C. α-Linolenic acid supplementation and conversion to n-3 long-chain polyunsaturated fatty acids in humans. *Prostaglandins Leukot. Essent. Fat Acids* **2009**, *80*, 85–91. [CrossRef] [PubMed]

35. Williams, C.; Burdge, G. Long-chain n-3 PUFA: Plant v. marine sources. *Proc. Nutr. Soc.* **2006**, *65*, 42–50. [CrossRef]

36. Calder, P.C. Omega-3 fatty acids and inflammatory processes: From molecules to man. *Biochem. Soc. Trans.* **2017**, *45*, 1105–1115. [CrossRef]

37. Serhan, C.; Hong, S.; Gronert, K.; Colgan, S.; Devchand, P.; Mirick, G.; Moussignac, R.-L. Resolvins: A family of bioactive products of omega-3 fatty acid transformation circuits initiated by aspirin treatment that counter proinflammation signals. *J. Exp. Med.* **2002**, *196*, 1025–1037. [CrossRef]

38. Nowak, J.Z. Anti-inflammatory pro-resolving derivatives of omega-3 and omega-6 polyunsaturated fatty acids. *Postępy Hig. Med. Dosw.* **2010**, *64*, 115–132.

39. Duvall, M.G.; Levy, B.D. DHA- and EPA-derived resolvins, protectins, and maresins in airway inflammation. *Eur. J. Pharmacol.* **2016**, *785*, 144–155. [CrossRef]

40. Lambertsen, K.L.; Biber, K.; Finsen, B. Inflammatory cytokines in experimental and human stroke. *Br. J. Pharmacol.* **2012**, *32*, 1677–1698. [CrossRef]

41. Bannenberg, G.; Serhan, C. Pro-resolving lipid mediators in the inflammatory response: An update. *Biochim. Biophys. Acta (BBA) Mol. Cell Biol. Lipids* **2010**, *1801*, 1260–1273. [CrossRef] [PubMed]

42. Xie, G.; Myint, P.K.; Zaman, M.J.S.; Li, Y.; Zhao, L.; Shi, P.; Ren, F.; Wu, Y. Relationship of serum interleukin-10 and its genetic variations with ischemic stroke in a chinese general population. *PLoS ONE* **2013**, *8*, e74126. [CrossRef] [PubMed]

43. Arponen, O.; Muuronen, A.; Taina, M.; Sipola, P.; Hedman, M.; Jäkälä, P.; Vanninen, R.; Pulkki, K.; Mustonen, P. Acute phase IL-10 plasma concentration associates with the high risk sources of cardiogenic stroke. *PLoS ONE* **2015**, *10*, e0120910. [CrossRef] [PubMed]

44. Oh, S.F.; Dona, M.; Fredman, G.; Krishnamoorthy, S.; Irimia, D.; Serhan, C.N. Resolvin E2 formation and impact in inflammation resolution. *J. Immunol.* **2012**, *188*, 4527–4534. [CrossRef] [PubMed]

45. Jenny, N.; Callas, P.; Judd, S.; McClure, L.; Kissela, B.; Zakai, N.; Cuchman, M. Inflammatory cytokines and schemic stroke risk: The REGARDS cohort. *Neurology* **2019**, *92*, e2375–e2384. [CrossRef]

46. Cherpokova, D.; Jouvene, C.C.; Libreros, S.; DeRoo, E.P.; Chu, L.; De La Rosa, X.; Norris, P.C.; Wagner, D.D.; Serhan, C.N. Resolvin D4 attenuates the severity of pathological thrombosis in mice. *Blood* **2019**, *134*, 1458–1468. [CrossRef] [PubMed]

47. Pirault, J.; Bäck, M. Lipoxin and resolvin receptors transducing the resolution of inflammation in cardiovascular disease. *Front Pharmacol.* **2018**, *9*, 1273. [CrossRef] [PubMed]

48. Elajami, T.K.; Colas, R.A.; Dalli, J.; Chiang, N.; Serhan, C.N.; Welty, F.K. Specialized proresolving lipid mediators in patients with coronary artery disease and their potential for clot remodeling. *FASEB J.* **2016**, *30*, 2792–2801. [CrossRef]

49. Fredman, G.; Spite, M. Specialized pro-resolving mediators in cardiovascular diseases. *Mol. Asp. Med.* **2017**, *58*, 65–71. [CrossRef]

50. Doran, A.C.; Meller, N.; McNamara, C.A. Role of smooth muscle cells in the initiation and early progression of atherosclerosis. *Arter. Thromb. Vasc. Biol.* **2008**, *28*, 812–819. [CrossRef]

51. Karagiannis, G.; Weile, J.; Bader, G.; Minta, J. Integrative pathway dissection of molecular mechanisms od moxLDL-induced vascular muscle phenotype transformation. *BMC Cardiovasc. Disord.* **2013**, *13*, 4. [CrossRef]

52. Arita, M.; Ohira, T.; Sun, Y.-P.; Elangovan, S.; Chiang, N.; Serhan, C.N. Resolvin E1 selectively interacts with leukotriene B4 receptor BLT1 and chemr23 to regulate inflammation. *J. Immunol.* **2007**, *178*, 3912–3917. [CrossRef] [PubMed]

53. Laguna-Fernandez, A.; Checa, A.; Carracedo, M.; Artiach, G.; Petri, M.; Baumgartner, R.; Forteza, M.J.; Jiang, X.; Andonova, T.; Waler, M.E.; et al. ERV1/ChemR23 signaling protects against atherosclerosis by modifying oxidized low-density lipoprotein uptake and phagocytosis in macrophages. *Circulation* **2018**, *138*, 1693–1705. [CrossRef] [PubMed]

54. Zuo, G.; Zhang, D.; Mu, R.; Shen, H.; Li, X.; Wang, Z.; Li, H.; Chen, G. Resolvin D2 protects against cerebral ischemia/reperfusion injury in rats. *Mol. Brain* **2018**, *11*, 1–13. [CrossRef]

55. Bäck, M. Omega-3 fatty acids in atherosclerosis and coronary artery disease. *Futur. Sci. OA* **2017**, *3*. [CrossRef]

56. Panigrahy, D.; Gartung, A.; Yang, J.; Yang, H.; Gilligan, M.M.; Sulciner, M.L.; Bhasin, S.S.; Bielenberg, D.R.; Chang, J.; Schmidt, B.A.; et al. Preoperative stimulation of resolution and inflammation blockade eradicates micrometastases. *J. Clin. Investig.* **2019**, *129*, 2964–2979. [CrossRef] [PubMed]

57. Dong, X.; Gao, J.; Zhang, C.Y.; Hayworth, C.; Frank, M.; Wang, Z. Neutrophil membrane-derived nanovesicles alleviate inflammation to protect mouse brain injury from ischemic stroke. *ACS Nano* **2019**, *13*, 1272–1283. [CrossRef] [PubMed]

58. Chiang, N.; Dalli, J.; Colas, R.A.; Serhan, C.N. Identification of resolvin D2 receptor mediating resolution of infections and organ protection. *J. Exp. Med.* **2015**, *212*, 1203–1217. [CrossRef]

59. Wang, C.-S.; Maruyama, C.L.; Easley, J.T.; Trump, B.G.; Baker, O.J. AT-RvD1 promotes resolution of inflammation in NOD/ShiLtJ mice. *Sci. Rep.* **2017**, *7*. [CrossRef]

60. Bacarin, C.C.; Mori, M.A.; Ferreira, E.D.F.; Romanini, C.V.; De Oliveira, R.M.W.; Milani, H. Fish oil provides robust and sustained memory recovery after cerebral ischemia: Influence of treatment regimen. *Physiol. Behav.* **2013**, *119*, 61–71. [CrossRef]

61. Xu, M.; Tan, B.; Zhou, W.; Wei, T.; Lai, W.; Tan, J.-W.; Dong, J. Resolvin D1, an endogenous lipid mediator for inactivation of inflammation-related signaling pathways in microglial cells, prevents lipopolysaccharide-induced inflammatory responses. *CNS Neurosci. Ther.* **2013**, *19*, 235–243. [CrossRef] [PubMed]

62. Murray, P.J.; Wynn, T.A. Obstacles and opportunities for understanding macrophage polarization. *J. Leukoc. Biol.* **2011**, *89*, 557–563. [CrossRef] [PubMed]

63. Nazimek, K.; Bryniarski, K. The biological activity of macrophages in health and disease. *Postępy Hig. Med. Dosw.* **2012**, *66*, 507–520. [CrossRef] [PubMed]

64. Akagi, D.; Chen, M.; Toy, R.; Chatterjee, A.; Conte, M.S. Systemic delivery of proresolving lipid mediators resolvin D 2 and maresin 1 attenuates intimal hyperplasia in mice. *FASEB J.* **2015**, *29*, 2504–2513. [CrossRef] [PubMed]

65. Eitos, E.; Rius, B.; Gonzalez-Periz, A.; Lopez-Vicario, C.; Moran-Salvador, E.; Martinez-Clemente, M.; Arroyo, V.; Claria, J. Resolvin D1 and its precursor docosahexaenoic acid promote resolution of adipose tissue inflammation by eliciting macrophage polarization towar dan M2-like phenotype. *J. Immunol.* **2011**, *187*, 5408–5418.

66. Hsiao, H.-M.; Sapinoro, R.E.; Thatcher, T.H.; Croasdell, A.; Levy, E.P.; Fulton, R.A.; Olsen, K.C.; Pollock, S.J.; Serhan, C.N.; Phipps, R.P.; et al. A novel anti-inflammatory and pro-resolving role for resolvin D1 in acute cigarette smoke-induced lung inflammation. *PLoS ONE* **2013**, *8*, e58258. [CrossRef]

67. Salic, K.; Morrison, M.C.; Verschuren, L.; Wielinga, P.Y.; Wu, L.; Kleemann, R.; Gjorstrup, P.; Kooistra, T. Resolvin E1 attenuates atherosclerosis in absence of cholesterol-lowering effects and on top of atorvastatin. *Atherosclerosis* **2016**, *250*, 158–165. [CrossRef] [PubMed]

68. Krashia, P.; Cordella, A.; Nobili, A.; La Barbera, L.; Federici, M.; Leuti, A.; Campanelli, F.; Natale, G.; Marino, G.; Calabrese, V.; et al. Blunting neuroinflammation with resolvin D1 prevents early pathology in a rat model of Parkinson's disease. *Nat. Commun.* **2019**, *10*, 1–19. [CrossRef]

69. Hasturk, H.; Abdallah, R.; Kantarci, A.; Nguyen, D.; Giordano, N.; Hamilton, J.; Van Dyke, T.E. Resolvin E1 (RvE1) attenuates atherosclerotic plaque formation in diet and inflammation-induced atherogenesis. *Arter. Thromb. Vasc. Biol.* **2015**, *35*, 1123–1133. [CrossRef]

70. Capó, X.; Martorell, M.; Busquets-Cortés, C.; Tejada, S.; Tur, J.A.; Pons, A.; Sureda, A. Resolvins as proresolving inflammatory mediators in cardiovascular disease. *Eur. J. Med. Chem.* **2018**, *153*, 123–130. [CrossRef]

71. Yokoyama, M.; Origasa, H.; Matsuzaki, M.; Matsuzawa, Y.; Saito, Y.; Ishikawa, Y.; Oikawa, S.; Sasaki, J.; Hishida, H.; Itakura, H.; et al. Effects of eicosapentaenoic acid on major coronary events in hypercholesterolaemic patients (JELIS): A randomised open-label, blinded endpoint analysis. *Lancet* **2007**, *369*, 1090–1098. [CrossRef]

72. Bhatt, D.L.; Steg, P.G.; Miller, M.; Brinton, E.A.; Jacobson, T.A.; Ketchum, S.B.; Doyle, R.T.; Juliano, R.A.; Jiao, L.; Granowitz, C.; et al. Cardiovascular risk reduction with icosapent ethyl for hypertriglyceridemia. *N. Engl. J. Med.* **2019**, *380*, 11–22. [CrossRef] [PubMed]

73. Risk and Prevention Study Collaborative Group; Roncaglioni, M.C.; Tombesi, M.; Avanzini, F.; Barlera, S.; Caimi, V.; Longoni, P.; Marzona, I.; Milani, V.; Silletta, M.G.; et al. n–3 fatty acids in patients with multiple cardiovascular risk factors. *N. Engl. J. Med.* **2013**, *368*, 1800–1808. [CrossRef] [PubMed]

74. Manson, J.E.; Cook, N.R.; Lee, I.-M.; Christen, W.; Bassuk, S.S.; Mora, S.; Gibson, H.; Albert, C.M.; Gordon, D.; Copeland, T.; et al. Marine n–3 fatty acids and prevention of cardiovascular disease and cancer. *N. Engl. J. Med.* **2019**, *380*, 23–32. [CrossRef]

3

Pathophysiology and Treatment of Stroke: Present Status and Future Perspectives

Diji Kuriakose[ID] **and Zhicheng Xiao** *

Development and Stem Cells Program, Monash Biomedicine Discovery Institute and Department of Anatomy and Developmental Biology, Monash University, Melbourne, VIC 3800, Australia; diji.kuriakose@monash.edu
* Correspondence: zhicheng.xiao@monash.edu

Abstract: Stroke is the second leading cause of death and a major contributor to disability worldwide. The prevalence of stroke is highest in developing countries, with ischemic stroke being the most common type. Considerable progress has been made in our understanding of the pathophysiology of stroke and the underlying mechanisms leading to ischemic insult. Stroke therapy primarily focuses on restoring blood flow to the brain and treating stroke-induced neurological damage. Lack of success in recent clinical trials has led to significant refinement of animal models, focus-driven study design and use of new technologies in stroke research. Simultaneously, despite progress in stroke management, post-stroke care exerts a substantial impact on families, the healthcare system and the economy. Improvements in pre-clinical and clinical care are likely to underpin successful stroke treatment, recovery, rehabilitation and prevention. In this review, we focus on the pathophysiology of stroke, major advances in the identification of therapeutic targets and recent trends in stroke research.

Keywords: stroke; pathophysiology; treatment; neurological deficit; recovery; rehabilitation

1. Introduction

Stroke is a neurological disorder characterized by blockage of blood vessels. Clots form in the brain and interrupt blood flow, clogging arteries and causing blood vessels to break, leading to bleeding. Rupture of the arteries leading to the brain during stroke results in the sudden death of brain cells owing to a lack of oxygen. Stroke can also lead to depression and dementia.

Until the International Classification of Disease 11 (ICD-11) was released in 2018, stroke was classified as a disease of the blood vessels. Under the previous ICD coding rationale, clinical data generated from stroke patients were included as part of the cardiovascular diseases chapter, greatly misrepresenting the severity and specific disease burden of stroke. Due to this misclassification within the ICD, stroke patients and researchers did not benefit from government support or grant funding directed towards neurological disease. After prolonged advocacy from a group of clinicians, the true nature and significance of stroke was acknowledged in the ICD-11; stroke was re-categorized into the neurological chapter [1]. The reclassification of stroke as a neurological disorder has led to more accurate documentation of data and statistical analysis, supporting improvements in acute healthcare and acquisition of research funding for stroke.

2. Epidemiology of Stroke

Stroke is the second leading cause of death globally. It affects roughly 13.7 million people and kills around 5.5 million annually. Approximately 87% of strokes are ischemic infarctions, a prevalence which increased substantially between 1990 and 2016, attributed to decreased mortality and improved clinical interventions. Primary (first-time) hemorrhages comprise the majority of strokes, with secondary (second-time) hemorrhages constituting an estimated 10–25% [2,3]. The incidence of stroke doubled in low-and-middle income countries over 1990–2016 but declined by 42% in high-income countries over the same period. According to the Global Burden of Disease Study (GBD), although the prevalence of stroke has decreased, the age of those affected, their sex and their geographic location mean that the socio-economic burden of stroke has increased over time [3].

Age-specific stroke: The incidence of stroke increases with age, doubling after the age of 55 years. However, in an alarming trend, strokes in people aged 20–54 years increased from 12.9% to 18.6% of all cases globally between 1990 and 2016. Nevertheless, age-standardized attributable death rates decreased by 36.2% over the same period [3–5]. The highest reported stroke incidence is in China, where it affects an estimated 331–378 individuals per 100,000 life years. The second-highest rate is in eastern Europe (181–218 per 100,000 life years) and the lowest in Latin America (85–100 per 100,000 life years) [3].

Gender-specific stroke: The occurrence of stroke in men and women also depends on age. It is higher at younger ages in women, whereas incidence increases slightly with older age in men. The higher risk for stroke in women is due to factors related to pregnancy, such as preeclampsia, contraceptive use and hormonal therapy, as well as migraine with aura. Atrial fibrillation increases stroke risk in women over 75 years by 20%. Based on the National Institutes of Health Stroke Scale (0 = no stroke, 1–4 = minor stroke, 5–15 = moderate stroke, 15–20 = moderate/severe stroke, 21–42 = severe stroke), mean stroke severity was estimated at 10 for women and 8.2 for men. Both brain infarction and intracerebral hemorrhage (ICH) are common in men, but cardioembolic stroke, a more severe form of stroke, is more prevalent among women. The fatality rate for stroke is also higher among women [5–7]. Women live longer than men, which is one reason for their higher incidence of stroke; another important concern is women's delay in accepting help for ongoing symptoms [8]. For men, the most common causes of stroke are tobacco smoking, excessive alcohol consumption, myocardial infarction and arterial disorders [9].

Geographic and racial variation: As noted earlier, stroke incidence varies considerably across the globe. A global population-based study of the prevalence of stroke and related risks examined demography, behavior, physical characteristics, medical history and laboratory reports, and revealed the contribution of exposure to air pollution and particulate matter to stroke mortality [10]. Another population-based study, conducted in north-eastern China, is thought to be broadly representative of the disease situation in developing countries. It found hypertension to be a statistically significant risk for stroke, specifically ischemic stroke [11]. A study conducted in the United States (US) also identified hypertension as a major cause of stroke and described geographical variation in symptomatic intensity in stroke sufferers. Insufficient physical activity, poor food habits and nicotine and alcohol consumption were considered added risks [12]. Differences in exposure to environmental pollutants, such as lead and cadmium, also influenced stroke incidences across regions. This study also revealed differences in stroke incidence between non-Hispanic white and black populations aged 40–50 years [13].

Socioeconomic variation: There is a strong inverse relationship between stroke and socioeconomic status, attributable to inadequate hospital facilities and post-stroke care among low-income populations [14]. A case study conducted in the US showed that people with high financial status had better stroke treatment options than deprived individuals [15]. A study in China linked low income and lack of health insurance to prevention of secondary stroke attack [16]. Research conducted in Austria associated level of education with take-up of treatments such as echocardiography and speech therapy; however, there was no difference in administration of thrombolysis, occupational therapy, physiotherapy or stroke care for secondary attack by socioeconomic status [17]. Similarly, in the Scottish healthcare system, basic treatments like thrombolysis were provided irrespective of the economic status of patients [18].

3. Pathophysiology of Stroke

Stroke is defined as an abrupt neurological outburst caused by impaired perfusion through the blood vessels to the brain. It is important to understand the neurovascular anatomy to study the clinical manifestation of the stroke. The blood flow to the brain is managed by two internal carotids anteriorly and two vertebral arteries posteriorly (the circle of Willis). Ischemic stroke is caused by deficient blood and oxygen supply to the brain; hemorrhagic stroke is caused by bleeding or leaky blood vessels.

Ischemic occlusions contribute to around 85% of casualties in stroke patients, with the remainder due to intracerebral bleeding. Ischemic occlusion generates thrombotic and embolic conditions in the brain [19]. In thrombosis, the blood flow is affected by narrowing of vessels due to atherosclerosis. The build-up of plaque will eventually constrict the vascular chamber and form clots, causing thrombotic stroke. In an embolic stroke, decreased blood flow to the brain region causes an embolism; the blood flow to the brain reduces, causing severe stress and untimely cell death (necrosis). Necrosis is followed by disruption of the plasma membrane, organelle swelling and leaking of cellular contents into extracellular space [20], and loss of neuronal function. Other key events contributing to stroke pathology are inflammation, energy failure, loss of homeostasis, acidosis, increased intracellular calcium levels, excitotoxicity, free radical-mediated toxicity, cytokine-mediated cytotoxicity, complement activation, impairment of the blood–brain barrier, activation of glial cells, oxidative stress and infiltration of leukocytes [21–25].

Hemorrhagic stroke accounts for approximately 10–15% of all strokes and has a high mortality rate. In this condition, stress in the brain tissue and internal injury cause blood vessels to rupture. It produces toxic effects in the vascular system, resulting in infarction [26]. It is classified into intracerebral and subarachnoid hemorrhage. In ICH, blood vessels rupture and cause abnormal accumulation of blood within the brain. The main reasons for ICH are hypertension, disrupted vasculature, excessive use of anticoagulants and thrombolytic agents. In subarachnoid hemorrhage, blood accumulates in the subarachnoid space of the brain due to a head injury or cerebral aneurysm (Figure 1) [27,28].

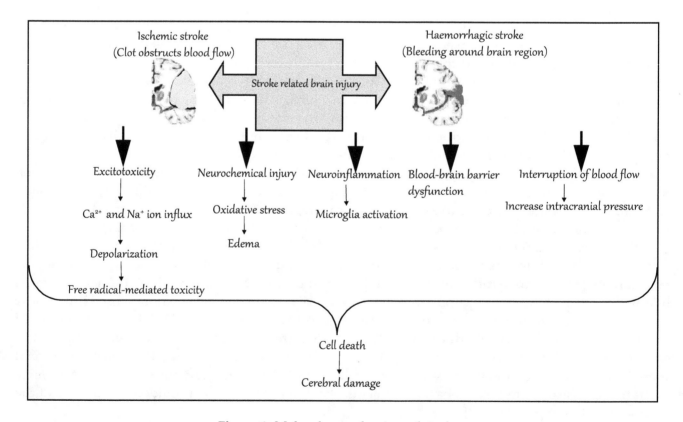

Figure 1. Molecular mechanism of stroke.

4. Risk Factors for Stroke

As noted earlier, the risk of stroke increases with age and doubles over the age of 55 years in both men and women. Risk is increased further when an individual has an existing medical condition like hypertension, coronary artery disease or hyperlipidemia. Nearly 60% of strokes are in patients with a history of transient ischemic attack (TIA). Some of the risk factors for stroke are modifiable, and some are non-modifiable (Figure 2).

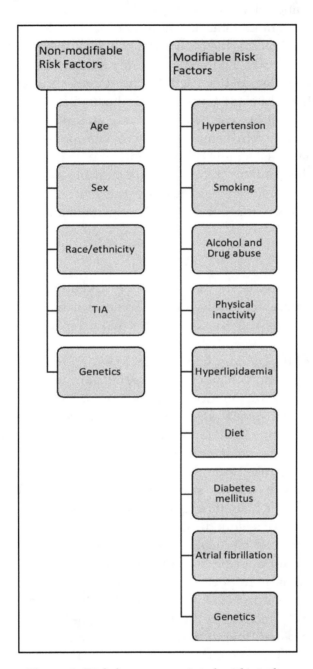

Figure 2. Risk factors associated with stroke.

4.1. Non-Modifiable Risk Factors

These include age, sex, ethnicity, TIA and hereditary characteristics. In the US in 2005, the average age of incidence of stroke was 69.2 years [2,29,30]. Recent research has indicated that people aged 20–54 years are at increasing risk of stroke, probably due to pre-existing secondary factors [31]. Women are at equal or greater risk of stroke than men, irrespective of age [32]. US research shows that Hispanic and black populations are at higher risk of stroke than white populations; notably, the incidence of hemorrhagic stroke is significantly higher in black people than in age-matched white populations [33–35].

Transient ischemic attack is classified as a mini stroke; the underlying mechanism is the same as for full-blown stroke. In TIA, the blood supply to part of the brain is blocked temporarily. It acts as a warning sign before the actual event, providing an opportunity to change lifestyle and commence medications to reduce the chance of stroke [36,37].

Genetics contribute to both modifiable and non-modifiable risk factors for stroke. Genetic risk is proportional to the age, sex and race of the individual [38,39], but a multitude of genetic mechanisms can increase the risk of stroke. Firstly, a parental or family history of stroke increases the chance of an individual developing this neurological disorder. Secondly, a rare single gene mutation can contribute to pathophysiology in which stroke is the primary clinical manifestation, such as in cerebral autosomal dominant arteriopathy. Thirdly, stroke can be one of many after-effects of multiple syndromes caused by genetic mutation, such as sickle cell anemia. Fourthly, some common genetic variants are associated with increased stroke risk, such as genetic polymorphism in 9p21 [40]. A genome-wide association study of stroke showed high heritability (around 40%) for large blood vessel disease, and low heritability (16.7%) for small vessel disorders. Recent evidence suggests that studying heritability will improve the understanding of stroke sub-types, improve patient management and enable earlier and more efficient prognosis [5,41].

4.2. Modifiable Risk Factors

These are of paramount importance, because timely and appropriate medical intervention can reduce the risk of stroke in susceptible individuals. The major modifiable risk factors for stroke are hypertension, diabetes, lack of physical exercise, alcohol and drug abuse, cholesterol, diet management and genetics.

Hypertension: It is one of the predominant risk factors for stroke. In one study, a blood pressure (BP) of at least 160/90 mmHg and a history of hypertension were considered equally important predispositions for stroke, with 54% of the stroke-affected population having these characteristics [42,43]. BP and prevalence of stroke are correlated in both hypertensive and normal individuals. A study reported that a 5–6 mm Hg reduction in BP lowered the relative risk of stroke by 42% [44]. Randomized trials of interventions to reduce hypertension in people aged 60+ have shown similar results, lowering the incidences of symptoms of stroke by 36% and 42%, respectively [45,46].

Diabetes: It doubles the risk of ischemic stroke and confers an approximately 20% higher mortality rate. Moreover, the prognosis for diabetic individuals after a stroke is worse than for non-diabetic patients, including higher rates of severe disability and slower recovery [47,48]. Tight regulation of glycemic levels alone is ineffective; medical intervention plus behavioral modifications could help decrease the severity of stroke for diabetic individuals [49].

Atrial fibrillation (AF): AF is an important risk factor for stroke, increasing risk two- to five-fold depending upon the age of the individual concerned [50]. It contributes to 15% of all strokes and produces more severe disability and higher mortality than non-AF-related strokes [51]. Research has shown that in AF, decreased blood flow in the left atrium causes thrombolysis and embolism in the brain. However, recent studies have contradicted this finding, citing poor evidence of sequential timing of incidence of AF and stroke, and noting that in some patients the occurrence of AF is recorded only after a stroke. In other instances, individuals harboring genetic mutations specific to AF can be affected by stroke long before the onset of AF [52,53]. Therefore, we need better methods of monitoring the heart rhythms that are associated with the vascular risk factors of AF and thromboembolism.

Hyperlipidemia: It is a major contributor to coronary heart disease, but its relationship to stroke is complicated. Total cholesterol is associated with risk of stroke, whereas high-density lipoprotein (HDL) decreases stroke incidence [54–56]. Therefore, evaluation of lipid profile enables estimation of the risk of stroke. In one study, low levels of HDL (<0.90 mmol/L), high levels of total triglyceride (>2.30 mmol/L) and hypertension were associated with a two-fold increase in the risk of stroke-related death in the population [55].

Alcohol and drug abuse: The relationship between stroke risk and alcohol intake follows a curvilinear pattern, with the risk related to the amount of alcohol consumed daily. Low to moderate consumption of alcohol (≤2 standard drinks daily for men and ≤1 for women) reduces stroke risk, whereas high intake increases it. In contrast, even low consumption of alcohol escalates the risk of hemorrhagic stroke [57–59]. Regular use of illegitimate substances such as cocaine, heroin, phencyclidine (PCP), lysergic acid diethylamide (LSD), cannabis/marijuana or amphetamines is related to increased risk of all subtypes of strokes [60]. Illicit drug use is a common predisposing factor for stroke among individuals aged below 35 years. US research showed that the proportion of illicit drug users among stroke patients aged 15–44 years was six times higher than among age-matched patients admitted with other serious conditions [61]. However, there is no strong evidence to confirm these findings, and the relationship between these drugs and stroke is anecdotal [62].

Smoking: Tobacco smoking is directly linked to increased risk of stroke. An average smoker has twice the chance of suffering from a stroke of a non-smoker. Smoking contributes to 15% of stroke-related mortality. Research suggests that an individual who stops smoking reduces the relative risk of stroke, while prolonged second-hand smoking confers a 30% elevation in the risk of stroke [63–65].

Insufficient physical inactivity and poor diet are associated with increased risk for stroke. Lack of exercise increases the chances of stroke attack in an individual. Insufficient physical activity is also linked to other health issues like high BP, obesity and diabetes, all conditions related to high stroke incidence [66,67]. Poor diet influences the risk of stroke, contributing to hypertension, hyperlipidemia, obesity and diabetes. Certain dietary components are well known to heighten risk; for example, excessive salt intake is linked to high hypertension and stroke. Conversely, a diet high in fruit and vegetables (notably, the Mediterranean diet) has been shown to decrease the risk of stroke [68–72].

5. Animal Models of Stroke

Animal models usually used for research include induced, spontaneous, negative and orphan models. In the induced model, a disease condition is induced in the animal with a view to studying the effects, whereas in the spontaneous model, an animal is selected with a similar disease state naturally present in the model. Negative animal models are used to study the resistance mechanisms underlying a particular disease condition. Orphan models are deployed to understand the pathology of a newly characterized disease in human subjects [73,74].

Many animal models have been developed to study the pathophysiology associated with stroke; they offer several advantages over studying stroke in humans or in vitro. The nature of stroke in humans is unpredictable, with diverse clinical manifestation and localization, whereas animal models are highly predictable and reproducible. Pathophysiological investigation often requires direct access to brain tissue, which is possible with animal models but not in humans. Moreover, current imaging techniques are unable to characterize events occurring within the first few minutes of a stroke. Finally, some aspects of stroke, such as vasculature and perfusion, cannot be studied in in vitro models [75]. Different stroke models used in animals are described in the session below (Table 1).

The intraluminal suture MCAo model: The middle cerebral artery (MCA) is vulnerable to ischemic insult and occlusion in humans, accounting for 70% of stroke-related disability. This disease model has been widely studied in rat and mouse models, with more than 2600 experiments conducted [76,77]. The MCAo procedure is minimally invasive; it involves occlusion of the carotid artery by insertion of a suture until it interrupts blood flow to the MCA. This procedure is applied for time periods such as 60 or 90 min or permanently, to induce infarction, and has a success rate of 88–100% in rats and mice [78]. The most commonly used animal for studying pre-clinical stroke is the Sprague–Dawley rat, which has a small infarct volume [79]. In mice, C57BL/6 and SV129 are commonly used to introduce MCA infarction. The reproducibility of the technique depends on a multitude of factors, such as the animal strain, suture diameter, body weight and age. The advantage of this model is that it mimics the human ischemic stroke and displays similar penumbra [80]. The MCAo model is appropriate for reproducing ischemic stroke and associated clinical manifestations such as neuronal cell death, cerebral inflammation and blood–brain barrier damage [75].

Table 1. Advantages and disadvantages of the stroke models.

Stroke Models	Advantages	Disadvantages
Intraluminal suture MCAo model	Mimics human ischemic stroke, Exhibits a penumbra, Highly reproducible, No craniectomy	Hyper-/hypothermia, Increased haemorrhage, Not suitable for thrombolysis studies
Craniotomy model	High long-term survival rates, Visual confirmation of successful MCAo	Highly invasive and procedural complications, Requires surgical skills
Photo-thrombosis model	Enables well-defined localization of an ischemic lesion, Highly reproducible, Less invasive	Causes early vasogenic edema, Not suitable for investigating neuroprotective agents
Endothelin-1 model	Less invasive, Induction of ischemic lesion in cortical regions, Low mortality	Duration of ischemia not controllable, Induction of astrocytosis and axonal sprouting
Embolic stroke model	Mimics the pathogenesis of human stroke	Low reproducibility of infarcts, Spontaneous recanalization
Neurorehabilitation	Rapid establishment of independence in activities of daily living Improves outcomes for cognitive, language, and motor skills	Develop cost-effective rehabilitative services Lack of in-depth studies on efficacy related to neurorehabilitation
Biomaterial testing	Reduction in lesion volume Bridge the lesion with neural tissue for neural reorganization Reduce secondary damage Improve neurological behaviour	Long-term experiments with the same biomaterial are challenging because of the degradation of material which might affect the treatment

Craniectomy model: This model uses a surgical procedure for inducing occlusion in the artery. In this technique, a neurological deficit can be induced in mice by electrocoagulation causing permanent insult or a microaneurysm until blood flow is interrupted. Alternatively, three-vessel occlusion is used, reducing the blood flow and resulting in damaged tissue. The infarct volume differs depending on whether the occlusion is permanent or transient [81–83]. A study conducted in neonatal P14–P18 rats mimicked pediatric stroke in a younger human population; a 3-h occlusion was performed to induce lesions affecting 40–50% of the brain [84]. Similarly, in P7 rats, oedema formation was observed in the MCA, followed by microglial infiltration. The P12 CB-17 is another animal model used for stroke research, mainly due to low variability in occlusion insult to the brain [85]. The other advantages of this model include reproducible infarct size and neurofunctional deficits, reduced mortality and visual ratification. The CB-17 model was successfully used to reproduce cerebral infarction and long-term survival rate, and to study ischemic reperfusion. Researchers showed that reperfusion supports neuron survival, rescues vascular phenotypes and is associated with functional recovery after stroke [86].

The Levine–Rice model: It involves histological examination and behavioral tests in rat pups, and it is used to study neonatal hypoxic-ischemic stroke [87]. In this model, a unilateral ligation is followed by reperfusion and recovery. Later, the animal is placed in a hypoxic chamber to understand neonatal stroke pathophysiology as well as regenerative and rehabilitative therapeutic possibilities. P7 rat animal models are commonly used to study the clinical manifestations of hypoxic-ischemic injury [88–90].

Photo-thrombosis model: This model is based on photo-oxidation of the vasculature leading to lesion formation in the cortex and striatum. In this method, the skull is irradiated with a photoactive dye that causes endothelial damage, intraparenchymal vessel aggregation and platelet stimulation in the affected area. It is injected intraperitoneally in mice and intravenously in rats [91]. This model is highly reproducible, with a low mortality rate and no surgery. The pathophysiology of this method is slightly different to that seen in human stroke due to little collateral blood flow or formation of ischemic penumbra. However, recent researchers modified the photothrombotic ischemia model to include hypoperfusion in an attempt to mimic penumbra. It has also been deployed in freely moving mice to evaluate the development of motor cortex ischemia and motor deficits. This model permits assessment of the ongoing infarction and improves our understanding of the neuronal insult and repair process [92,93].

Endothelin-1 model: Endothelin-1 (ET-1): ET-1 is a small peptide molecule produced by smooth muscle cells and the endothelium. It is a paracrine factor that restricts the vascular system through cell-specific receptors. Ischemic lesion is induced by stereotaxic injection of ET-1 directly into the exposed MCA in the intracerebral or cortex region [94]. ET-1 administration was observed to cause 70–90% reduction in cerebral blood flow, followed by reperfusion [95]. This technique is minimally invasive, has a low death rate and can be applied to deep and superficial brain regions. It is appropriate for long-term lesion studies, and the lesion size can be controlled by regulating ET-1 concentration, which is critical for reproducibility [95]. ET-1 is expressed by both neurons and astrocytes, which may decrease the stringency of interpretation of neuronal dysfunction in stroke [96]. A study in juvenile P21 rats used ET-1 to induce focal lesion in the striatum [97]. Similarly, aged P12 and P25 rats showed neuronal damage and lesion formation after injection of ET-1 into the hippocampus [98].

The embolic stroke model: It includes microsphere, macrosphere and thromboembolic models. The microsphere model involves introduction of spheres of diameter 20–50 μm into the circulatory system using a microcatheter to form multifocal infarcts [99]. Macrospheres are 100–400 μm in diameter and introduced into the intracerebral artery (ICA) to produce reproducible lesions in the MCA [100]. In the thromboembolic model, thrombin is directly injected to form clots in the ICA or MCA. The volume of the infarct depends upon the size of the clot formed [101]. This model closely resembles the type of stroke seen in humans. Prior study of clots induced by this model in mice have showed that they are mainly comprised of polymerized fibrin with few cells and platelets present, and 75% of clots exhibit platelet/fibrin build-up and deposition of neutrophils, monocytes and erythrocytes [102].

Neurorehabilitation in animal models: Various rehabilitative devices and forced training strategies have been deployed in stroke-affected animals to study neurological behavior. Robotic and electric devices have also been developed for training purposes in animal models to evaluate the functionality and effectiveness of the rehabilitation process. Similarly, forced exercise regimes, such as running on a treadmill or task-oriented motor training, are used to study rehabilitation scope in humans. Housing environments that provide social, motor and sensory stimuli and support cell engraftment, creating a more realistic approximation of human treatment, can be tested using animal models [103–105].

Animal models in biomaterial testing: Animal models have been well characterized for the study of brain tissues via brain atlases (http://www.med.harvard.edu/AANLIB/, https://portal.brain-map.org) for the required species. Stereotaxic techniques are utilized to introduce biomaterials or cells into particular coordinates of the target tissue. Microlesions can be studied precisely, and targeted localization can be confirmed using magnetic resonance imaging (MRI)-based lesion cartography [106–108].

6. Prevention and Treatment Strategies for Stroke

Stroke prevention involves modifying risk factors within a population or individuals, while stroke management depends on treating its pathophysiology. Despite an enormous amount of research into stroke over the last two decades, no simple means of treating or preventing all the clinical causes of stroke has been established. The overall direction of current stroke research is to generate novel therapies that modulate factors leading to primary and secondary stroke. Recent and current strategies for stroke prevention and treatment are discussed below (Figure 3).

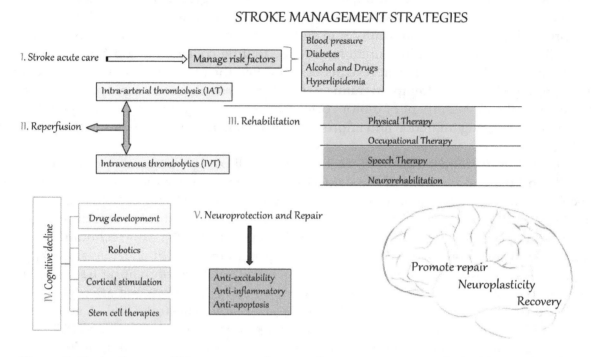

Figure 3. Stroke therapy. This represents the overall process to manage the incidence of stroke.

Excitotoxicity: Neuronal death is a key manifestation of stroke. A key reason for this phenomenon is neuronal depolarization and inability to maintain membrane potential within the cell. This process is mediated by glutamate receptors N-methyl-D-aspartate (NMDA) and α-amino-3-hydroxy-5-methyl-4-isoxazolepropionic acid (AMPA), which were among the first neuroprotective agents tested in stroke prevention. However, the untimely release of glutamate overpowers the system that removes glutamate from the cell and causes abnormal release of NMDA and AMPA molecules, leading to uninhibited calcium influx and protein damage. As a result, these agents have not been shown to reduce neuronal death in human subjects. Targeting the molecular pathways downstream of excitotoxicity signaling, rather than directly targeting glutamatergic signaling, might reduce the side effects of the process [109,110].

Gamma aminobutyric acid (GABA) agonists: Clomethiazole is a GABA agonist that has been tested for its ability to improve stroke symptoms in patients, but failed to reduce the toxicity induced by the glutamate receptor [111].

Sodium (Na^+) channel blockers: Na^+ channel blockers have been used as neuroprotective agents in various animal models of stroke. They prevent neuronal death and reduce white matter damage. Many voltage-gated Na^+ channel blockers have been tested in clinical trials, but most have proved to be ineffective [112]. Mexiletine is a neuroprotectant and Na^+ channel blocker that proved effective in grey and white matter ischemic stroke, though further evaluation is required to confirm its role [113]. Lubeluzole was shown to reduce mortality in stroke in initial clinical trials, but successive trials failed to reproduce similar outcomes. Similarly, sipatrigine is a Na^+ and Ca^{2+} channel blocker which failed in a Phase II clinical trial in stroke patients. Amiodarone was shown to aggravate brain injury due to defective transportation and accumulation of Na^+ ions in the brain after stroke [114].

Calcium (Ca^{2+}) channel blockers: Voltage-dependent Ca^{2+} ion channel blockers have been shown to decrease the ischemic insult in animal models of brain injury. The Ca^{2+} ion chelator DP-b99 proved efficient and safe in Phase I and II clinical trials when administered to stroke patients. Similarly, Phase II trials significantly improved clinical symptoms in stroke patients treated within 12 h of onset [115].

In another study, Ca^{2+} channel blockers reduced the risk of stroke by 13.5% in comparison to diuretics and β-blockers [116].

Antioxidants: Reactive oxygen species produced in the normal brain are balanced by antioxidants generated in a responsive mechanism. However, in the ischemic stroke model, excess production of free radicals and inactivation of detoxifying agents cause redox disequilibrium. This phenomenon leads to oxidative stress, followed by neuronal injury. Therefore, antioxidants are employed in treatment of acute stroke to inhibit or scavenge free radical production and degrade free radicals in the system. In one study, antioxidant AEOL 10,150 (manganese (III) meso-tetrakis (di-N-ethylimidazole) porphyrin) effectively regulated the gene expression profiles specific to inflammation and stress response to decrease the ischemic damage and reperfusion in stroke patients [117]. In another, deferoxamine was shown to regulate the expression of hypoxia-inducible factor-1, a transcriptional factor regulated by oxygen levels, which in turn switched on other genes like vascular endothelial growth factor and erythropoietin. This mechanism, studied in an animal stroke model, proved beneficial in reducing lesion size and improving sensorimotor capabilities [118,119]. Similarly, NXY-059 compound acts as a scavenger to eliminate free radicals and decrease neurological deficits. The Stroke-Acute-Ischemic-NXY-Treatment-I (SAINT) clinical trial showed the efficacy and safety of NXY-059, but SAINT II failed to reproduce the positive effect of this drug in stroke patients [120,121]. In another study, researchers employed intravenous injection of antioxidants directly into mice brains to understand the benefits of route of administration. This method reduced neurological defects, but had minimal influence on brain damage [122].

6.1. Reperfusion

The intravenous thrombolytics (IVT): The IVT treatment paradigm was originally developed to treat coronary thrombolysis but was found to be effective in treating stroke patients. The efficiency of thrombolytic drugs depends on factors including the age of the clot, the specificity of the thrombolytic agent for fibrin and the presence and half-life of neutralizing antibodies [123]. The drugs used in IVT treatment aim to promote fibrinolysin formation, which catalyzes the dissolution of the clot blocking the cerebral vessel. The most effective IVT drug, recombinant tissue plasminogen activator (rt-PA, or alteplase), was developed from research conducted by the US National Institute of Neurological Disorders and Stroke (NINDS) [124]. However, European Cooperative Acute Stroke Study (ECASS and ECASS II) researchers were unable to reproduce NINDS' results. Later, it was found that this drug was effective in reducing clot diameter in stroke patients within three hours of incidence. The Safe Implementation of Thrombolysis in Stroke Monitoring Study (SITS-MOST) confirmed the efficacy and safety of alteplase within the designated time frame [125]. Another category of thrombolytics, consisting of fibrin and non-fibrin drugs, is used for treatment of stroke symptoms. Fibrin activators like alteplase, reteplase and tenecteplase convert plasminogen to plasmin directly, whereas non-fibrin activators like the drugs streptokinase and staphylokinase do so indirectly [123].

Intra-arterial thrombolysis (IAT): IAT is another approach designed to combat acute stroke. This treatment is most effective in the first six hours of onset of MCA occlusion, and requires experienced clinicians and angiographic techniques [115]. Prolyse in Acute Cerebral Thromboembolism II (PROACT II) and Middle Cerebral Artery Embolism Local Fibrinolytic Intervention (MELT) were randomized clinical trials (RCTs) undertaken to test the efficacy and safety of a recombinant pro-urokinase drug [126,127], but did not produce any data useful for stroke treatment. Thrombolytics and glycoprotein IIb/IIIa antagonists were combined in two small clinical trials; this approach was helpful in treating atherosclerotic occlusions but less effective for cardioembolism [128,129]. The Interventional Management of Stroke (IMS) III trial tested IVT and IAT together to assess the benefits of combining rapid administration of therapy (IVT) and a superior recanalization methodology for faster relief (IAT) [130]. The IMS III trial was fruitful with bridging therapy (combination of IVT and IAT) as compared to IVT alone. There was an increase of 69.6% in the recanalization rate using bridging therapy in stroke patients [131,132].

Fibrinogen-depleting agents: Research has found a strong correlation between high fibrinogen levels in stroke patients and poor diagnosis for clinical outcomes. Fibrinogen-depleting agents decrease blood plasma levels of fibrinogen, hence reduce blood thickness and increase blood flow. They also remove the blood clot in the artery and restore blood flow in the affected regions of the brain. However, although some RCTs of defibrinogen therapy identified beneficial effects of fibrinogen-depleting agents in stroke patients, others failed to show positive effects on clinical outcomes after stroke [133]. Moreover, some studies reported bleeding after treatment with defibrinogen agents. Ancrod is a defibrinogenating agent derived from snake venom that has been studied for its ability to treat ischemic stroke within three hours of onset [134]. The European Stroke Treatment with Ancrod Trial (ESTAT) concluded that controlled administration of ancrod at 70 mg/dL fibrinogen was efficacious and safe, and achieved lower prevalence of ICH than observed at lower fibrinogen levels [135].

6.2. Others

Antihypertensive therapy: Hypertension is a risk factor for stroke. There are many reasons for high BP in stroke, including a history of hypertension, acute neuroendocrine stimulation, increased intracranial pressure, stress linked to hospital admission and intermittent painful spells [136]. Correct treatment of high BP during stroke is uncertain due to contradictory outcomes of clinical studies. Some research shows positive correlations between high BP and stroke-related mortality, hematoma expansion or intracerebral damage, suggesting that high BP should be treated. In other studies, low BP levels led to tissue perfusion and increased lesion size, thereby worsening the clinical outcome [137,138]. The multi-center Acute Candesartan Cilexetil Therapy in Stroke Survivors (ACCESS) Phase II study proved that taking medication (candesartan) for BP during stroke was safe, with no orchestrated cerebrovascular events reported due to hypotension. Similar research has been performed with antihypertensive drugs, such as the Continue Or Stop post Stroke Antihypertensives Collaborative Study (COSSACS) to study the efficacy of antihypertensive therapy in stroke; the Control of Hypertension and Hypotension Immediately Post Stroke (CHHIPS) study, designed to determine the cut-off value for BP during an attack; and the Scandinavian Candesartan Acute Stroke Trial (SCAST), which aimed to measure the effectiveness of the drug candesartan on stroke and cardiovascular disease [115,139]. In the COSSACS study, continuing antihypertensive drugs for a two-week period produced no extra harm as compared to stopping it and might be associated with reduced two-week mortality in patients with ischemic stroke [140]. The CHHIPS study demonstrated that a relatively moderate reduction in blood pressure lowered the mortality rate [141], whereas the SCAST study suggested that a careful BP-lowering treatment was associated with a higher risk of poor clinical outcome [142].

Glucose management: Hyperglycemia (elevated blood glucose) is common in stroke patients, so targeting blood glucose levels is an efficient stroke management strategy. Hyperglycemia > 6.0 mmol/L (108 mg/dL) is observed in most stroke patients; it initiates lipid peroxidation and cell lysis in compromised tissue, leading to stroke complications. An experimental study conducted in a rat model of collagenase-induced ICH found that hyperglycemia worsens edema formation and increases cell death, accelerating the course of ischemic injury. Increased blood glucose level is also associated with progression of infarction, reduced recanalization and poor clinical outcome [143]. Continuous glucose monitoring systems have been deployed to reduce stroke-related risks in both diabetic and non-diabetic stroke patients [144].

Antiplatelet therapy: This therapy is used for acute ischemic stroke management and for prevention of stroke incidence. It is also vital in controlling non-cardioembolic ischemic stroke and TIA. Antiplatelet agents like aspirin, clopidogrel and ticagrelor are the most widely used drugs administered to stroke sufferers within the first few days of attack [145]. Dual antiplatelet therapy, which involves a combination of clopidogrel, prasugrel or ticagrelor with aspirin, has become popular; many studies have tested the efficacy and safety of this dual therapy. It has been claimed that clopidogrel and aspirin combination therapy is most beneficial if introduced within 24 h of stroke and continued for 4–12 weeks [146].

Stem cell therapy: It offers promising therapeutic opportunities, safety and efficacy to stroke patients. Research on embryonic stem cells, mesenchymal cells and induced pluripotent stem cells has assessed their potential for tissue regeneration, maintenance, migration and proliferation, rewiring of neural circuitry and physical and behavioral rejuvenation [147]. Recently, a new type of mesenchymal stem cells (MSCs), called multilineage differentiating stress-enduring (Muse) cells, has been found in connective tissue. These cells offer great regenerative capacity and have been tested as a stroke treatment. After intravenous transplantation of Muse cells in a mouse model, they were found to engraft into the damaged host tissue and differentiate to provide functional recovery in the host [148]. Neovascularization is another mode of action of cell therapies in stroke; studies conducted in vitro and in vivo have shown that transplanted cells promote angiogenesis [149,150]. Furthermore, multiple stroke studies have reported that MSCs stimulate neurogenesis; this was confirmed in human embryonic neural stem cells using BrdU-labelling [151,152]. Stem cell therapy enhances the proliferation of neural stem cells and neuritogenesis [153]. Careful experimental design and clinical trials of stem cell therapies are likely to usher in a new era of treatment for stroke by promoting neurogenesis, rebuilding neural networks and boosting axonal growth and synaptogenesis.

Neural repair: This is an alternative therapy to neuroprotection. It is used to rejuvenate the tissue when the damage is already done and is therefore not time-bound but is most effective when administered 24 h after stroke attack. Many animal models have been used in attempts to stimulate neurogenesis and initiate the neuronal repair process [154]. Neural repair utilizes stem cell therapy to initiate repair mechanisms through cell integration into the wound or use of neurotrophic factors to block neuronal growth inhibitors. These cells may be channeled to any injured region to facilitate greater synaptic connectivity. Clinical trials using neural stem cells have proven beneficial in stroke patients. However, trials of myelin-associated glycoprotein, neurite outgrowth inhibitor (NOGO) proteins and chondroitin sulphate proteoglycans have shown these agents to be insufficiently effective; more clinical trials are required to increase treatment efficacy [155]. Biological intrusions may foster regeneration of newer cells, improve axonal guidance and enhance neural circuitry. Pharmacological and immunological interventions may target receptors to provide signaling cues for regeneration or block inhibitory factors in stroke-affected regions of the brain [156].

Rehabilitation: Stroke can leave individuals with short- and long-term disabilities. Daily activities like walking and toileting are often affected, and sensorimotor and visual impairment are common. Rehabilitation aims to reinforce the functional independence of people affected by stroke [157]. It includes working with patients and families to provide supportive services and post-stroke guidance after 48 h of stroke attack in stable patients. Stroke rehabilitation may involve physical, occupational, speech and/or cognitive therapy. It is designed to assist patients to recover problem-solving skills, access social and psychological support, improve their mobility and achieve independent living. Rehabilitation may also include neurobiological tasks designed to lessen the impact of cognitive dysfunction and induce synaptic plasticity, as well as long-term potentiation [158,159]. Neuromodulators play a vital role in triggering expression of specific genes that promote axon regeneration, dendritic spine development, synapse formation and cell replacement therapy. Task-oriented approaches, like arm training and walking, help stroke patients to manage their physical disability, and visual computer-assisted gaming activities have been used to enhance visuomotor neuronal plasticity [160].

7. Trends in Stroke Research

The incidence of stroke-related emergencies has decreased substantially over recent years due to improved understanding of the pathophysiology of stroke and identification of new drugs designed to treat the multitude of possible targets. Technological advancements like telestroke [161] and mobile stroke [162] units have reduced mortality and morbidity. Therefore, stroke management systems should include post-stroke care facilities on top of existing primary care and access to occupational, speech or any physical therapy following hospital discharge. Hospitals should develop standardized policies to handle emergencies in a timely fashion to avoid casualties and prevent secondary stroke [163]. Recently, the role of physiotherapists has emerged as an important aspect of post-stroke care management. Physiotherapists have initiated clinical trials of stroke recovery processes and rehabilitation therapy sessions. One ongoing study includes a strategy to manage disability by improving mobility using treadmill exercise, electromechanical device therapy and circuit class therapy [164,165]. Stroke Recovery and Rehabilitation Roundtables bring physiotherapists and other experts together to recommend research directions and produce guidance for the post-stroke healthcare system. Optimized delivery of stroke care systems and access to rehabilitation services are the future of healthcare for stroke [166].

Animal models used in stroke research reflect only a portion of the consequences of the condition in human subjects. Moreover, experiments conducted within a single laboratory are often constrained in terms of their research output. In vivo animal models of stroke should include aged populations to maximize their relevance, but most recent studies involve young and adult animals. Stroke studies should be conducted in both male and female subjects to exclude gender bias, and should take account of other confounders like hypertension, diabetes and obesity. All these issues make stroke research complex and expensive, and imply that it should be carried out collaboratively, across multiple labs. Ideally, an international multicenter platform for clinical trials would be established to increase the validity of research outcomes with respect to efficacy, safety, translational value, dose–response relationships and proof-of-principle. This strategy will help to overcome the current hurdles in transforming laboratory data into therapeutics for stroke.

Advancements in stem cell technologies and genomics have led to regenerative therapy to rebuild neural networks and repair damaged neurons due to ischemic insult [167,168]. The WIP1 gene is a regulator of Wnt signaling and a promising target for drug development. Studies in mice models showed that knockdown of WIP1 downregulates the stroke functional recovery process after injury, and that the presence of this gene regulates neurogenesis through activation of β-Catenin/Wnt signaling [169]. Similarly, NB-3 (contactin-6) plays a vital role in neuroprotection, as shown by knockdown of NB-3 in mice after stroke attack. NB-3-deficient mice had increased brain damage after MCAo, which also affected neurite outgrowth and neuronal survival rate. NB-3 is believed to have therapeutic benefits for ischemic insult [170]. Therefore, WIP1 and NB-3 are promising candidates for future drug trials. This is a vast field, and more research must be conducted in the coming years to enable the development of therapeutic drugs.

Numerous natural compounds have proven to be beneficial for stroke prevention and treatment. They can be synthesized at a lower cost than synthetic compounds and offer competitive efficacy and safety. Honokiol is a natural product that showed neuroprotective effects in animal models, and appears to have a role in reducing oxidative stress and inhibiting inflammatory responses [171]. Gastrodin, a compound extracted from *Gastrodia elata*, is a promising candidate in stroke treatment. In a mouse model, it improved neurogenesis and activated β-Catenin-dependent Wnt signaling to provide neuroprotection after ischemic insult. It also has antioxidative effects which protects the neural progenitor cells from neuron functional impairment. Gastrodin's safety has been proved in clinical trials, hence it is an option for stroke management in the coming years [172].

The Utstein methodology is a process of standardizing and reporting research on out-of-hospital stroke and defining the essential elements of management tools. Its growing popularity led to the establishment of the Global Resuscitation Alliance (GRA), an organization that governs best practices. The primary aim of GRA is to facilitate stroke care from pre-hospital admission to rehabilitation and recovery. It has developed 10 guidelines to ensure smooth transitioning of services during and after attack. It has implemented a stroke registry, public awareness and educational programs, promoted techniques for early stroke recognition by first responders, sought to optimize prehospital and in-hospital stroke care, advocated the use of advanced neuroimaging techniques and promoted a culture of excellence. The Utstein community has developed comprehensive plans to improve early diagnosis and treatment of stroke patients globally [173].

Future clinical trials should aim not only to determine the efficacy and safety of drugs but to characterize recovery and clinical outcomes. Clinical trials of pharmacological therapies for post-stroke recovery should adhere to the following guidelines [174]. Patients should be enrolled within two weeks of stroke whenever possible. Studies should include sampling from a multicenter platform and include global scale criteria for data analysis. The underlying mechanism of action of the tested drugs on target molecules should be thoroughly understood. Secondary measurements like day-to-day progress of recovery, length of rehabilitation, treatment endpoint analysis and any other compounding factors should also be recorded. Overall, research on stoke management has advanced rapidly in recent years and is certain to make additional valuable discoveries through the application of new technologies in hypothesis-driven clinical trials.

8. Translational Challenges for the Current Stroke Therapeutic Strategies

Stroke research has seen fundamental advancements over recent years. The improvements in the selection of animal models, imaging techniques and methodological progress have led to immense drug targets and therapeutic interventions. In spite of this, the subsequent clinical trials failed to prove pre-clinical outcomes. Recanalization therapy showed some promising results in the clinical trials but only a small section of stroke patients benefited from this treatment [175]. Hence, the translational potential of stroke research is still under-investigated.

The key challenges that hinder the smooth transition of pre-clinical research into successful drugs include relevant endpoint selection, confounding diseases models like hypertension and diabetes, modelling age and gender effects in stroke patients, development of medical devices, investigating medical conditions that co-exist during stroke incidence, reproducibility of pre-clinical stroke research data and modelling functional and behavioral outcome [176–178]. Multiple causality of the stroke occurrence is another problem that is often over-looked. Homogeneity in stroke models to exhibit the broad spectrum of stroke pathophysiology associated with ischemic lesions or cortical or intracerebral damage is critical. Therefore, stroke animal models that target specific causes of stroke should be included. Latent interaction between comorbidities and stroke treatment should be identified to increase the safety and efficacy of the clinical outcome [179]. Short-term experimental trials often result in failed therapeutic development due to false-negative outcomes in the clinical settings [180]. Understanding the functional and behavioral output which might mislead true recovery is problematic in clinical trials wherein animal models have greater ability to mask the functional benefits [181]. This affects the affecting translational capability of the research. Adapting a combined approach to model recovery and rehabilitation is also important for successful transition.

One of the other problems with the clinical trials for stroke is the lack of efficient data management. The impact of large data generated from numerous clinical experiments is over-whelming and there should be a standardized system to manage such data. Moreover, these data should be deposited into a public data repository for easy access.

Industry and academic corroborations in stroke research are critical to improve the translational value [182]. A consensus between industry and academic interests is vital for successful transition. The industry collaborations are mostly monetary driven and have time constraints which might compromise the pre-clinical study protocol design, appropriate sample sizes and overestimation of treatment effects. IP protection and publication of research data may discord between these groups. A multicenter approach, long-term collaborations, effective project management, use of advanced methodologies and establishment of functional endpoints will probably advance the translational roadblocks in stroke research [183].

9. Conclusions

Stroke is the second leading cause of death and contributor to disability worldwide and has significant economic costs. Thus, more effective therapeutic interventions and improved post-stroke management are global health priorities. The last 25 years of stroke research has brought considerable progress with respect to animal experimental models, therapeutic drugs, clinical trials and post-stroke rehabilitation studies, but large gaps of knowledge about stroke treatment remain. Despite our increased understanding of stroke pathophysiology and the large number of studies targeting multiple pathways causing stroke, the inability to translate research into clinical settings has significantly hampered advances in stroke research. Most research has focused on restoring blood flow to the brain and minimizing neuronal deficits after ischemic insult. The major challenges for stroke investigators are to characterize the key mechanisms underlying therapies, generate reproducible data, perform multicenter pre-clinical trials and increase the translational value of their data before proceeding to clinical studies.

Author Contributions: Conceptualization, D.K.; writing—original draft preparation, D.K.; writing—review and editing, Z.X.; funding acquisition, Z.X. All authors have read and agreed to the published version of the manuscript.

References

1.   Shakir, R. The struggle for stroke reclassification. *Nat. Rev. Neurol.* **2018**, *14*, 447–448. [CrossRef]
2.   Roger, V.L.; Go, A.S.; Lloyd-Jones, D.M.; Adams, R.J.; Berry, J.D.; Brown, T.M.; Carnethon, M.R.; Dai, S.; de Simone, G.; Ford, E.S.; et al. Heart disease and stroke statistics–2011 update: A report from the American Heart Association. *Circulation* **2011**, *123*, e18–e209. [CrossRef]
3.   Collaborators, G.S. Global, regional, and national burden of stroke, 1990-2016: A systematic analysis for the Global Burden of Disease Study 2016. *Lancet Neurol.* **2019**, *18*, 439–458.
4.   Kelly-Hayes, M. Influence of age and health behaviors on stroke risk: Lessons from longitudinal studies. *J. Am. Geriatr. Soc.* **2010**, *58*, S325–S328. [CrossRef]
5.   Boehme, A.K.; Esenwa, C.; Elkind, M.S. Stroke Risk Factors, Genetics, and Prevention. *Circ. Res.* **2017**, *120*, 472–495. [CrossRef]
6.   Appelros, P.; Stegmayr, B.; Terént, A. Sex differences in stroke epidemiology: A systematic review. *Stroke* **2009**, *40*, 1082–1090. [CrossRef]
7.   Reeves, M.J.; Bushnell, C.D.; Howard, G.; Gargano, J.W.; Duncan, P.W.; Lynch, G.; Khatiwoda, A.; Lisabeth, L. Sex differences in stroke: Epidemiology, clinical presentation, medical care, and outcomes. *Lancet Neurol.* **2008**, *7*, 915–926. [CrossRef]
8.   Stuart-Shor, E.M.; Wellenius, G.A.; DelloIacono, D.M.; Mittleman, M.A. Gender differences in presenting and prodromal stroke symptoms. *Stroke* **2009**, *40*, 1121–1126. [CrossRef]
9.   Girijala, R.L.; Sohrabji, F.; Bush, R.L. Sex differences in stroke: Review of current knowledge and evidence. *Vasc. Med.* **2017**, *22*, 135–145. [CrossRef]
10.   Chen, J.C. Geographic determinants of stroke mortality: Role of ambient air pollution. *Stroke* **2010**, *41*, 839–841. [CrossRef]
11.   Zhang, F.L.; Guo, Z.N.; Wu, Y.H.; Liu, H.Y.; Luo, Y.; Sun, M.S.; Xing, Y.Q.; Yang, Y. Prevalence of stroke and associated risk factors: A population based cross sectional study from northeast China. *BMJ Open* **2017**, *7*, e015758. [CrossRef] [PubMed]
12.   Kiefe, C.I.; Williams, O.D.; Bild, D.E.; Lewis, C.E.; Hilner, J.E.; Oberman, A. Regional disparities in the incidence of elevated blood pressure among young adults: The CARDIA study. *Circulation* **1997**, *96*, 1082–1088. [CrossRef] [PubMed]
13.   Ishii, M. The sixth report of the Joint National Committee on Prevention, Detection, Evaluation, and Treatment of High Blood Pressure, and 1999 World Health Organization-International Society of Hypertension Guidelines for the Management of Hypertension. *Nihon Rinsho* **2000**, *58*, 267–275.
14.   Addo, J.; Ayerbe, L.; Mohan, K.M.; Crichton, S.; Sheldenkar, A.; Chen, R.; Wolfe, C.D.; McKevitt, C. Socioeconomic status and stroke: An updated review. *Stroke* **2012**, *43*, 1186–1191. [CrossRef]
15.   Sandel, M.E.; Wang, H.; Terdiman, J.; Hoffman, J.M.; Ciol, M.A.; Sidney, S.; Quesenberry, C.; Lu, Q.; Chan, L. Disparities in stroke rehabilitation: Results of a study in an integrated health system in northern California. *PM R* **2009**, *1*, 29–40. [CrossRef]

16. Wang, Y.L.; Wu, D.; Nguyen-Huynh, M.N.; Zhou, Y.; Wang, C.X.; Zhao, X.Q.; Liao, X.L.; Liu, L.P.; Wang, Y.J.; The Prevention of Recurrences of Stroke Study in China (PRESS-China) Investigators. Antithrombotic management of ischaemic stroke and transient ischaemic attack in China: A consecutive cross-sectional survey. *Clin. Exp. Pharmacol. Physiol.* **2010**, *37*, 775–781.

17. Arrich, J.; Müllner, M.; Lalouschek, W.; Greisenegger, S.; Crevenna, R.; Herkner, H. Influence of socioeconomic status and gender on stroke treatment and diagnostics. *Stroke* **2008**, *39*, 2066–2072. [CrossRef]

18. Kerr, G.D.; Higgins, P.; Walters, M.; Ghosh, S.K.; Wright, F.; Langhorne, P.; Stott, D.J. Socioeconomic status and transient ischaemic attack/stroke: A prospective observational study. *Cerebrovasc. Dis.* **2011**, *31*, 130–137. [CrossRef]

19. Musuka, T.D.; Wilton, S.B.; Traboulsi, M.; Hill, M.D. Diagnosis and management of acute ischemic stroke: Speed is critical. *CMAJ* **2015**, *187*, 887–893. [CrossRef] [PubMed]

20. Broughton, B.R.; Reutens, D.C.; Sobey, C.G. Apoptotic mechanisms after cerebral ischemia. *Stroke* **2009**, *40*, e331–e339. [CrossRef]

21. Woodruff, T.M.; Thundyil, J.; Tang, S.C.; Sobey, C.G.; Taylor, S.M.; Arumugam, T.V. Pathophysiology, treatment, and animal and cellular models of human ischemic stroke. *Mol. Neurodegener.* **2011**, *6*, 11. [CrossRef] [PubMed]

22. Gelderblom, M.; Leypoldt, F.; Steinbach, K.; Behrens, D.; Choe, C.U.; Siler, D.A.; Arumugam, T.V.; Orthey, E.; Gerloff, C.; Tolosa, E.; et al. Temporal and spatial dynamics of cerebral immune cell accumulation in stroke. *Stroke* **2009**, *40*, 1849–1857. [CrossRef] [PubMed]

23. Suh, S.W.; Shin, B.S.; Ma, H.; Van Hoecke, M.; Brennan, A.M.; Yenari, M.A.; Swanson, R.A. Glucose and NADPH oxidase drive neuronal superoxide formation in stroke. *Ann. Neurol.* **2008**, *64*, 654–663. [CrossRef]

24. Qureshi, A.I.; Ali, Z.; Suri, M.F.; Shuaib, A.; Baker, G.; Todd, K.; Guterman, L.R.; Hopkins, L.N. Extracellular glutamate and other amino acids in experimental intracerebral hemorrhage: An in vivo microdialysis study. *Crit. Care Med.* **2003**, *31*, 1482–1489. [CrossRef] [PubMed]

25. Wang, J.; Fields, J.; Zhao, C.; Langer, J.; Thimmulappa, R.K.; Kensler, T.W.; Yamamoto, M.; Biswal, S.; Doré, S. Role of Nrf2 in protection against intracerebral hemorrhage injury in mice. *Free Radic. Biol. Med.* **2007**, *43*, 408–414. [CrossRef]

26. Flaherty, M.L.; Woo, D.; Haverbusch, M.; Sekar, P.; Khoury, J.; Sauerbeck, L.; Moomaw, C.J.; Schneider, A.; Kissela, B.; Kleindorfer, D.; et al. Racial variations in location and risk of intracerebral hemorrhage. *Stroke* **2005**, *36*, 934–937. [CrossRef] [PubMed]

27. Testai, F.D.; Aiyagari, V. Acute hemorrhagic stroke pathophysiology and medical interventions: Blood pressure control, management of anticoagulant-associated brain hemorrhage and general management principles. *Neurol. Clin.* **2008**, *26*, 963–985. [CrossRef]

28. Aronowski, J.; Zhao, X. Molecular pathophysiology of cerebral hemorrhage: Secondary brain injury. *Stroke* **2011**, *42*, 1781–1786. [CrossRef]

29. Mozaffarian, D.; Benjamin, E.J.; Go, A.S.; Arnett, D.K.; Blaha, M.J.; Cushman, M.; Das, S.R.; de Ferranti, S.; Després, J.P.; Fullerton, H.J.; et al. Executive Summary: Heart Disease and Stroke Statistics–2016 Update: A Report From the American Heart Association. *Circulation* **2016**, *133*, 447–454. [CrossRef]

30. Roger, V.L.; Go, A.S.; Lloyd-Jones, D.M.; Benjamin, E.J.; Berry, J.D.; Borden, W.B.; Bravata, D.M.; Dai, S.; Ford, E.S.; Fox, C.S.; et al. Executive summary: Heart disease and stroke statistics—2012 update: A report from the American Heart Association. *Circulation* **2012**, *125*, 188–197.

31. George, M.G.; Tong, X.; Kuklina, E.V.; Labarthe, D.R. Trends in stroke hospitalizations and associated risk factors among children and young adults, 1995–2008. *Ann. Neurol.* **2011**, *70*, 713–721. [CrossRef]

32. Kapral, M.K.; Fang, J.; Hill, M.D.; Silver, F.; Richards, J.; Jaigobin, C.; Cheung, A.M.; Investigators of the Registry of the Canadian Stroke Network. Sex differences in stroke care and outcomes: Results from the Registry of the Canadian Stroke Network. *Stroke* **2005**, *36*, 809–814. [CrossRef] [PubMed]

33. Cruz-Flores, S.; Rabinstein, A.; Biller, J.; Elkind, M.S.; Griffith, P.; Gorelick, P.B.; Howard, G.; Leira, E.C.; Morgenstern, L.B.; Ovbiagele, B.; et al. Racial-ethnic disparities in stroke care: The American experience: A statement for healthcare professionals from the American Heart Association/American Stroke Association. *Stroke* **2011**, *42*, 2091–2116. [CrossRef] [PubMed]

34. Kleindorfer, D.; Broderick, J.; Khoury, J.; Flaherty, M.; Woo, D.; Alwell, K.; Moomaw, C.J.; Schneider, A.; Miller, R.; Shukla, R.; et al. The unchanging incidence and case-fatality of stroke in the 1990s: A population-based study. *Stroke* **2006**, *37*, 2473–2478. [CrossRef]

35. Zahuranec, D.B.; Brown, D.L.; Lisabeth, L.D.; Gonzales, N.R.; Longwell, P.J.; Eden, S.V.; Smith, M.A.; Garcia, N.M.; Morgenstern, L.B. Differences in intracerebral hemorrhage between Mexican Americans and non-Hispanic whites. *Neurology* **2006**, *66*, 30–34. [CrossRef] [PubMed]

36. Ferro, J.M.; Falcão, I.; Rodrigues, G.; Canhão, P.; Melo, T.P.; Oliveira, V.; Pinto, A.N.; Crespo, M.; Salgado, A.V. Diagnosis of transient ischemic attack by the nonneurologist. A validation study. *Stroke* **1996**, *27*, 2225–2229. [CrossRef]

37. Easton, J.D.; Saver, J.L.; Albers, G.W.; Alberts, M.J.; Chaturvedi, S.; Feldmann, E.; Hatsukami, T.S.; Higashida, R.T.; Johnston, S.C.; Kidwell, C.S.; et al. Definition and evaluation of transient ischemic attack: A scientific statement for healthcare professionals from the American Heart Association/American Stroke Association Stroke Council; Council on Cardiovascular Surgery and Anesthesia; Council on Cardiovascular Radiology and Intervention; Council on Cardiovascular Nursing; and the Interdisciplinary Council on Peripheral Vascular Disease. The American Academy of Neurology affirms the value of this statement as an educational tool for neurologists. *Stroke* **2009**, *40*, 2276–2293.

38. Seshadri, S.; Beiser, A.; Pikula, A.; Himali, J.J.; Kelly-Hayes, M.; Debette, S.; DeStefano, A.L.; Romero, J.R.; Kase, C.S.; Wolf, P.A. Parental occurrence of stroke and risk of stroke in their children: The Framingham study. *Circulation* **2010**, *121*, 1304–1312. [CrossRef]

39. Touzé, E.; Rothwell, P.M. Sex differences in heritability of ischemic stroke: A systematic review and meta-analysis. *Stroke* **2008**, *39*, 16–23. [CrossRef]

40. Matarin, M.; Brown, W.M.; Singleton, A.; Hardy, J.A.; Meschia, J.F.; For the ISGS Investigators. Whole genome analyses suggest ischemic stroke and heart disease share an association with polymorphisms on chromosome 9p21. *Stroke* **2008**, *39*, 1586–1589. [CrossRef]

41. Bevan, S.; Traylor, M.; Adib-Samii, P.; Malik, R.; Paul, N.L.; Jackson, C.; Farrall, M.; Rothwell, P.M.; Sudlow, C.; Dichgans, M.; et al. Genetic heritability of ischemic stroke and the contribution of previously reported candidate gene and genomewide associations. *Stroke* **2012**, *43*, 3161–3167. [CrossRef] [PubMed]

42. O'Donnell, M.J.; Xavier, D.; Liu, L.; Zhang, H.; Chin, S.L.; Rao-Melacini, P.; Rangarajan, S.; Islam, S.; Pais, P.; McQueen, M.J.; et al. Risk factors for ischaemic and intracerebral haemorrhagic stroke in 22 countries (the INTERSTROKE study): A case-control study. *Lancet* **2010**, *376*, 112–123. [CrossRef]

43. Lewington, S.; Clarke, R.; Qizilbash, N.; Peto, R.; Collins, R.; Collaboration, P.S. Age-specific relevance of usual blood pressure to vascular mortality: A meta-analysis of individual data for one million adults in 61 prospective studies. *Lancet* **2002**, *360*, 1903–1913. [PubMed]

44. Collins, R.; Peto, R.; MacMahon, S.; Hebert, P.; Fiebach, N.H.; Eberlein, K.A.; Godwin, J.; Qizilbash, N.; Taylor, J.O.; Hennekens, C.H. Blood pressure, stroke, and coronary heart disease. Part 2, Short-term reductions in blood pressure: Overview of randomised drug trials in their epidemiological context. *Lancet* **1990**, *335*, 827–838. [CrossRef]

45. Prevention of Stroke by Antihypertensive Drug Treatment in Older Persons with Isolated Systolic Hypertension. Final results of the Systolic Hypertension in the Elderly Program (SHEP). SHEP Cooperative Research Group. *JAMA* **1991**, *265*, 3255–3264. [CrossRef]

46. Staessen, J.A.; Fagard, R.; Thijs, L.; Celis, H.; Arabidze, G.G.; Birkenhäger, W.H.; Bulpitt, C.J.; de Leeuw, P.W.; Dollery, C.T.; Fletcher, A.E.; et al. Randomised double-blind comparison of placebo and active treatment for older patients with isolated systolic hypertension. The Systolic Hypertension in Europe (Syst-Eur) Trial Investigators. *Lancet* **1997**, *350*, 757–764. [CrossRef]

47. Vermeer, S.E.; Sandee, W.; Algra, A.; Koudstaal, P.J.; Kappelle, L.J.; Dippel, D.W.; Dutch TIA Trial Study Group. Impaired glucose tolerance increases stroke risk in nondiabetic patients with transient ischemic attack or minor ischemic stroke. *Stroke* **2006**, *37*, 1413–1417. [CrossRef]

48. Banerjee, C.; Moon, Y.P.; Paik, M.C.; Rundek, T.; Mora-McLaughlin, C.; Vieira, J.R.; Sacco, R.L.; Elkind, M.S. Duration of diabetes and risk of ischemic stroke: The Northern Manhattan Study. *Stroke* **2012**, *43*, 1212–1217. [CrossRef]

49. Lukovits, T.G.; Mazzone, T.M.; Gorelick, T.M. Diabetes mellitus and cerebrovascular disease. *Neuroepidemiology* **1999**, *18*, 1–14. [CrossRef]

50. Wolf, P.A.; Abbott, R.D.; Kannel, W.B. Atrial fibrillation as an independent risk factor for stroke: The Framingham Study. *Stroke* **1991**, *22*, 983–988. [CrossRef]

51. Romero, J.R.; Morris, J.; Pikula, A. Stroke prevention: Modifying risk factors. *Ther. Adv. Cardiovasc. Dis.* **2008**, *2*, 287–303. [CrossRef] [PubMed]

52. Brambatti, M.; Connolly, S.J.; Gold, M.R.; Morillo, C.A.; Capucci, A.; Muto, C.; Lau, C.P.; Van Gelder, I.C.; Hohnloser, S.H.; Carlson, M.; et al. Temporal relationship between subclinical atrial fibrillation and embolic events. *Circulation* **2014**, *129*, 2094–2099. [CrossRef]

53. Disertori, M.; Quintarelli, S.; Grasso, M.; Pilotto, A.; Narula, N.; Favalli, V.; Canclini, C.; Diegoli, M.; Mazzola, S.; Marini, M.; et al. Autosomal recessive atrial dilated cardiomyopathy with standstill evolution associated with mutation of Natriuretic Peptide Precursor A. *Circ. Cardiovasc. Genet.* **2013**, *6*, 27–36. [CrossRef] [PubMed]

54. Iribarren, C.; Jacobs, D.R.; Sadler, M.; Claxton, A.J.; Sidney, S. Low total serum cholesterol and intracerebral hemorrhagic stroke: Is the association confined to elderly men? The Kaiser Permanente Medical Care Program. *Stroke* **1996**, *27*, 1993–1998. [CrossRef]

55. Denti, L.; Cecchetti, A.; Annoni, V.; Merli, M.F.; Ablondi, F.; Valenti, G. The role of lipid profile in determining the risk of ischemic stroke in the elderly: A case-control study. *Arch. Gerontol. Geriatr.* **2003**, *37*, 51–62. [CrossRef]

56. Iso, H.; Jacobs, D.R.; Wentworth, D.; Neaton, J.D.; Cohen, J.D. Serum cholesterol levels and six-year mortality from stroke in 350,977 men screened for the multiple risk factor intervention trial. *N. Engl. J. Med.* **1989**, *320*, 904–910. [CrossRef]

57. Gill, J.S.; Zezulka, A.V.; Shipley, M.J.; Gill, S.K.; Beevers, D.G. Stroke and alcohol consumption. *N. Engl. J. Med.* **1986**, *315*, 1041–1046. [CrossRef]

58. Hillbom, M.; Numminen, H.; Juvela, S. Recent heavy drinking of alcohol and embolic stroke. *Stroke* **1999**, *30*, 2307–2312. [CrossRef] [PubMed]

59. Klatsky, A.L.; Armstrong, M.A.; Friedman, G.D.; Sidney, S. Alcohol drinking and risk of hospitalization for ischemic stroke. *Am. J. Cardiol.* **2001**, *88*, 703–706. [CrossRef]

60. Esse, K.; Fossati-Bellani, M.; Traylor, A.; Martin-Schild, S. Epidemic of illicit drug use, mechanisms of action/addiction and stroke as a health hazard. *Brain Behav.* **2011**, *1*, 44–54. [CrossRef]

61. Kaku, D.A.; Lowenstein, D.H. Emergence of recreational drug abuse as a major risk factor for stroke in young adults. *Ann. Intern. Med.* **1990**, *113*, 821–827. [CrossRef]

62. Brust, J.C. Neurologic complications of substance abuse. *J. Acquir. Immune Defic. Syndr.* **2002**, *31*, S29–S34. [CrossRef] [PubMed]

63. Bhat, V.M.; Cole, J.W.; Sorkin, J.D.; Wozniak, M.A.; Malarcher, A.M.; Giles, W.H.; Stern, B.J.; Kittner, S.J. Dose-response relationship between cigarette smoking and risk of ischemic stroke in young women. *Stroke* **2008**, *39*, 2439–2443. [CrossRef] [PubMed]

64. Song, Y.M.; Cho, H.J. Risk of stroke and myocardial infarction after reduction or cessation of cigarette smoking: A cohort study in korean men. *Stroke* **2008**, *39*, 2432–2438. [CrossRef] [PubMed]

65. Shinton, R.; Beevers, G. Meta-analysis of relation between cigarette smoking and stroke. *BMJ* **1989**, *298*, 789–794. [CrossRef]

66. Zhou, M.L.; Zhu, L.; Wang, J.; Hang, C.H.; Shi, J.X. The inflammation in the gut after experimental subarachnoid hemorrhage. *J. Surg. Res.* **2007**, *137*, 103–108. [CrossRef] [PubMed]

67. Manson, J.E.; Colditz, G.A.; Stampfer, M.J.; Willett, W.C.; Krolewski, A.S.; Rosner, B.; Arky, R.A.; Speizer, F.E.; Hennekens, C.H. A prospective study of maturity-onset diabetes mellitus and risk of coronary heart disease and stroke in women. *Arch. Intern. Med.* **1991**, *151*, 1141–1147. [CrossRef] [PubMed]

68. Larsson, S.C.; Orsini, N.; Wolk, A. Dietary potassium intake and risk of stroke: A dose-response meta-analysis of prospective studies. *Stroke* **2011**, *42*, 2746–2750. [CrossRef]

69. Estruch, R.; Ros, E.; Martínez-González, M.A. Mediterranean diet for primary prevention of cardiovascular disease. *N. Engl. J. Med.* **2013**, *369*, 676–677. [CrossRef]

70. Appel, L.J.; Brands, M.W.; Daniels, S.R.; Karanja, N.; Elmer, P.J.; Sacks, F.M.; Association, A.H. Dietary approaches to prevent and treat hypertension: A scientific statement from the American Heart Association. *Hypertension* **2006**, *47*, 296–308. [CrossRef]

71. Li, X.Y.; Cai, X.L.; Bian, P.D.; Hu, L.R. High salt intake and stroke: Meta-analysis of the epidemiologic evidence. *CNS Neurosci. Ther.* **2012**, *18*, 691–701. [CrossRef] [PubMed]

72. He, J.; Ogden, L.G.; Vupputuri, S.; Bazzano, L.A.; Loria, C.; Whelton, P.K. Dietary sodium intake and subsequent risk of cardiovascular disease in overweight adults. *JAMA* **1999**, *282*, 2027–2034. [CrossRef] [PubMed]

73. Fagundes, D.J.; Omar, T.M. Animal disease model: Choice's criteria and current animals specimens. *Acta Cir. Bras.* **2004**, *19*, 59–65. [CrossRef]

74. Rollin, B.E. *The Experimental Animal in Biomedical Research: Care, Husbandry and Well-Being: An Overview by Species*; Kesel, M.L., Ed.; CRC Press: Boston, MA, USA, 1995.

75. Fluri, F.; Schuhmann, M.K.; Kleinschnitz, C. Animal models of ischemic stroke and their application in clinical research. *Drug Des. Devel. Ther.* **2015**, *9*, 3445–3454. [PubMed]

76. Bogousslavsky, J.; Van Melle, G.; Regli, F. The Lausanne Stroke Registry: Analysis of 1,000 consecutive patients with first stroke. *Stroke* **1988**, *19*, 1083–1092. [CrossRef] [PubMed]

77. Howells, D.W.; Porritt, M.J.; Rewell, S.S.; O'Collins, V.; Sena, E.S.; van der Worp, H.B.; Traystman, R.J.; Macleod, M.R. Different strokes for different folks: The rich diversity of animal models of focal cerebral ischemia. *J. Cereb. Blood Flow Metab.* **2010**, *30*, 1412–1431. [CrossRef] [PubMed]

78. Liu, S.; Zhen, G.; Meloni, B.P.; Campbell, K.; Winn, H.R. Rodent stroke model guidelines for preclinical stroke trials (1st edition). *J. Exp. Stroke Transl. Med.* **2009**, *2*, 2–27. [CrossRef] [PubMed]

79. VE, O.C.; GA, D.; MR, M.; DW, H. Animal models of stroke versus clinical stroke: Comparison of infarct size, cause, location, study design, and efficacy of experimental therapies. In *Animal Models for the Study of Human Disease*; Michael Conn, P., Ed.; Academic Press: Waltham, MA, USA, 2013; pp. 531–568.

80. Connolly, E.S.; Winfree, C.J.; Stern, D.M.; Solomon, R.A.; Pinsky, D.J. Procedural and strain-related variables significantly affect outcome in a murine model of focal cerebral ischemia. *Neurosurgery* **1996**, *38*, 523–531, discussion 532. [PubMed]

81. Popa-Wagner, A.; Schröder, E.; Schmoll, H.; Walker, L.C.; Kessler, C. Upregulation of MAP1B and MAP2 in the rat brain after middle cerebral artery occlusion: Effect of age. *J. Cereb. Blood Flow Metab.* **1999**, *19*, 425–434. [CrossRef] [PubMed]

82. Sugimori, H.; Yao, H.; Ooboshi, H.; Ibayashi, S.; Iida, M. Krypton laser-induced photothrombotic distal middle cerebral artery occlusion without craniectomy in mice. *Brain Res. Brain Res. Protoc.* **2004**, *13*, 189–196. [CrossRef] [PubMed]

83. McAuley, M.A. Rodent models of focal ischemia. *Cerebrovasc. Brain Metab. Rev.* **1995**, *7*, 153–180.

84. Derugin, N.; Ferriero, D.M.; Vexler, Z.S. Neonatal reversible focal cerebral ischemia: A new model. *Neurosci. Res.* **1998**, *32*, 349–353. [CrossRef]

85. Tsuji, M.; Ohshima, M.; Taguchi, A.; Kasahara, Y.; Ikeda, T.; Matsuyama, T. A novel reproducible model of neonatal stroke in mice: Comparison with a hypoxia-ischemia model. *Exp. Neurol.* **2013**, *247*, 218–225. [CrossRef] [PubMed]

86. Tachibana, M.; Ago, T.; Wakisaka, Y.; Kuroda, J.; Shijo, M.; Yoshikawa, Y.; Komori, M.; Nishimura, A.; Makihara, N.; Nakamura, K.; et al. Early Reperfusion After Brain Ischemia Has Beneficial Effects Beyond Rescuing Neurons. *Stroke* **2017**, *48*, 2222–2230. [CrossRef] [PubMed]

87. Rumajogee, P.; Bregman, T.; Miller, S.P.; Yager, J.Y.; Fehlings, M.G. Rodent Hypoxia-Ischemia Models for Cerebral Palsy Research: A Systematic Review. *Front. Neurol.* **2016**, *7*, 57. [CrossRef] [PubMed]

88. Giraud, A.; Guiraut, C.; Chevin, M.; Chabrier, S.; Sébire, G. Role of Perinatal Inflammation in Neonatal Arterial Ischemic Stroke. *Front. Neurol.* **2017**, *8*, 612. [CrossRef]

89. Kim, H.; Koo, Y.S.; Shin, M.J.; Kim, S.Y.; Shin, Y.B.; Choi, B.T.; Yun, Y.J.; Lee, S.Y.; Shin, H.K. Combination of Constraint-Induced Movement Therapy with Electroacupuncture Improves Functional Recovery following Neonatal Hypoxic-Ischemic Brain Injury in Rats. *Biomed. Res. Int.* **2018**, *2018*, 8638294. [CrossRef]

90. Gennaro, M.; Mattiello, A.; Pizzorusso, T. Rodent Models of Developmental Ischemic Stroke for Translational Research: Strengths and Weaknesses. *Neural Plast.* **2019**, *2019*, 5089321. [CrossRef]

91. Watson, B.D.; Dietrich, W.D.; Busto, R.; Wachtel, M.S.; Ginsberg, M.D. Induction of reproducible brain infarction by photochemically initiated thrombosis. *Ann. Neurol.* **1985**, *17*, 497–504. [CrossRef]

92. Hu, X.; Wester, P.; Brännström, T.; Watson, B.D.; Gu, W. Progressive and reproducible focal cortical ischemia with or without late spontaneous reperfusion generated by a ring-shaped, laser-driven photothrombotic lesion in rats. *Brain Res. Brain Res. Protoc.* **2001**, *7*, 76–85. [CrossRef]

93. Yu, C.L.; Zhou, H.; Chai, A.P.; Yang, Y.X.; Mao, R.R.; Xu, L. Whole-scale neurobehavioral assessments of photothrombotic ischemia in freely moving mice. *J. Neurosci. Methods* **2015**, *239*, 100–107. [CrossRef] [PubMed]

94. Robinson, M.J.; Macrae, I.M.; Todd, M.; Reid, J.L.; McCulloch, J. Reduction of local cerebral blood flow to pathological levels by endothelin-1 applied to the middle cerebral artery in the rat. *Neurosci. Lett.* **1990**, *118*, 269–272. [CrossRef]

95. Biernaskie, J.; Corbett, D.; Peeling, J.; Wells, J.; Lei, H. A serial MR study of cerebral blood flow changes and lesion development following endothelin-1-induced ischemia in rats. *Magn. Reson. Med.* **2001**, *46*, 827–830. [CrossRef] [PubMed]

96. del Zoppo, G.J.; Schmid-Schönbein, G.W.; Mori, E.; Copeland, B.R.; Chang, C.M. Polymorphonuclear leukocytes occlude capillaries following middle cerebral artery occlusion and reperfusion in baboons. *Stroke* **1991**, *22*, 1276–1283. [CrossRef]

97. Saggu, R. Characterisation of endothelin-1-induced intrastriatal lesions within the juvenile and adult rat brain using MRI and 31P MRS. *Transl. Stroke Res.* **2013**, *4*, 351–367. [CrossRef]

98. Tsenov, G.; Mátéffyová, A.; Mares, P.; Otáhal, J.; Kubová, H. Intrahippocampal injection of endothelin-1: A new model of ischemia-induced seizures in immature rats. *Epilepsia* **2007**, *48*, 7–13. [CrossRef]

99. Hossmann, K.A. Cerebral ischemia: Models, methods and outcomes. *Neuropharmacology* **2008**, *55*, 257–270. [CrossRef]

100. Gerriets, T.; Li, F.; Silva, M.D.; Meng, X.; Brevard, M.; Sotak, C.H.; Fisher, M. The macrosphere model: Evaluation of a new stroke model for permanent middle cerebral artery occlusion in rats. *J. Neurosci. Methods* **2003**, *122*, 201–211. [CrossRef]

101. Overgaard, K.; Sereghy, T.; Boysen, G.; Pedersen, H.; Høyer, S.; Diemer, N.H. A rat model of reproducible cerebral infarction using thrombotic blood clot emboli. *J. Cereb. Blood Flow Metab.* **1992**, *12*, 484–490. [CrossRef]

102. Smith, W.S.; Sung, G.; Starkman, S.; Saver, J.L.; Kidwell, C.S.; Gobin, Y.P.; Lutsep, H.L.; Nesbit, G.M.; Grobelny, T.; Rymer, M.M.; et al. Safety and efficacy of mechanical embolectomy in acute ischemic stroke: Results of the MERCI trial. *Stroke* **2005**, *36*, 1432–1438. [CrossRef]

103. Zhao, S.; Zhao, M.; Xiao, T.; Jolkkonen, J.; Zhao, C. Constraint-induced movement therapy overcomes the intrinsic axonal growth-inhibitory signals in stroke rats. *Stroke* **2013**, *44*, 1698–1705. [CrossRef] [PubMed]

104. Hicks, A.U.; Lappalainen, R.S.; Narkilahti, S.; Suuronen, R.; Corbett, D.; Sivenius, J.; Hovatta, O.; Jolkkonen, J. Transplantation of human embryonic stem cell-derived neural precursor cells and enriched environment after cortical stroke in rats: Cell survival and functional recovery. *Eur. J. Neurosci.* **2009**, *29*, 562–574. [CrossRef] [PubMed]

105. Vigaru, B.; Lambercy, O.; Graber, L.; Fluit, R.; Wespe, P.; Schubring-Giese, M.; Luft, A.; Gassert, R. A small-scale robotic manipulandum for motor training in stroke rats. *IEEE Int. Conf. Rehabil. Robot.* **2011**, *2011*, 5975349. [PubMed]

106. Modo, M.; Crum, W.R.; Gerwig, M.; Vernon, A.C.; Patel, P.; Jackson, M.J.; Rose, S.; Jenner, P.; Iravani, M.M. Magnetic resonance imaging and tensor-based morphometry in the MPTP non-human primate model of Parkinson's disease. *PLoS ONE* **2017**, *12*, e0180733. [CrossRef]

107. Nitzsche, B.; Frey, S.; Collins, L.D.; Seeger, J.; Lobsien, D.; Dreyer, A.; Kirsten, H.; Stoffel, M.H.; Fonov, V.S.; Boltze, J. A stereotaxic, population-averaged T1w ovine brain atlas including cerebral morphology and tissue volumes. *Front. Neuroanat.* **2015**, *9*, 69. [CrossRef]

108. Modo, M.M.; Jolkkonen, J.; Zille, M.; Boltze, J. Future of Animal Modeling for Poststroke Tissue Repair. *Stroke* **2018**, *49*, 1099–1106. [CrossRef]

109. Sutherland, B.A.; Minnerup, J.; Balami, J.S.; Arba, F.; Buchan, A.M.; Kleinschnitz, C. Neuroprotection for ischaemic stroke: Translation from the bench to the bedside. *Int. J. Stroke* **2012**, *7*, 407–418. [CrossRef]

110. Hoyte, L.; Barber, P.A.; Buchan, A.M.; Hill, M.D. The rise and fall of NMDA antagonists for ischemic stroke. *Curr. Mol. Med.* **2004**, *4*, 131–136. [CrossRef]

111. Wahlgren, N.G.; Bornhov, S.; Sharma, A.; Cederin, B.; Rosolacci, T.; Ashwood, T.; Claesson, L.; CLASS Study Group. The clomethiazole acute stroke study (CLASS): Efficacy results in 545 patients classified as total anterior circulation syndrome (TACS). *J. Stroke Cerebrovasc. Dis.* **1999**, *8*, 231–239. [CrossRef]

112. Carter, A.J. The importance of voltage-dependent sodium channels in cerebral ischaemia. *Amino Acids* **1998**, *14*, 159–169. [CrossRef]

113. Hewitt, K.E.; Stys, P.K.; Lesiuk, H.J. The use-dependent sodium channel blocker mexiletine is neuroprotective against global ischemic injury. *Brain Res.* **2001**, *898*, 281–287. [CrossRef]

114. Kotoda, M.; Hishiyama, S.; Ishiyama, T.; Mitsui, K.; Matsukawa, T. Amiodarone exacerbates brain injuries after hypoxic-ischemic insult in mice. *BMC Neurosci.* **2019**, *20*, 62. [CrossRef] [PubMed]

115. Segura, T.; Calleja, S.; Jordan, J. Recommendations and treatment strategies for the management of acute ischemic stroke. *Expert Opin. Pharmacother.* **2008**, *9*, 1071–1085. [CrossRef] [PubMed]

116. Angeli, F.; Verdecchia, P.; Reboldi, G.P.; Gattobigio, R.; Bentivoglio, M.; Staessen, J.A.; Porcellati, C. Calcium channel blockade to prevent stroke in hypertension: A meta-analysis of 13 studies with 103,793 subjects. *Am. J. Hypertens.* **2004**, *17*, 817–822. [CrossRef]

117. Bowler, R.P.; Sheng, H.; Enghild, J.J.; Pearlstein, R.D.; Warner, D.S.; Crapo, J.D. A catalytic antioxidant (AEOL 10150) attenuates expression of inflammatory genes in stroke. *Free Radic. Biol. Med.* **2002**, *33*, 1141–1152. [CrossRef]

118. Ono, S.; Hishikawa, T.; Ogawa, T.; Nishiguchi, M.; Onoda, K.; Tokunaga, K.; Sugiu, K.; Date, I. Effect of deferoxamine-activated hypoxia inducible factor-1 on the brainstem following subarachnoid haemorrhage. In *Cerebral Vasospasm*; Acta Neurochirurgica Supplement, Volume 104; Springer: Vienna, Austria, 2008; pp. 69–73.

119. Mu, D.; Chang, Y.S.; Vexler, Z.S.; Ferriero, D.M. Hypoxia-inducible factor 1alpha and erythropoietin upregulation with deferoxamine salvage after neonatal stroke. *Exp. Neurol.* **2005**, *195*, 407–415. [CrossRef]

120. Shuaib, A.; Lees, K.R.; Lyden, P.; Grotta, J.; Davalos, A.; Davis, S.M.; Diener, H.C.; Ashwood, T.; Wasiewski, W.W.; Emeribe, U.; et al. NXY-059 for the treatment of acute ischemic stroke. *N. Engl. J. Med.* **2007**, *357*, 562–571. [CrossRef]

121. Lees, K.R.; Zivin, J.A.; Ashwood, T.; Davalos, A.; Davis, S.M.; Diener, H.C.; Grotta, J.; Lyden, P.; Shuaib, A.; Hårdemark, H.G.; et al. NXY-059 for acute ischemic stroke. *N. Engl. J. Med.* **2006**, *354*, 588–600. [CrossRef]

122. Shirley, R.; Ord, E.N.; Work, L.M. Oxidative Stress and the Use of Antioxidants in Stroke. *Antioxidants* **2014**, *3*, 472–501. [CrossRef]

123. Barreto, A.D. Intravenous thrombolytics for ischemic stroke. *Neurotherapeutics* **2011**, *8*, 388–399. [CrossRef]

124. The National Institute of Neurological Disorders and Stroke rt-PA Stroke Study Group. Tissue plasminogen activator for acute ischemic stroke. *N. Engl. J. Med.* **1995**, *333*, 1581–1587. [CrossRef] [PubMed]

125. Külkens, S.; Hacke, W. Thrombolysis with alteplase for acute ischemic stroke: Review of SITS-MOST and other Phase IV studies. *Expert Rev. Neurother.* **2007**, *7*, 783–788. [CrossRef] [PubMed]

126. Furlan, A.; Higashida, R.; Wechsler, L.; Gent, M.; Rowley, H.; Kase, C.; Pessin, M.; Ahuja, A.; Callahan, F.; Clark, W.M.; et al. Intra-arterial prourokinase for acute ischemic stroke. The PROACT II study: A randomized controlled trial. Prolyse in Acute Cerebral Thromboembolism. *JAMA* **1999**, *282*, 2003–2011. [CrossRef] [PubMed]

127. Ogawa, A.; Mori, E.; Minematsu, K.; Taki, W.; Takahashi, A.; Nemoto, S.; Miyamoto, S.; Sasaki, M.; Inoue, T.; The MELT Japan Study Group. Randomized trial of intraarterial infusion of urokinase within 6 hours of middle cerebral artery stroke: The middle cerebral artery embolism local fibrinolytic intervention trial (MELT) Japan. *Stroke* **2007**, *38*, 2633–2639. [CrossRef]

128. Abou-Chebl, A.; Bajzer, C.T.; Krieger, D.W.; Furlan, A.J.; Yadav, J.S. Multimodal therapy for the treatment of severe ischemic stroke combining GPIIb/IIIa antagonists and angioplasty after failure of thrombolysis. *Stroke* **2005**, *36*, 2286–2288. [CrossRef]

129. Qureshi, A.I.; Harris-Lane, P.; Kirmani, J.F.; Janjua, N.; Divani, A.A.; Mohammad, Y.M.; Suarez, J.I.; Montgomery, M.O. Intra-arterial reteplase and intravenous abciximab in patients with acute ischemic stroke: An open-label, dose-ranging, phase I study. *Neurosurgery* **2006**, *59*, 789–796; discussion 796–787. [CrossRef]

130. Investigators, I.I.T. The Interventional Management of Stroke (IMS) II Study. *Stroke* **2007**, *38*, 2127–2135. [CrossRef]

131. Mazighi, M.; Meseguer, E.; Labreuche, J.; Amarenco, P. Bridging therapy in acute ischemic stroke: A systematic review and meta-analysis. *Stroke* **2012**, *43*, 1302–1308. [CrossRef]

132. Jung, S.; Stapf, C.; Arnold, M. Stroke unit management and revascularisation in acute ischemic stroke. *Eur. Neurol.* **2015**, *73*, 98–105. [CrossRef]

133. Chen, J.; Sun, D.; Liu, M.; Zhang, S.; Ren, C. Defibrinogen Therapy for Acute Ischemic Stroke: 1332 Consecutive Cases. *Sci. Rep.* **2018**, *8*, 9489. [CrossRef]

134. Hao, Z.; Liu, M.; Counsell, C.; Wardlaw, J.M.; Lin, S.; Zhao, X. Fibrinogen depleting agents for acute ischaemic stroke. *Cochrane Database Syst. Rev.* **2012**. [CrossRef] [PubMed]

135. Levy, D.E.; Trammel, J.; Wasiewski, W.W.; For the Ancrod Stroke Program (ASP) Study Team. Ancrod for acute ischemic stroke: A new dosing regimen derived from analysis of prior ancrod stroke studies. *J. Stroke Cerebrovasc. Dis.* **2009**, *18*, 23–27. [CrossRef] [PubMed]

136. Carlberg, B.; Asplund, K.; Hägg, E. Factors influencing admission blood pressure levels in patients with acute stroke. *Stroke* **1991**, *22*, 527–530. [CrossRef] [PubMed]

137. Ohwaki, K.; Yano, E.; Nagashima, H.; Hirata, M.; Nakagomi, T.; Tamura, A. Blood pressure management in acute intracerebral hemorrhage: Relationship between elevated blood pressure and hematoma enlargement. *Stroke* **2004**, *35*, 1364–1367. [CrossRef]

138. Owens, W.B. Blood pressure control in acute cerebrovascular disease. *J. Clin. Hypertens.* **2011**, *13*, 205–211. [CrossRef]

139. Schrader, J.; Lüders, S.; Kulschewski, A.; Berger, J.; Zidek, W.; Treib, J.; Einhäupl, K.; Diener, H.C.; Dominiak, P.; On behalf of the ACCESS Study Group. The ACCESS Study: Evaluation of Acute Candesartan Cilexetil Therapy in Stroke Survivors. *Stroke* **2003**, *34*, 1699–1703. [CrossRef]

140. Robinson, T.G.; Potter, J.F.; Ford, G.A.; Bulpitt, C.J.; Chernova, J.; Jagger, C.; James, M.A.; Knight, J.; Markus, H.S.; Mistri, A.K.; et al. Effects of antihypertensive treatment after acute stroke in the Continue or Stop Post-Stroke Antihypertensives Collaborative Study (COSSACS): A prospective, randomised, open, blinded-endpoint trial. *Lancet Neurol.* **2010**, *9*, 767–775. [CrossRef]

141. Potter, J.; Mistri, A.; Brodie, F.; Chernova, J.; Wilson, E.; Jagger, C.; James, M.; Ford, G.; Robinson, T. Controlling hypertension and hypotension immediately post stroke (CHHIPS)–a randomised controlled trial. *Health Technol. Assess.* **2009**, *13*, 1–73. [CrossRef]

142. Hankey, G.J. Lowering blood pressure in acute stroke: The SCAST trial. *Lancet* **2011**, *377*, 696–698. [CrossRef]

143. Lindsberg, P.J.; Roine, R.O. Hyperglycemia in acute stroke. *Stroke* **2004**, *35*, 363–364. [CrossRef]

144. Wada, S.; Yoshimura, S.; Inoue, M.; Matsuki, T.; Arihiro, S.; Koga, M.; Kitazono, T.; Makino, H.; Hosoda, K.; Ihara, M.; et al. Outcome Prediction in Acute Stroke Patients by Continuous Glucose Monitoring. *J. Am. Heart Assoc.* **2018**, *7*. [CrossRef] [PubMed]

145. Hackam, D.G.; Spence, J.D. Antiplatelet Therapy in Ischemic Stroke and Transient Ischemic Attack. *Stroke* **2019**, *50*, 773–778. [CrossRef] [PubMed]

146. Stringberg, A.; Camden, R.; Qualls, K.; Naqvi, S.H. Update on Dual Antiplatelet Therapy for Secondary Stroke Prevention. *Mo. Med.* **2019**, *116*, 303–307.

147. Borlongan, C.V.; Koutouzis, T.K.; Jorden, J.R.; Martinez, R.; Rodriguez, A.I.; Poulos, S.G.; Freeman, T.B.; McKeown, P.; Cahill, D.W.; Nishino, H.; et al. Neural transplantation as an experimental treatment modality for cerebral ischemia. *Neurosci. Biobehav. Rev.* **1997**, *21*, 79–90. [CrossRef]

148. Park, Y.J.; Niizuma, K.; Mokin, M.; Dezawa, M.; Borlongan, C.V. Cell-Based Therapy for Stroke: Musing With Muse Cells. *Stroke* **2020**, *51*, 2854–2862. [CrossRef]

149. Aizman, I.; Vinodkumar, D.; McGrogan, M.; Bates, D. Cell Injury-Induced Release of Fibroblast Growth Factor 2: Relevance to Intracerebral Mesenchymal Stromal Cell Transplantations. *Stem Cells Dev.* **2015**, *24*, 1623–1634. [CrossRef]

150. Dao, M.; Tate, C.C.; McGrogan, M.; Case, C.C. Comparing the angiogenic potency of naïve marrow stromal cells and Notch-transfected marrow stromal cells. *J. Transl. Med.* **2013**, *11*, 81. [CrossRef] [PubMed]

151. Bao, X.; Wei, J.; Feng, M.; Lu, S.; Li, G.; Dou, W.; Ma, W.; Ma, S.; An, Y.; Qin, C.; et al. Transplantation of human bone marrow-derived mesenchymal stem cells promotes behavioral recovery and endogenous neurogenesis after cerebral ischemia in rats. *Brain Res.* **2011**, *1367*, 103–113. [CrossRef] [PubMed]

152. Yoo, S.W.; Kim, S.S.; Lee, S.Y.; Lee, H.S.; Kim, H.S.; Lee, Y.D.; Suh-Kim, H. Mesenchymal stem cells promote proliferation of endogenous neural stem cells and survival of newborn cells in a rat stroke model. *Exp. Mol. Med.* **2008**, *40*, 387–397. [CrossRef]

153. Aizman, I.; Tate, C.C.; McGrogan, M.; Case, C.C. Extracellular matrix produced by bone marrow stromal cells and by their derivative, SB623 cells, supports neural cell growth. *J. Neurosci. Res.* **2009**, *87*, 3198–3206. [CrossRef] [PubMed]

154. Chopp, M.; Li, Y.; Zhang, Z.G. Mechanisms underlying improved recovery of neurological function after stroke in the rodent after treatment with neurorestorative cell-based therapies. *Stroke* **2009**, *40*, S143–S145. [CrossRef]

155. Cramer, S.C.; Abila, B.; Scott, N.E.; Simeoni, M.; Enney, L.A.; Investigators, M.S. Safety, pharmacokinetics, and pharmacodynamics of escalating repeat doses of GSK249320 in patients with stroke. *Stroke* **2013**, *44*, 1337–1342. [CrossRef]

156. Emerick, A.J.; Neafsey, E.J.; Schwab, M.E.; Kartje, G.L. Functional reorganization of the motor cortex in adult rats after cortical lesion and treatment with monoclonal antibody IN-1. *J. Neurosci.* **2003**, *23*, 4826–4830. [CrossRef] [PubMed]

157. Patel, A.T.; Duncan, P.W.; Lai, S.M.; Studenski, S. The relation between impairments and functional outcomes poststroke. *Arch. Phys. Med. Rehabil.* **2000**, *81*, 1357–1363. [CrossRef] [PubMed]

158. Dobkin, B.H. *The Clinical Science of Neurologic Rehabilitation*; Oxford University Press: New York, NY, USA, 2003.

159. Dobkin, B.H. Strategies for stroke rehabilitation. *Lancet Neurol.* **2004**, *3*, 528–536. [CrossRef]

160. Iacoboni, M.; Woods, R.P.; Brass, M.; Bekkering, H.; Mazziotta, J.C.; Rizzolatti, G. Cortical mechanisms of human imitation. *Science* **1999**, *286*, 2526–2528. [CrossRef] [PubMed]

161. Akbik, F.; Hirsch, J.A.; Chandra, R.V.; Frei, D.; Patel, A.B.; Rabinov, J.D.; Rost, N.; Schwamm, L.H.; Leslie-Mazwi, T.M. Telestroke-the promise and the challenge. Part one: Growth and current practice. *J. Neurointerv. Surg.* **2017**, *9*, 357–360. [CrossRef]

162. Bowry, R.; Parker, S.; Rajan, S.S.; Yamal, J.M.; Wu, T.C.; Richardson, L.; Noser, E.; Persse, D.; Jackson, K.; Grotta, J.C. Benefits of Stroke Treatment Using a Mobile Stroke Unit Compared With Standard Management: The BEST-MSU Study Run-In Phase. *Stroke* **2015**, *46*, 3370–3374. [CrossRef]

163. Association, A.H. *New Recommendations for Stroke Systems of Care to Improve Patient Outcomes*; ScienceDaily: Rockville, MD, USA, 2019.

164. Arienti, C.; Lazzarini, S.G.; Pollock, A.; Negrini, S. Rehabilitation interventions for improving balance following stroke: An overview of systematic reviews. *PLoS ONE* **2019**, *14*, e0219781. [CrossRef]

165. Bonini-Rocha, A.C.; de Andrade, A.L.S.; Moraes, A.M.; Gomide Matheus, L.B.; Diniz, L.R.; Martins, W.R. Effectiveness of Circuit-Based Exercises on Gait Speed, Balance, and Functional Mobility in People Affected by Stroke: A Meta-Analysis. *PM R* **2018**, *10*, 398–409. [CrossRef]

166. Eng, J.J.; Bird, M.L.; Godecke, E.; Hoffmann, T.C.; Laurin, C.; Olaoye, O.A.; Solomon, J.; Teasell, R.; Watkins, C.L.; Walker, M.F. Moving stroke rehabilitation research evidence into clinical practice: Consensus-based core recommendations from the Stroke Recovery and Rehabilitation Roundtable. *Int. J. Stroke* **2019**, *14*, 766–773. [CrossRef] [PubMed]

167. Kalladka, D.; Sinden, J.; Pollock, K.; Haig, C.; McLean, J.; Smith, W.; McConnachie, A.; Santosh, C.; Bath, P.M.; Dunn, L.; et al. Human neural stem cells in patients with chronic ischaemic stroke (PISCES): A phase 1, first-in-man study. *Lancet* **2016**, *388*, 787–796. [CrossRef]

168. Macrae, I.M.; Allan, S.M. Stroke: The past, present and future. *Brain Neurosci. Adv.* **2018**, *2*, 2398212818810689. [CrossRef] [PubMed]

169. Qiu, C.W.; Liu, Z.Y.; Hou, K.; Liu, S.Y.; Hu, Y.X.; Zhang, L.; Zhang, F.L.; Lv, K.Y.; Kang, Q.; Hu, W.Y.; et al. Wip1 knockout inhibits neurogenesis by affecting the Wnt/β-catenin signaling pathway in focal cerebral ischemia in mice. *Exp. Neurol.* **2018**, *309*, 44–53. [CrossRef]

170. Huang, X.; Sun, J.; Zhao, T.; Wu, K.W.; Watanabe, K.; Xiao, Z.C.; Zhu, L.L.; Fan, M. Loss of NB-3 aggravates cerebral ischemia by impairing neuron survival and neurite growth. *Stroke* **2011**, *42*, 2910–2916. [CrossRef]

171. Zhang, P.; Liu, X.; Zhu, Y.; Chen, S.; Zhou, D.; Wang, Y. Honokiol inhibits the inflammatory reaction during cerebral ischemia reperfusion by suppressing NF-κB activation and cytokine production of glial cells. *Neurosci. Lett.* **2013**, *534*, 123–127. [CrossRef]

172. Qiu, C.W.; Liu, Z.Y.; Zhang, F.L.; Zhang, L.; Li, F.; Liu, S.Y.; He, J.Y.; Xiao, Z.C. Post-stroke gastrodin treatment ameliorates ischemic injury and increases neurogenesis and restores the Wnt/β-Catenin signaling in focal cerebral ischemia in mice. *Brain Res.* **2019**, *1712*, 7–15. [CrossRef]

173. Rudd, A.G.; Bladin, C.; Carli, P.; De Silva, D.A.; Field, T.S.; Jauch, E.C.; Kudenchuk, P.; Kurz, M.W.; Lærdal, T.; Ong, M.; et al. Utstein recommendation for emergency stroke care. *Int. J. Stroke* **2020**, *15*, 555–564. [CrossRef]

174. Chollet, F.; Cramer, S.C.; Stinear, C.; Kappelle, L.J.; Baron, J.C.; Weiller, C.; Azouvi, P.; Hommel, M.; Sabatini, U.; Moulin, T.; et al. Pharmacological therapies in post stroke recovery: Recommendations for future clinical trials. *J. Neurol.* **2014**, *261*, 1461–1468. [CrossRef]

175. Khandelwal, P.; Yavagal, D.R.; Sacco, R.L. Acute Ischemic Stroke Intervention. *J. Am. Coll. Cardiol.* **2016**, *67*, 2631–2644. [CrossRef]

176. Boltze, J.; Ayata, C. Challenges and Controversies in Translational Stroke Research—An Introduction. *Transl. Stroke Res.* **2016**, *7*, 355–357. [CrossRef] [PubMed]

177. Endres, M.; Engelhardt, B.; Koistinaho, J.; Lindvall, O.; Meairs, S.; Mohr, J.P.; Planas, A.; Rothwell, N.; Schwaninger, M.; Schwab, M.E.; et al. Improving outcome after stroke: Overcoming the translational roadblock. *Cerebrovasc. Dis.* **2008**, *25*, 268–278. [CrossRef] [PubMed]

178. Zerna, C.; Hill, M.D.; Boltze, J. Towards Improved Translational Stroke Research: Progress and Perspectives of the Recent National Institute of Neurological Disorders and Stroke Consensus Group Meeting. *Stroke* **2017**, *48*, 2341–2342. [CrossRef] [PubMed]

179. Boltze, J.; Nitzsche, F.; Jolkkonen, J.; Weise, G.; Pösel, C.; Nitzsche, B.; Wagner, D.C. Concise Review: Increasing the Validity of Cerebrovascular Disease Models and Experimental Methods for Translational Stem Cell Research. *Stem Cells* **2017**, *35*, 1141–1153. [CrossRef] [PubMed]

180. Fisher, M.; Feuerstein, G.; Howells, D.W.; Hurn, P.D.; Kent, T.A.; Savitz, S.I.; Lo, E.H.; Group, S. Update of the stroke therapy academic industry roundtable preclinical recommendations. *Stroke* **2009**, *40*, 2244–2250. [CrossRef]

181. Boltze, J.; Lukomska, B.; Jolkkonen, J.; For the MEMS–IRBI Consortium. Mesenchymal stromal cells in stroke: Improvement of motor recovery or functional compensation? *J. Cereb. Blood Flow Metab.* **2014**, *34*, 1420–1421. [CrossRef]

182. Boltze, J.; Wagner, D.C.; Barthel, H.; Gounis, M.J. Academic-industry Collaborations in Translational Stroke Research. *Transl. Stroke Res.* **2016**, *7*, 343–353. [CrossRef]

183. Wang, L.; Plump, A.; Ringel, M. Racing to define pharmaceutical R&D external innovation models. *Drug Discov. Today* **2015**, *20*, 361–370.

4

Adjunctive Therapy Approaches for Ischemic Stroke: Innovations to Expand Time Window of Treatment

Talia Knecht [1,2,†], Jacob Story [1,†], Jeffrey Liu [1,3], Willie Davis [1], Cesar V. Borlongan [4] and Ike C. dela Peña [1,*]

[1]   Department of Pharmaceutical and Administrative Sciences, Loma Linda University School of Pharmacy, Loma Linda, CA 92350, USA; knecht.talia@gmail.com (T.K.); jstory512@gmail.com (J.S.); jefliu@llu.edu (J.L.); wldavis@llu.edu (W.D.)

[2]   Department of Psychology, University of California, San Diego, CA 92093, USA

[3]   Department of Neuroscience, University of California, Riverside, CA 92521, USA

[4]   Department of Neurosurgery and Brain Repair, Center of Excellence for Aging and Brain Repair, University of South Florida College of Medicine, Tampa, FL 33612, USA; cborlong@health.usf.edu

*   Correspondence: idelapena@llu.edu;

†   These authors contributed equally to this work.

Abstract: Tissue plasminogen activator (tPA) thrombolysis remains the gold standard treatment for ischemic stroke. A time-constrained therapeutic window, with the drug to be given within 4.5 h after stroke onset, and lethal side effects associated with delayed treatment, most notably hemorrhagic transformation (HT), limit the clinical use of tPA. Co-administering tPA with other agents, including drug or non-drug interventions, has been proposed as a practical strategy to address the limitations of tPA. Here, we discuss the pharmacological and non-drug approaches that were examined to mitigate the complications—especially HT—associated with delayed tPA treatment. The pharmacological treatments include those that preserve the blood-brain barrier (e.g., atovarstatin, batimastat, candesartan, cilostazol, fasudil, minocycline, etc.), enhance vascularization and protect the cerebrovasculature (e.g., coumarin derivate IMM-H004 and granulocyte-colony stimulating factor (G-CSF)), and exert their effects through other modes of action (e.g., oxygen transporters, ascorbic acid, etc.). The non-drug approaches include stem cell treatments and gas therapy with multi-pronged biological effects. Co-administering tPA with the abovementioned therapies showed promise in attenuating delayed tPA-induced side effects and stroke-induced neurological and behavioral deficits. Thus, adjunctive treatment approach is an innovative therapeutic modality that can address the limitations of tPA treatment and potentially expand the time window for ischemic stroke therapy.

Keywords: tissue plasminogen activator; hemorrhage; blood-brain barrier; stem cell; matrix metalloproteinase (MMP)

1. Introduction

Stroke persists as one of the most prolific killers of Americans, and poses a considerable threat to millions of others worldwide [1]. The therapeutic options for this disease are limited, and most of the currently used medications show limited efficacy in restoring lost neurological functions. Furthermore, there is but one Food and Drug Administration (FDA)-approved drug for stroke, namely, tissue plasminogen activator (tPA), which presents significant limitations: a time-constrained therapeutic window (the drug must be given within 4.5 h from stroke onset), and adverse side effects associated with delayed treatment of the drug, most notably hemorrhagic transformation (HT) [2]. These hurdles of tPA treatment result in a mere 3 percent of ischemic stroke patients actually benefiting from tPA therapy [3–5]. As a result of the scarcity of effective therapies and other unmet clinical needs for stroke, preclinical and clinical research for novel stroke interventions have been initiated.

An assortment of drugs ranging from those that augment neurogenesis [6] and other thrombolytic agents [7,8] have been tested with poor clinical results. As reperfusion with tPA continues to be regarded as the gold standard treatment for ischemic stroke, a considerable clinical dilemma at hand is identifying strategies that will enhance the therapeutic time window for tPA therapy and curtail the adverse effects (especially HT) of tPA treatment [9]. Therefore, identifying interventions that will address the aforementioned impediments of tPA therapy is as important as developing new drugs for acute ischemic stroke [9]. Expanding the thrombolytic time window for ischemic stroke treatment via combination therapy will not only minimize the complications or detrimental side effects of delayed tPA treatment, but also allow the time window of neuroplasticity to remain open for a longer period of time, likely resulting in improved recovery and functional outcomes post-treatment.

2. Adjunctive Treatment to Expand Therapeutic Time Window for tPA

Disruption of the blood-brain barrier (BBB), damage to microvessels, and the toxic and non-thrombolytic actions of tPA have been suggested as the mechanisms underlying delayed tPA-induced complications, especially HT [8,10–13]. Pharmacological and non-drug interventions that counter the above events and target the molecules that contribute to BBB disruption, promote vascularization, etc., are logical treatments that could be given along with tPA to prevent such complications. Moreover, treatments with multi-pronged therapeutic effects are ideal in view of the complex mechanisms of stroke and delayed tPA-induced HT [9,14]. In the following sections, we discuss the pharmacological and non-drug treatments that have been examined to attenuate the complications, especially HT, of delayed tPA treatment. We focus on interventions that have been tested in experimental animal models, whereby delayed tPA treatment has been defined as >4.5 h after stroke onset. When available, data describing the performance of these agents in clinical studies are also discussed. These adjunctive treatments, their effects, and proposed mechanisms of action are shown in Figure 1 and summarized in Tables 1 and 2.

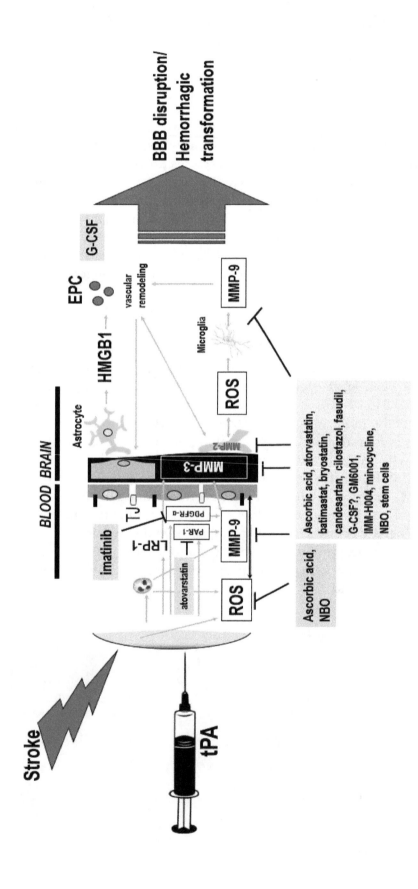

Figure 1. Proposed molecular targets of adjunctive treatments to enhance therapeutic window of tissue plasminogen activator (tPA) treatment. Acute stroke may cause injury to endothelial cells causing release of free radicals and pro-inflammatory cytokines. The signaling actions of tPA on the neurovascular unit may also increase blood-brain barrier (BBB) leakage, neurovascular cell death, and hemorrhagic transformation (HT). Moreover, the HT that ensues after delayed tPA treatment has been attributed to increased reperfusion and the effect of tPA on metalloproteinase (MMP) activity and other signaling pathways, including lipoprotein receptor-related protein (LRP), protease-activated receptor (PAR1), and PDGRF-α signaling. Ascorbic acid, normobaric oxygen (NBO) attenuates delayed tPA-induced complications in preclinical stroke models via inhibition of ROS production and BBB protection. Atovarstatin, minocycline, cilostazol, GM6001, fasudil, candesartan, bryostatin, and IMM-H004 reduces the HT by preserving the BBB through their actions on various MMPs and tight junction proteins. Granulocyte-colony stimulating factor (G-CSF) and IMM-H004 may reduce the HT by enhancing neurovascularization in addition to restoring BBB integrity. Imatinib reduces HT through the PDGRF-α receptor, while atovarstatin exerts its therapeutic benefits via inhibition of PAR1. Stem cells may also exert multi-pronged effects including BBB protection via its actions on various matrix metalloproteinases (MMPs). Abbreviations: EPC, endothelial progenitor cell; G-CSF, granulocyte-colony stimulating factor; HMGB1, high-mobility-group-box-1; ROS, reactive oxygen species; LRP, lipoprotein receptor-related protein; PAR1, protease-activated receptor; PDGFR-α, platelet-derived growth factor α-receptor (PDGFR-α); NBO, normobaric oxygen.

Table 1. Pharmacological adjunctive treatments to extend therapeutic window for ischemic stroke treatment.

Adjunctive Treatment (Dosage, Mode and Timing of Treatment)	Species & Stroke Model	tPA Dose, Mode & Timing of Treatment	Parameter/Molecular Target	Outcome	Timing of Evaluation	Ref.
Ascorbic acid (500 mg, p.o.) 5 h post stroke	Male rats; MCA cauterization	1 mg/kg, i.v., 5 h post stroke	infarct volume / brain edema / brain permeability / MMP-9 / Sensorimotor functions	decreased / decreased / decreased / decreased / improved	48 h post stroke	[15]
Atovarstatin (First dose: 20 mg/kg 4 h after stroke, Second dose: 20 mg/kg at 24 h after the first dose, s.c.)	Male Wistar rats; embolic	10 mg/kg, i.v., 6 h post stroke	HT / infarct volume / neurological functions / thrombolysis and vascular patency / ICAM-1 / PAR-1 / Collagen type IV / MMP-9	decreased / improved / increased / reduced / reduced / reduced / increased	7 h 30 h post stroke	[16]
Batimastat (MMP inhibitor; 50 mg/kg; i.p., 3 and 6 h after stroke)	Male spontaneously hypertensive rats; embolic	10 mg/kg, i.v., 6 h post stroke	HT / infarct volume / neurological functions / Mortality	decreased / decreased / improved / decreased	24 h post stroke	[17]
Bryostatin (PKC modulator; 2.5 mg/kg, i.v., alongside tPA)	Female SD rats, 18–20 mo old; embolic	5 mg/kg, i.v., 6 h post stroke	HT / infarct volume / MMP-9 / MMP-2 / PKCε / PKCα / PKCδ	decreased / not changed / decreased / not changed / increased / not changed / not changed	24 h post stroke	[18]
Candesartan (AT1R blocker; 1 mg/kg, i.v., 3 h after stroke)	Male Wistar rats (330–350 g); embolic	10 mg/kg, i.v., 6 h post stroke	HT / infarct volume / MMP-9 / MMP-2 / MMP-3 / NF-κB / TNF-α / p-eNOS	decreased / not changed / not changed / not changed / decreased / decreased / decreased / decreased	24 h post stroke	[19]

Table 1. Cont.

Adjunctive Treatment (Dosage, Mode and Timing of Treatment)	Species & Stroke Model	tPA Dose, Mode & Timing of Treatment	Parameter/Molecular Target	Outcome	Timing of Evaluation	Ref.
Cilostazol (PDEIII-inhibitor; 10 mg/kg, i.p., before tPA)	Male ddY (22–26 g) 4 weeks old; intraluminal filament/reperfusion	10 mg/kg, i.v., 6 h post stroke, before reperfusion	HT infarct volume MMP-9 claudin 5 locomotor behavior	decreased decreased decreased enhanced improved	18 h post reperfusion 7 days post stroke	[17]
Dodecafluoropentane emulsion (DDFPe) nanodroplets 0.3 mL/kg, i.v. 1 h after stroke, and 5 additional doses at 90 min intervals	New Zealand male or female rabbits; 3.4 to 4.7 kg/bw; Embolic	0.9 mg/kg tPA, 9 h after last DDFPe dose	stroke volume neurological functions	decreased improved	24 h post stroke	[20]
Fasudil (ROCK inhibitor; 3 mg/kg, i.p., before tPA)	Male SD rats (250–330 g); intraluminal filament/reperfusion	10 mg/kg, i.v., 6 h post stroke, after reperfusion	HT infarct volume MMP-9 (in vitro) locomotor behavior	decreased not changed decreased improved	18 h post reperfusion 7 days post stroke	[21]
G-CSF (300 µg/kg, i.v., alongside tPA)	Male SD rats, (200–250 g), 9–10 weeks old; intraluminal filament/reperfusion	10 mg/kg, i.v., post stroke, before reperfusion	HT infarct volume neurological functions Ang-1 Ang-2 CD34 eNOS VEGFR2 vWF	decreased not changed improved not changed increased increased increased increased increased	24 h post drug treatment	[22]
GM6001 (MMP inhibitor; 100 mg/kg, i.p., alongside tPA)	Male ddY mice (22–30 g) 4 weeks old; intraluminal filament/reperfusion	10 mg/kg, i.v., 6 h post stroke, after reperfusion	HT infarct volume MMP-9 claudin (in vitro, in vivo) occludin (in vitro, in vivo) ZO-1 (in vitro, in vivo)	decreased not examined decreased not changed enhanced enhanced	48 h post stroke/reperfusion	[23]
Imatinib (PDGFR-α antagonist; 200 mg/kg, i.v., at 1 h after ischemia)	C57BL/6J mice, 10 weeks old, photothrombotic induction of MCAO	10 mg/kg, i.v., 5 h after stroke	HT	decreased	24 h post stroke	[24]

Table 1. *Cont.*

Adjunctive Treatment (Dosage, Mode and Timing of Treatment)	Species & Stroke Model	tPA Dose, Mode & Timing of Treatment	Parameter/Molecular Target	Outcome	Timing of Evaluation	Ref.
IMM-H004 (Coumarin derivative; 6 mg/kg, i.v., alongside tPA)	Male SD rats (300–320 g); embolic; Male SD rats (260–280 g); intraluminal filament/reperfusion	10 mg/kg, i.v., post stroke	HT	decreased	18 h post stroke	[25]
			infarct volume	decreased	24 h post stroke	
			neurological functions	improved	1, 2, 3 days post stroke	
			HT	decreased		
			infarct volume	decreased		
			neurological functions	improved	24 h post stroke	
			pro-MMP-9	decreased	1–7 days post stroke	
			Akt (in vitro)	decreased		
			Ang-1	increased	24 h post stroke/reperfusion	
			CD31	increased		
			CD31 + Ki67	increased	7 days post stroke/reperfusion	
			MMP-2	not co-localized in astrocytes		
			occludin	decreased		
			Tie2	increased		
Minocycline (antibiotic; 3 mg/kg, intravenous (i.v.), 4 h after stroke)	Male SHR; embolic	10 mg/kg, i.v., 6 h post stroke	HT	decreased	24 h post stroke	[26]
			infarct volume	decreased		
			MMP-9 (plasma)	decreased		

Abbreviations: tPA, tissue plasminogen activator; SHR, spontaneously hypertensive rat; HT, hemorrhagic transformation; PDEIII, phosphodiesterase III; MMP, matrix metalloproteinase; ZO, zonula occludens; ROCK, Rho-associated protein kinase; SD, Sprague Dawley; AT1R, angiotensin II type 1 receptor; MCAO, middle cerebral artery occlusion; NF-κB, nuclear factor NF-κB; TNF-α, tumor necrosis factor; eNOS, endothelial nitric oxide synthase; ICAM-1, Intercellular Adhesion Molecule 1; PAR-1, Protease-activated receptor-1; PKC, protein kinase C, Akt or protein kinase B, Ang, angiotensin, CD, cluster of differentiation; Tie, tyrosine kinase with Ig and EGF, G-CSF, granulocyte–colony stimulating factor; VEGFR2, vascular endothelial growth factor receptor 2; vWF, Von Willebrand factor.

Table 2. Non-drug adjunctive treatments to extend therapeutic window for ischemic stroke treatment.

Adjunctive Treatment (Dosage, Mode and Timing of Treatment)	Species & Stroke Model	tPA Dose, Mode & Timing of Treatment	Parameter/Molecular Target	Outcome	Timing of Evaluation	Ref.
Neural stem cells (1 day post stroke) + minocycline	Aged mice Intraluminal filament model	10 mg/kg, i.v., 6 h post stroke	neurological functions mortality	improved reduced	48 h post stroke	[27]
Normobaric oxygen (100% O_2)	Male Sprague-Dawley rats (290–320 g) suture occlusion, and reperfusion	10 mg/kg, i.v., 5 and 7 h post stroke, 15 min prior to reperfusion	HT infarct volume brain edema BBB disruption MMP-9 Occludin Claudin-5 neurological deficits mortality	reduced reduced reduced reduced reduced enhanced enhanced reduced decreased	24 h post stroke	[28]

Abbreviations: BBB, blood-brain barrier; HT, hemorrhagic transformation; MMP, matrix metalloproteinase.

3. Pharmacological Approaches to Extend Thrombolytic Time Window for Ischemic Stroke Treatment

The HT following delayed tPA treatment can be curtailed by an intervention that could help preserve the integrity of the BBB. Of note, stabilizing the BBB after stroke has been suggested to enhance the overall efficacy of tPA reperfusion therapy [11]. In light of the participation of metalloproteinases (MMPs) in the disruption of the BBB [8,10–13], targeting various MMPs has been explored. Moreover, preserving endothelial tight junction proteins (TJP) has also been considered, given that TJPs comprise the basic structure of the BBB [21,29,30]. Examples of pharmacological agents that exert therapeutic benefits by preserving the BBB are atovarstatin, batimastat, bryostatin, candesartan, cilostazol, fasudil, minocycline, etc. Vascular disruption plays a key role in intracerebral hemorrhage resulting in BBB leakage [31]. Thus, in addition to restoring BBB integrity, enhancing neovascularization or blood vessel formation is a logical strategy to counteract delayed tPA-induced HT. Angiogenesis, or the formation of new blood vessels, is also initiated in the ischemic region post vascular occlusion and contributes to improvements following infarction and neuronal recovery [32]. The pharmacological agents investigated to attenuate side effects of delayed tPA treatment by enhancing vascularization and protecting the cerebrovasculature include the coumarin derivative IMM-H004 and granulocyte-colony stimulating factor (G-CSF). Also, considering the role of free radicals in the complications associated with delayed tPA treatment, the effects of antioxidants have also been investigated [15]. The potential of oxygen transporters, which are promising stroke treatments based on preclinical studies, has also been recently explored for their ability to enhance the therapeutic window of tPA [20].

3.1. Ascorbic Acid

That glutathione and ascorbic acid (AA) levels decrease and free radical formation increases after ischemic brain injury (IBI) indicate the potential of AA supplementation to improve outcomes after IBI [33]. Ascorbic acid, or vitamin C, which could preserve endothelial function against ischemic oxidative injury in diabetes and counteract the formation of free radicals in the brain parenchyma, may attenuate the adverse effects of delayed tPA treatment [15]. In rats subjected to permanent middle cerebral artery occlusion (MCAO) and administered with low dose tPA (1 mg/kg, intravenous (i.v.)) and oral vitamin C (500 mg/kg) at 5 h after stroke, infarct volume and edema were reduced at 48 h post stroke, in comparison with rats given tPA only [15]. MMP-9 formation is triggered by oxidative stress which, in turn, promotes BBB damage after ischemia-reperfusion. The increase in MMP-9 levels and BBB disruption due to delayed tPA treatment were reduced by vitamin C administration [15]. Thus, vitamin C supplementation attenuates some of the deleterious side effects of delayed tPA therapy and exerts neuroprotection, indicating its potential as an adjunctive treatment to expand the limited therapeutic window of tPA. While vitamin C supplementation has been shown to improve stroke volumes, its impact on HT has not yet been determined.

3.2. Atorvastatin

The pleiotropic (e.g., antithrombotic, anti-inflammatory, and BBB-preserving) effects of statins make them attractive co-treatments to reduce the complications of delayed tPA treatment, as well as to extend the therapeutic window of the drug [16]. Atorvastatin, administered at 4 h after embolic stroke in rats, was found to attenuate the embolus size at the origin of the middle cerebral artery, improve microvascular patency, and decrease infarct volume in animals treated with tPA at 6 h after stroke. Moreover, the combination therapy did not increase the incidence of HT. The tPA-induced increase of protease-activated receptor-1, intercellular adhesion molecule-1, and MMP-9 were decreased by atovarstatin. Atovarstatin also reduced cerebral microvascular platelet, neutrophil, and fibrin deposition. It has been proposed that atorvastatin-induced reduction of delayed tPA-potentiated adverse cerebrovascular events contributed to the neuroprotective effect of the drug [16]. The latter has been attributed to the thrombolytic efficacy of atovarstatin, which leads to enhanced cerebrovascular patency and integrity [16].

3.3. Batimastat (BB-94)

Batimastat is a broad-spectrum MMP inhibitor [17]. Treatment with batamistat (50 mg/kg, intraperitoneal (i.p.)), in spontaneously hypertensive rats subjected to embolic stroke was shown to significantly reduce the volume of delayed tPA (6 h post stroke)-associated cerebral hemorrhage [17]. However, the specific MMP members and pathways involved in the therapeutic effect of batimastat were not explored. Moreover, despite the reduction in hemorrhage, no remarkable attenuation of neurological deficits post stroke was observed in batimastat-treated animals. Time- and dose-response studies are warranted to determine the optimal treatment regimen of batimastat with tPA in experimental stroke models.

3.4. Bryostatin

The efficacy of the protein kinase C (PKC) modulator bryostatin (2.5 mg/kg; i.v.), given 2 h post MCAO to reduce delayed tPA (5 mg/kg, i.v.)-induced cerebral swelling, hemorrhage, and mortality at 24 h post MCAO in rats was investigated [18]. Notably, bryostatin decreased ischemic brain injury in aged female rats [34]. In rats subjected to delayed tPA treatment, bryostatin attenuated the HT and BBB disruption, and decreased MMP-9 expression while upregulating PKCε expression [18]. The bryostatin-mediated decrease in MMP-9 has been suggested to produce outcome improvements post-stroke. Moreover, bryostatin-induced upregulation of PKCε was also hypothesized to decrease damage to TJPs within the BBB and reduce the HT [18]. PKCε regulation of MMP-9 was also proposed to play an important role in the beneficial effect of bryostatin to reduce delayed tPA-induced hemorrhage and BBB disruption [18].

3.5. Candesartan

Candesartan blocks the angiotensin II type 1 receptor and prevents injury due to ischemic stroke [19]. Early treatment with candesartan (1 mg/kg, at 3 h after stroke onset) has been shown to decrease the brain hemorrhage and improve neurological outcomes in animals subjected to embolic strokes and given tPA (10 mg/kg, i.v.) at 6 h after stroke [19]. However, the combination therapy increased MMP-9 levels although it decreased MMP-3 levels. The intracranial bleeding after tPA treatment in stroked mice was also decreased in MMP-3-null, but not MMP-9-null mice compared to wild-type controls [35]. In view of the above findings, it was proposed that activation of MMP-9 alone is not enough to increase the incidence of hemorrhage in embolic stroke. Nevertheless, the combination therapy decreased nuclear factor kappa-B (NF-κB) expression, which has been shown to mediate MMP-3 expression in endothelial cells after tPA treatment, and also to decrease TNF-α expression following activation of NF-κB. Subjects given candesartan also showed enhancement in the activation of endothelial nitric oxide synthase, an enzyme required for vascular function and homeostasis [36].

3.6. Cilostazol

Cilostazol is used for the treatment of intermittent claudication [37]. Combination treatment with cilostazol (10 mg/kg; i.v.) and tPA (10 mg/kg, i.v.) at 6 h post stroke after reperfusion in mice has been shown to reduce HT, brain edema, morbidity and mortality, and neurological deficits at 18 h and 7 days after the reperfusion [30]. Cilostazol treatment also attenuated delayed tPA-induced upregulation of MMP-9 activity and counteracted the decrease in expression of claudin-5 [30], an essential molecule for the assembly of tight junctions between microvascular endothelial cells [38]. In vitro, cilostazol prevented the tPA-induced damage on endothelial cells and pericytes via its effects on cyclic adenosine monophosphate (cAMP) activity [30]. It remains to be known whether the neurovascular protective effects of the cilostazol persist for longer time periods post-stroke.

3.7. Dodecafluoropentane Emulsion (DDFPe) Nanodroplets

Dodecafluoropentane emulsion (DDFPe) is an oxygen-transporting perfluorocarbon given i.v. shown to provide neuroprotection in rabbits subjected to ischemic stroke [20]. The efficacy of DDFPe (0.3 mL/kg) to enhance the time window for tPA treatment was examined in rabbits which underwent embolic stroke procedures [20]. DDFPe treatment has been shown to reduce the neurological deficits and stroke volumes at 24 h post stroke in rabbits given tPA (0.9 mg/kg, given 9 h after stroke) [20]. Improved oxygen transport without the need for red blood cell flow has been proposed as the mechanism underlying the therapeutic efficacy of DDFPe [20]. The impact of DDFPe treatment on HT associated with delayed tPA administration has not yet been studied.

3.8. Fasudil

Fasudil has been marketed in Japan for the treatment of cerebral vasospasms occurring after subarachnoid hemorrhage [39]. It is a Rho kinase inhibitor initially described as an intracellular calcium antagonist. Fasudil (3 mg/kg, i.p.) has been shown to decrease HT at 18 h post reperfusion in mice subjected to 6-h MCAO and treated with tPA (10 mg/kg, i.v.) [21]. It also remarkably decreased mortality and improved locomotor activity in stroked animals at 7 days after the reperfusion. Fasudil treatment, however, did not exert neuroprotection when compared with controls and tPA-alone treatment group [21]. The in vitro studies showed that fasudil prevented the tPA-induced injury to human brain microvascular endothelial cells (HBMECs) via reduction of MMP-9 activity [21]. The lactate dehydrogenase assays also revealed that fasudil prevented tPA-induced damage by protecting the endothelial cells [21]. Exploring the long-term neurovascular protective effects of fasudil, the molecular mechanisms in delayed tPA-induced HT, and also the optimum doses of the drug when combined with tPA are worthwhile future research endeavors [21].

3.9. Granulocyte Colony-Stimulating Factor (G-CSF)

Granulocyte-colony stimulating factor (G-CSF) is an FDA-approved medical countermeasure to promote survival in patients exposed to myelosuppressive doses of radiation. Functionally, it is a cytokine which regulates the survival, proliferation, and differentiation of hematopoietic stem cells and hematopoietic progenitor cells [40]. G-CSF (300 µg/kg, i.v.) treatment has been shown to reduce delayed (6 h post MCAO) tPA (10 mg/kg, i.v.)-induced HT [22]. It also increased levels of angiogenesis marker Ang-2 but not Ang-1, vasculogenesis marker vWF, phosphorylated-eNOS, and endothelial progenitor cell (EPC) markers cluster of differentiation (CD) 34+ and vascular endothelial growth factor receptor (VEGFR)-2 in the ischemic hemispheres of stroked rats compared with rats given tPA treatment only. The neurological deficits at 24 h post drug treatment were also improved by G-CSF treatment. It has been proposed that G-CSF reduces delayed tPA-induced HT and enhances the neurological outcomes post stroke via angiogenic and vasculogenic activities of G-CSF, proliferative or regenerative actions of G-CSF-recruited EPCs, or both [22]. Although completion of vascularization typically requires several days, drugs that promote vascularization in stroke may accelerate the process and promote preservation of a patent vasculature against tPA-induced HT. Notably, a clinical study found that while the growth factors (GFs) vascular endothelial growth factor (VEGF), Ang-1 and G-CSF enhanced recanalization; Ang-1 but not VEGF or G-CSF enhanced HT [41]. High serum levels of G-CSF correlated with improved functional outcomes even at 90 days post treatment [41]. These results highlight the potential of G-CSF to reduce delayed tPA treatment-associated complications.

3.10. Ilomastat (GM6001)

GM6001 attaches to the active sites of MMPs and prevents the conversion of pro-MMPs to active forms of matrix-degrading MMPs [42]. GM6001 (100 mg/kg, i.p.) treatment in mice subjected to filamental MCAO and delayed tPA (10 mg/kg, i.v.) therapy (6 h post stroke) remarkably decreased tPA-induced elevation in brain hemoglobin, indicating that the drug reduced delayed tPA-associated

HT [23]. GM6001 treatment also reduced tPA-elevated MMP-9 at 42 h after the reperfusion, and the degradation of occludin and ZO-1 but not claudin-5 expression [23]. Moreover, GM6001 also increased the survival rate and the reduction in locomotor activity in animals at 7 days after ischemia and reperfusion [23]. In vitro studies showed that GM6001 countered tPA-induced damage in endothelial cells and the decrease in transendothelial electrical resistance [23]. Considering that GM6001 inhibited tumor necrosis factor-α (TNF-α) converting enzyme (TACE) expression and that increased levels of TNF-α correlates with intracerebral hemorrhage in animal models [43], the interaction between GM6001 and these molecules needs to be explored.

3.11. Imatinib

Imatinib is a platelet-derived growth factor α-receptor (PDGFR-α) inhibitor approved by the FDA for the treatment of chronic myelogenous leukemia and other cancers. The drug, given orally at a high dose of 200 mg/kg, at 1 h after ischemia via photothrombosis, was observed to reduce the extent of HT after delayed (5 h post stroke) treatment with tPA [24]. It also reduced the cerebrovascular permeability and stroke lesion volume. As it was given at 1 h post stroke, it remains to be known whether it is also effective in reducing complications associated with delayed tPA treatment when given at later time-points after stroke [24].

3.12. IMM-H004, a Coumarin Derivative

IMM-H004 is a coumarin derivative which belongs to a class of organic heterocyclic compounds with numerous biological effects [44]. In rats subjected to embolic stroke and given tPA (10 mg/kg, i.v., 6 h post stroke), IMM-H004 (6 mg/kg, i.v.) treatment decreased the hemorrhage, infarction volume, and cerebral edema [25]. IMM-H004 also reduced tPA-mediated HT and enhancement of ischemic infarction in rats subjected to stroke via the intraluminal filament method. Decreasing MMP-9/MMP-2, promoting co-localization of MMP-2 with astrocytes and IgG leakage, and increasing occludin levels were the mechanisms proposed to underlie the efficacy of IMM-H004. Moreover, IMM-H004 promoted vascularization and increased cerebral perfusion at 7 days post stroke by improving the integrity of vascular endothelial cells. The in vitro studies revealed that IMM-H004 increased levels of ATP and the protein kinase A (PKA) and PI3K-dependent activation of Akt in HBMECs and PC12 cells, suggesting the involvement of cAMP/PKA and PI3K/Akt signaling pathways [25]. Thus, IMM-H004 may attenuate delayed tPA-induced HT by enhancing neurovascularization along with preventing BBB disruption [25].

3.13. Minocycline

Clinically used for the treatment of acne vulgaris, minocycline (3 mg/kg, i.v., at 4 h post stroke) has been shown to reduce infarction and attenuate the brain hemorrhage observed 24 h after embolic stroke [26] in animals treated with tPA (10 mg/kg, i.v., at 6 h post stroke). As a potent MMP inhibitor [45], minocycline decreased plasma MMP-9 levels which coincided with volumes of infarction and hemorrhage [26]. It remains to be known whether brain MMP-9 levels are also reduced by minocycline and whether MMP-9 levels correlate with the extent of infarction and hemorrhage [26]. In an exploratory trial to measure safety and efficacy of minocycline when given in combination with tPA [46], 60% of patients given a loading dose of minocycline within a 6-h time window followed by maintenance dosing for 3 days showed no incidence of intracerebral hemorrhage. Subjects given tPA in the minocycline trial also showed lower plasma MMP-9 levels [47]. Other clinical trials in different populations have been started and are awaiting results [48].

4. Non-Drug Adjuvants to Extend Thrombolytic Time Window for Ischemic Stroke Treatment

Expanding the time window for thrombolysis may not only be achieved through pharmacological means, but also through non-drug strategies [9]. The multi-pronged effects of stem cells indicate their worth as treatments to attenuate the complications associated with delayed tPA treatment [9,49,50].

Gas therapy, which has been considered as a logical ischemic stroke treatment, has also been examined for its potential application to counter delayed tPA treatment-associated outcomes [28]. Other non-drug strategies are well-described techniques, such as brain imaging and endovascular procedures, that have been shown clinically to visualize stroke pathology and treatment efficacy, as well as to help extend the therapeutic window for tPA treatment in ischemic stroke [9,51–53].

4.1. Minocycline and Neural Stem Cells

Minocycline has been previously shown to reduce hemorrhage associated with delayed tPA treatment [17]. Intracranial transplantation of neural stem cells (hNSCs) has also been demonstrated to mitigate the BBB damage caused by ischemic stroke [54]. In mice subjected to MCAO followed by reperfusion and given tPA at 6 h post stroke, minocycline reduced the mortality associated with delayed tPA treatment, especially in aged mice [27]. Moreover, significant attenuation of delayed tPA-induced pathophysiology was observed in mice treated with minocycline and intracranially transplanted with hNSCs at 24 h post stroke [27]. Thus, the combination therapy of tPA and minocycline, and stem cell transplantation could not only mitigate delayed tPA-induced side effects, but also enhance neuroplasticity post stroke.

Other types of stem cells have also been investigated and have shown promise in mitigating the complications associated with tPA treatment. Mesenchymal stem cells (MSCs) which have been shown to reduce stroke volume and behavioral deficits in stroke models (for review, [55]), also reduced incidence of hemorrhage and improved behavioral dysfunctions in rats subjected to tPA (1 h 30 min post stroke, after reperfusion) treatment [56]. The treatment also reduced MMP-9 levels in the combination tPA + MSC group, compared with tPA alone-treated subjects [56]. MSCs may inhibit endothelial dysfunction to suppress hemorrhagic events and facilitate functional outcome. The combination MSCs and tPA therapy may also produce early behavioral recovery. Bone marrow stromal cells (BMSCs) have also been shown to improve functional outcomes in animal models of stroke as well as stroke patients [57]. The mechanism of action has been ascribed to the neurotrophic factors secreted by differentiated BMSCs (e.g., neural, glial, and endothelial cell types). Liu et al. [58] showed that intracerebral BMSC transplantation attenuated the MMP activation and subsequent neurovascular unit destruction caused by tPA treatment (1 h 30 min after MCAO and reperfusion). The authors suggested that the protective effect of BMSCs may be useful for reducing the damage of exogenous tPA in acute thrombolytic therapy for ischemic stroke patients. Considering that MSCs or other types of stem cells may exist endogenously, a better understanding of the therapeutic effects of minocycline or other drugs on both endogenous and exogenous stem cells may optimize such combination therapy.

4.2. Normobaric Hyperoxia (NBO) and Hyperbaric Oxygen (HBO) Therapy

NBO treatment affords neuroprotection when initiated early after ischemia onset [59]. Previous studies showed that NBO can protect the BBB against ischemic damage through inhibition of reactive oxygen species (ROS) production and MMP-9 induced damage of TJPs in stroked rats [60]. Early NBO treatment (100% O_2) was found to attenuate the MMP-9 induction in the ischemic microvessels of tPA-treated rats (tPA given at 3, 5, and 7 h MCAO) [28]. It also prevented the loss of occludin and claudin-5 due to delayed (5 and 7 h MCAO) tPA treatment. Importantly, NBO reduced the HT, brain edema, infarction volume, and mortality in tPA-treated rats. Neurological functions were also improved in rats subjected to NBO plus tPA. It was suggested that NBO could increase tPA's therapeutic window for ischemic stroke to at least 7 h. Rationally designed clinical studies with well-defined patient populations are required to validate whether NBO is a viable, safe, and efficacious adjunctive treatment for ischemic stroke [28]. Similarly, the documented therapeutic effects of HBO against experimental stroke [61,62] and in the clinic [63,64] warrant studies on its efficacy in combating tPA-induced complications.

4.3. Others

Brain imaging has been used to determine patient subgroups with increased risk for hemorrhage and poor clinical outcomes profile [51]. This technique has guided treatment decisions and consequently improved tPA's therapeutic time window with acceptable safety. Previous trials also demonstrated that endovascular procedures, for example intra-arterial thrombectomy, improved stroke outcomes in patients who received intravenous thrombolysis. In contrast with thrombolysis alone, thrombectomy combined with thrombolysis enhanced functional outcomes and reduced mortality in patients with ischemic stroke [52,53].

5. Summary and Conclusions

While we have only included in this review the preclinical studies which specified delayed tPA treatment as >4.5 h post stroke onset, it is noteworthy that some other drugs also attenuated HT and other complications associated with tPA treatment initiated at <4.5 h after stroke (e.g., annexin A2, fingolimod, progesterone, progranulin, uric acid, etc.) in animal models [12–14]. Nevertheless, considering that the studies mentioned in this paper are mostly preclinical studies, caution is needed when interpreting the results. As the effects of drug or non-drug interventions were examined in specific groups of animals (i.e., male or female only and/or old or young animals), the influence of age and gender on post-stroke outcomes, specifically delayed tPA-induced HT, needs to be explored. Moreover, rigorous preclinical studies are warranted in view of the clinical finding that erythropoietin, a vascular protective agent, did not reduce but rather increased HT occurrence [65].

Preclinical studies should also focus on interventions that exert neuroprotection in addition to attenuating HT. Notably, a recent meta-analysis involving 6756 participants in the nine clinical trials of intravenous alteplase versus controls showed that the increase in the occurrence of HT has been caused by a number of factors, including stroke severity [66]. Thus, in light of the role that stroke severity plays in HT, interventions given alongside tPA should also exert neuroprotection and accelerate the salvage of brain tissue after stroke.

Because tPA is essential for reperfusion therapy, finding the right dosage and timing of initiating treatment in relation to tPA is important to enhance possible clinical application of the combined therapy. Specifically, it is very difficult to estimate the precise time of stroke onset to administer the drugs in combination with tPA in the clinics. The FDA standards require assurance that any intervention (i.e., drugs) that are given alongside tPA should not block the fibrinolytic activity of tPA [65]. Nevertheless, to identify the appropriate targets and surmise interactions that could enhance the benefits of thrombolytic therapy, it is also imperative that we completely comprehend the exact mechanisms of tPA-induced HT and the other detrimental effects associated with delayed tPA treatment. Moreover, examining long-term efficacy of the combination therapy is also prudent to determine the worth of the drug when given as a treatment to curtail effects of delayed tPA treatment. Long-term efficacy assessments should include examining motor behavior functions not only a few days, but even months after drug treatment in view of the Stroke Treatment Academic Industry Roundtable (STAIR) guidelines [67,68]. In addition, when contemplating combination therapy with stem cells, the Stem cell Therapeutics as an Emerging Paradigm for Stroke (STEPS) recommendation may be helpful in translating these novel therapies to the clinic [69].

Enhancing tPA's time window via combination therapy will not only significantly improve HT and other side effects associated with delayed tPA therapy, but will also result in enhancement of the risk–benefit ratio for thrombolytic therapy and increase the number of patients eligible for tPA therapy. An expanded treatment window will also allow the time window of neuroplasticity to remain open for a longer period resulting in better recovery and functional outcomes post-treatment. Another potential, significant clinical application of this strategy is the treatment of "wake-up strokes", a case where patients awaken with stroke symptoms, which poses a significant challenge for acute stroke providers [70]. Combining tPA with interventions that could enhance its therapeutic time window is a reasonable strategy to treat patients with wake-up strokes.

At the time of writing, efforts are still underway to discover other fibrinolytics or thrombolytic drugs with better reperfusion efficacy than tPA [14,71,72]. Nevertheless, it is equally important to also explore logical and effective approaches that could improve the only FDA-approved stroke therapy [9]. As mentioned in this review, combining tPA with drugs and non-drug interventions is one approach that could circumvent the adverse outcomes associated with delayed tPA therapy, and thus, enhance the time window of tPA treatment.

Acknowledgments: The authors thank the research support from the American Heart Association (16POST27520023) and the Loma Linda University School of Pharmacy (LLUSP-360033).

Author Contributions: Talia Knecht and Jacob Story wrote the manuscript. Jeffrey Liu assisted in gathering data. Willie Davis, Cesar Borlongan, and Ike dela Peña provided input and supervised the editing of the manuscript.

References

1. Koton, S.; Schneider, A.L.; Rosamond, W.D.; Shahar, E.; Sang, Y.; Gottesman, R.F.; Coresh, J. Stroke incidence and mortality trends in US communities, 1987 to 2011. *JAMA* **2014**, *312*, 259–268. [CrossRef] [PubMed]
2. NINDS rt-PA Stroke Study Group. Intracerebral hemorrhage after intravenous tPA therapy for ischemic stroke. *Stroke* **1997**, *28*, 2109–2118.
3. Go, A.S.; Mozaffarian, D.; Roger, V.L.; Benjamin, E.J.; Berry, J.D.; Blaha, M.J.; Dai, S.; Ford, E.S.; Fox, C.S.; Franco, S.; et al. American Heart Association Statistics Committee and Stroke Statistics Subcommittee. Heart disease and stroke statistics—2014 update: A report from the American Heart Association. *Circulation* **2014**, *129*, e28–e292. [CrossRef] [PubMed]
4. Graham, G.D. Tissue plasminogen activator for acute ischemic stroke in clinical practice: A meta-analysis of safety data. *Stroke* **2003**, *34*, 2847–2850. [CrossRef] [PubMed]
5. Yip, T.R.; Demaerschalk, B.M. Estimated cost savings of increased use of intravenous tissue plasminogen activator for acute ischemic stroke in Canada. *Stroke* **2007**, *38*, 1952–1955. [CrossRef] [PubMed]
6. Greenberg, D.A. Neurogenesis and stroke. *CNS Neurol. Disord. Drug Targets* **2007**, *6*, 321–325. [CrossRef] [PubMed]
7. Adams, H.; Adams, R.; Del Zoppo, G.; Goldstein, L.B.; Stroke Council of the American Heart Association; American Stroke Association. Guidelines for the early management of patients with ischemic stroke: 2005 guidelines update a scientific statement from the Stroke Council of the American Heart Association/American Stroke Association. *Stroke* **2005**, *36*, 916–923. [PubMed]
8. Wang, X.; Tsuji, K.; Lee, S.R.; Ning, M.; Furie, K.L.; Buchan, A.M.; Lo, E.H. Mechanisms of hemorrhagic transformation after tissue plasminogen activator reperfusion therapy for ischemic stroke. *Stroke* **2004**, *35*, 2726–2730. [CrossRef] [PubMed]
9. Dela Peña, I.C.; Borlongan, C.V.; Shen, G.; Davis, W. Strategies to Extend Thrombolytic Time Window for Ischemic Stroke Treatment: An Unmet Clinical Need. *J. Stroke* **2017**, *19*, 50–60. [CrossRef] [PubMed]
10. Rosell, A.; Foerch, C.; Murata, Y.; Lo, E.H. Mechanisms and markers for hemorrhagic transformation after stroke. *Acta Neurochir. Suppl.* **2008**, *105*, 173–178. [PubMed]
11. Wang, W.; Li, M.; Chen, Q.; Wang, J. Hemorrhagic transformation after tissue plasminogen activator reperfusion therapy for ischemic stroke: Mechanisms, models, and biomarkers. *Mol. Neurobiol.* **2015**, *52*, 1572–1579. [CrossRef] [PubMed]
12. Jickling, G.C.; Liu, D.Z.; Stamova, B.; Ander, B.P.; Zhan, X.; Lu, A.; Sharp, F.R. Hemorrhagic transformation after ischemic stroke in animals and humans. *J. Cereb. Blood Flow Metab.* **2014**, *34*, 185–199. [CrossRef] [PubMed]
13. Lapchak, P.A. Hemorrhagic transformation following ischemic stroke: Significance, causes, and relationship to therapy and treatment. *Curr. Neurol. Neurosci. Rep.* **2002**, *2*, 38–43. [CrossRef] [PubMed]
14. Kanazawa, M.; Takahashi, T.; Nishizawa, M.; Shimohata, T. Therapeutic strategies to attenuate hemorrhagic transformation after tissue plasminogen activator treatment for acute ischemic stroke. *J. Atheroscler. Thromb.* **2017**, *24*, 240–253. [CrossRef] [PubMed]

15. Allahtavakoli, M.; Amin, F.; Esmaeeli-Nadimi, A.; Shamsizadeh, A.; Kazemi-Arababadi, M.; Kennedy, D. Ascorbic acid reduces the adverse effects of delayed daministration of tissue plasminogen activator in a rat stroke model. *Basic Clin. Pharmacol. Toxicol.* **2015**, *117*, 335–339. [CrossRef] [PubMed]

16. Zhang, L.; Chopp, M.; Jia, L.; Cui, Y.; Lu, M.; Zhang, Z.G. Atorvastatin extends the therapeutic window for tPA to 6 h after the onset of embolic stroke in rats. *J. Cereb. Blood Flow Metab.* **2009**, *29*, 1816–1824. [CrossRef] [PubMed]

17. Sumii, T.; Lo, E.H. Involvement of matrix metalloproteinase in thrombolysis-associated hemorrhagic transformation after embolic focal ischemia in rats. *Stroke* **2002**, *33*, 831–836. [CrossRef] [PubMed]

18. Tan, Z.; Lucke-Wold, B.P.; Logsdon, A.F.; Turner, R.C.; Tan, C.; Li, X.; Hongpaison, J.; Alkon, D.L.; Simpkins, J.W.; Rosen, C.L.; et al. Bryostatin extends tPA time window to 6 h following middle cerebral artery occlusion in aged female rats. *Eur. J. Pharmacol.* **2015**, *764*, 404–412. [CrossRef] [PubMed]

19. Ishrat, T.; Pillai, B.; Ergul, A.; Hafez, S.; Fagan, S.C. Candesartan reduces the hemorrhage associated with delayed tissue plasminogen activator treatment in rat embolic stroke. *Neurochem. Res.* **2013**, *38*, 2668–2677. [CrossRef] [PubMed]

20. Culp, W.C.; Brown, A.T.; Lowery, J.D.; Arthur, M.C.; Roberson, P.K.; Skinner, R.D. Dodecafluoropentane emulsion extends window for tPA therapy in a rabbit stroke model. *Mol. Neurobiol.* **2015**, *52*, 979–984. [CrossRef] [PubMed]

21. Ishiguro, M.; Kawasaki, K.; Suzuki, Y.; Ishizuka, F.; Mishiro, K.; Egashira, Y.; Ikegaki, I.; Tsuruma, K.; Shimazawa, M.; Yoshimura, S.; et al. A Rho kinase (ROCK) inhibitor, fasudil, prevents matrix metalloproteinase-9-related hemorrhagic transformation in mice treated with tissue plasminogen activator. *Neuroscience* **2012**, *220*, 302–312. [CrossRef] [PubMed]

22. Dela Peña, I.C.; Yoo, A.; Tajiri, N.; Acosta, S.A.; Ji, X.; Kaneko, Y.; Borlongan, C.V. Granulocyte colony-stimulating factor attenuates delayed tPA-induced hemorrhagic transformation in ischemic stroke rats by enhancing angiogenesis and vasculogenesis. *J. Cereb. Blood Flow Metab.* **2015**, *35*, 338–346. [CrossRef] [PubMed]

23. Mishiro, K.; Ishiguro, M.; Suzuki, Y.; Tsuruma, K.; Shimazawa, M.; Hara, H. A broad-spectrum matrix metalloproteinase inhibitor prevents hemorrhagic complications induced by tissue plasminogen activator in mice. *Neuroscience* **2012**, *205*, 39–48. [CrossRef] [PubMed]

24. Su, E.J.; Fredriksson, L.; Geyer, M.; Folestad, E.; Cale, J.; Andrae, J.; Gao, Y.; Pietras, K.; Mann, K.; Yepes, M.; et al. Activation of PDGF-CC by tissue plasminogen activator impairs blood-brain barrier integrity during ischemic stroke. *Nat. Med.* **2008**, *14*, 731–737. [CrossRef] [PubMed]

25. Zuo, W.; Chen, J.; Zhang, S.; Tang, J.; Liu, H.; Zhang, D.; Chen, N. IMM-H004 prevents toxicity induced by delayed treatment of tPA in a rat model of focal cerebral ischemia involving PKA-and PI3K-dependent Akt activation. *Eur. J. Neurosci.* **2014**, *39*, 2107–2118. [CrossRef] [PubMed]

26. Murata, Y.; Rosell, A.; Scannevin, R.H.; Rhodes, K.J.; Wang, X.; Lo, E.H. Extension of the thrombolytic time window with minocycline in experimental stroke. *Stroke* **2008**, *39*, 3372–3377. [CrossRef] [PubMed]

27. Eckert, A.D.; Hamblin, M.; Lee, J.P. Neural Stem Cells Reduce Symptomatic Inflammation and Mortality in Aged Stroke Mice following Delayed tPA Treatment. *FASEB J.* **2017**, *31*, 693–696.

28. Liang, J.; Qi, Z.; Liu, W.; Wang, P.; Shi, W.; Dong, W.; Ji, X.; Luo, Y.; Liu, K.J. Normobaric hyperoxia slows blood-brain barrier damage and expands the therapeutic time window for tissue-type plasminogen activator treatment in cerebral ischemia. *Stroke* **2015**, *46*, 1344–1351. [CrossRef] [PubMed]

29. Ballabh, P.; Braun, A.; Nedergaard, M. The blood-brain barrier: An overview: Structure, regulation, and clinical implications. *Neurobiol. Dis.* **2004**, *16*, 1–13. [CrossRef] [PubMed]

30. Ishiguro, M.; Mishiro, K.; Fujiwara, Y.; Chen, H.; Izuta, H.; Tsuruma, K.; Shimazawa, M.; Yoshimura, S.; Satoh, M.; Iwama, T.; et al. Phosphodiesterase-III inhibitor prevents hemorrhagic transformation induced by focal cerebral ischemia in mice treated with tPA. *PLoS ONE* **2010**, *5*. [CrossRef] [PubMed]

31. Keep, R.F.; Zhou, N.; Xiang, J.; Andjelkovic, A.V.; Hua, Y.; Xi, G. Vascular disruption and blood-brain barrier dysfunction in intracerebral hemorrhage. *Fluids Barriers CNS* **2014**, *11*, 18. [CrossRef] [PubMed]

32. Thiyagarajan, M.; Fernández, J.A.; Lane, S.M.; Griffin, J.H.; Zlokovic, B.V. Activated protein C promotes neovascularization and neurogenesis in post-ischemic brain via protease activated receptor 1. *J. Neurosci.* **2008**, *28*, 12788–12797. [CrossRef] [PubMed]

33. Ullegaddi, R.; Powers, H.J.; Gariballa, S.E. Antioxidant supplementa-tion with or without B-group vitamins after acute ischemic stroke: A randomized controlled trial. *JPEN J. Parenter Enter. Nutr.* **2006**, *30*, 108–114. [CrossRef] [PubMed]

34. Tan, Z.; Turner, R.C.; Leon, R.L.; Li, X.; Hongpaisan, J.; Zheng, W.; Logsdon, A.F.; Naser, Z.J.; Alkon, D.L.; Rosen, C.L.; et al. Bryostatin improves survival and reduces ischemic brain injury in aged rats after acute ischemic stroke. *Stroke* **2013**, *44*, 3490–3497. [CrossRef] [PubMed]

35. Suzuki, Y.; Nagai, N.; Umemura, K.; Collen, D.; Lijnen, H.R. Stromelysin-1 (MMP-3) is critical for intracranial bleeding after t-PA treatment of stroke in mice. *J. Thromb. Haemost.* **2007**, *5*, 1732–1739. [CrossRef] [PubMed]

36. Huang, Z.; Huang, P.L.; Ma, J.; Meng, W.; Ayata, C.; Fishman, M.C.; Moskowitz, M.A. Enlarged infarcts in endothelial nitric oxide synthase knockout mice are attenuated by nitro-L-arginine. *J. Cereb. Blood Flow Metab.* **1996**, *16*, 981–987. [CrossRef] [PubMed]

37. Matsumoto, M. Cilostazol in secondary prevention of stroke: Impact of the cilostazol stroke prevention study. *Atheroscler. Suppl.* **2005**, *6*, 33–40. [CrossRef] [PubMed]

38. Koto, T.; Takubo, K.; Ishida, S.; Shinoda, H.; Inoue, M.; Tsubota, K.; Okada, Y.; Ikeda, E. Hypoxia disrupts the barrier function of neural blood vessels through changes in the expression of claudin-5 in endothelial cells. *Am. J. Pathol.* **2007**, *170*, 1389–1397. [CrossRef] [PubMed]

39. Shibuya, M.; Suzuki, Y.; Sugita, K.; Saito, I.; Sasaki, T.; Takakura, K.; Nagata, I.; Kikuchi, H.; Takemae, T.; Hidaka, H.; et al. Effect of AT877 on cerebral vasospasm after aneurismal subarachnoid hemorrhage. Results of a prospective placebo-controlled double-blind trial. *J. Neurosurg.* **1992**, *76*, 571–577. [CrossRef] [PubMed]

40. Hartung, T. Anti-inflammatory effects of granulocyte colony-stimulating factor. *Curr. Opin. Hematol.* **1998**, *5*, 221–225. [CrossRef] [PubMed]

41. Sobrino, T.; Millán, M.; Castellanos, M.; Blanco, M.; Brea, D.; Dorado, L.; Rodríguez-González, R.; Rodríguez-Yáñez, M.; Serena, J.; Leira, R.; et al. Association of growth factors with arterial recanalization and clinical outcome in patients with ischemic stroke treated with tPA. *J. Thromb. Haemost.* **2010**, *8*, 1567–1574. [CrossRef] [PubMed]

42. Hao, J.L.; Nagano, T.; Nakamura, M.; Kumagai, N.; Mishima, H.; Nishida, T. Galardin inhibits collagen degradation by rabbit keratocytes by inhibiting the activation of pro-matrix metalloproteinases. *Exp. Eye Res.* **1999**, *68*, 565–572. [CrossRef] [PubMed]

43. Mayne, M.; Ni, W.; Yan, H.J.; Xue, M.; Johnston, J.B.; Del Bigio, M.R.; Peeling, J.; Power, C. Antisense oligodeoxynucleotide inhibition of tumor necrosis factor-alpha expression is neuroprotective after intracerebral hemorrhage. *Stroke* **2001**, *32*, 240–248. [CrossRef] [PubMed]

44. Fylaktakidou, K.C.; Hadjipaclou-Litina, D.; Litinas, K.E.; Nicolaides, D.N. Natural and synthetic coumarin derivatives with anti-inflammatory/antioxidant activities. *Curr. Pharm. Des.* **2004**, *30*, 3813–3833. [CrossRef]

45. Machado, L.S.; Kozak, A.; Ergul, A.; Hess, D.; Borlongan, C.V.; Fagan, S.C. Delayed minocycline inhibits ischemia-activated matrix metalloproteinases 2 and 9 after experimental stroke. *BMC Neurosci.* **2006**, *7*, 56. [CrossRef] [PubMed]

46. Fagan, S.C.; Waller, J.L.; Nichols, F.T.; Edwards, D.J.; Pettigrew, L.C.; Clark, W.M.; Hall, C.E.; Switzer, J.A.; Ergul, A.; Hess, D.C. Minocycline to improve neurologic outcome in stroke (MINOS): A dose-finding study. *Stroke* **2010**, *41*, 2283–2287. [CrossRef] [PubMed]

47. Switzer, J.A.; Hess, D.C.; Ergul, A.; Waller, J.L.; Machado, L.S.; Portik-Dobos, V.; Pettigrew, L.C.; Clark, W.M.; Fagan, S.C. Matrix metalloproteinase-9 in an exploratory trial of intravenous minocycline for acute ischemic stroke. *Stroke* **2011**, *42*, 2633–2635. [CrossRef] [PubMed]

48. Blacker, D.J.; Prentice, D.; Alvaro, A.; Bates, T.R.; Bynevelt, M.; Kelly, A.; Kho, L.K.; Kohler, E.; Hankey, G.J.; Thompson, A.; et al. Reducing haemorrhagic transformation after thrombolysis for stroke: A strategy utilising minocycline. *Stroke Res. Treat.* **2013**, *2013*. [CrossRef] [PubMed]

49. Borlongan, C.V. Bone marrow stem cell mobilization in stroke: A 'bonehead' may be good after all! *Leukemia* **2011**, *25*, 1674–1686. [CrossRef] [PubMed]

50. Dela Peña, I.; Antoine, A.; Reyes, S.; Hernandez, D.; Acosta, S.; Pabon, M.; Tajiri, N.; Kaneko, Y.; Borlongan, C.V. Stem cell-based neuroprotective strategies in stroke. In *Neural Stem Cells in Health and Disease*; Shetty, A., Ed.; World Scientific: Singapore, 2015; pp. 371–408.

51. Bentley, P.; Ganesalingam, J.; Carlton Jones, A.L.; Mahady, K.; Epton, S.; Rinne, P.; Sharma, P.; Halse, O.; Mehta, A.; Rueckert, D. Prediction of stroke thrombolysis outcome using CT brain machine learning. *Neuroimage Clin.* **2014**, *4*, 635–640. [CrossRef] [PubMed]

52. Berkhemer, O.A.; Fransen, P.S.; Beumer, D.; van den Berg, L.A.; Lingsma, H.F.; Yoo, A.J.; Schonewille, W.J.; Vos, J.A.; Nederkoorn, P.J.; Wermer, M.J.; et al. A randomized trial of intraarterial treatment for acute ischemic stroke. *N. Engl. J. Med.* **2014**, *372*, 1009–1018. [CrossRef] [PubMed]

53. Minnerup, J.; Wersching, H.; Teuber, A.; Wellmann, J.; Eyding, J.; Weber, R.; Reimann, G.; Weber, W.; Krause, L.U.; Kurth, T.; et al. Outcome after thrombectomy and intravenous thrombolysis in patients with acute ischemic stroke: A prospective observational study. *Stroke* **2016**, *47*, 1584–1592. [CrossRef] [PubMed]

54. Huang, L.; Wong, S.; Snyder, E.Y.; Hamblin, M.H.; Lee, J.P. Human neural stem cells rapidly ameliorate symptomatic inflammation in early-stage ischemic-reperfusion cerebral injury. *Stem Cell Res. Ther.* **2014**, *5*. [CrossRef] [PubMed]

55. Anderson, J.D.; Pham, M.T.; Contreras, Z.; Hoon, M.; Fink, K.; Johansson, H.J.; Rossignol, J.; Dunbar, G.L.; Showalter, M.; Fiehn, O.; et al. Mesenchymal stem cell-based therapy for ischemic stroke. *Chin. Neurosurg. J.* **2016**, *2*. [CrossRef]

56. Nakazaki, M.; Sasaki, M.; Kataoka-Sasaki, Y.; Oka, S.; Namioka, T.; Namioka, A.; Onodera, R.; Suzuki, J.; Sasaki, Y.; Nagahama, H.; et al. Intravenous infusion of mesenchymal stem cells inhibits intracranial hemorrhage after recombinant tissue plasminogen activator therapy for transient middle cerebral artery occlusion in rats. *J. Neurosurg.* **2017**, *6*, 1–10. [CrossRef] [PubMed]

57. Bang, O.Y.; Lee, J.S.; Lee, P.H.; Lee, G. Autologous mesenchymal stem cell transplantation in stroke patients. *Ann. Neurol.* **2005**, *57*, 874–882. [CrossRef] [PubMed]

58. Liu, N.; Deguchi, K.; Yamashita, T.; Liu, W.; Ikeda, Y.; Abe, K. Intracerebral transplantation of bone marrow stromal cells ameliorates tissue plasminogen activator-induced brain damage after cerebral ischemia in mice detected by in vivo and ex vivo optical imaging. *J. Neurosci. Res.* **2012**, *90*, 2086–2093. [CrossRef] [PubMed]

59. Singhal, A.B. A review of oxygen therapy in ischemic stroke. *Neurol. Res.* **2007**, *29*, 173–183. [CrossRef] [PubMed]

60. Liu, W.; Sood, R.; Chen, Q.; Sakoglu, U.; Hendren, J.; Cetin, O.; Miyake, M.; Liu, K.J. Normobaric hyperoxia inhibits NADPH oxidase-mediated matrix metalloproteinase-9 induction in cerebral microvessels in experimental stroke. *J. Neurochem.* **2008**, *107*, 1196–1205. [CrossRef] [PubMed]

61. Chang, C.F.; Niu, K.C.; Hoffer, B.J.; Wang, Y.; Borlongan, C.V. Hyperbaric oxygen therapy for treatment of postischemic stroke in adult rats. *Exp. Neurol.* **2000**, *166*, 298–306. [CrossRef] [PubMed]

62. Hu, Q.; Manaenko, A.; Bian, H.; Guo, Z.; Huang, J.L.; Guo, Z.N.; Yang, P.; Tang, J.; Zhang, J.H. Hyperbaric Oxygen reduces infarction volume and hemorrhagic transformation through ATP/NAD+/Sirt1 pathway in hyperglycemic middle cerebral artery occlusion rats. *Stroke* **2017**, *48*, 1655–1664. [CrossRef] [PubMed]

63. Zhai, W.W.; Sun, L.; Yu, Z.Q.; Chen, G. Hyperbaric oxygen therapy in experimental and clinical stroke. *Med. Gas Res.* **2016**, *6*, 111–118. [PubMed]

64. Boussi-Gross, R.; Golan, H.; Volkov, O.; Bechor, Y.; Hoofien, D.; Beeri, M.S.; Ben-Jacob, E.; Efrati, S. Improvement of memory impairments in poststroke patients by hyperbaric oxygen therapy. *Neuropsychology* **2015**, *29*, 610–621. [CrossRef] [PubMed]

65. Ehrenreich, H.; Weissenborn, K.; Prange, H.; Schneider, D.; Weimar, C.; Wartenberg, K.; Schellinger, P.D.; Bohn, M.; Becker, H.; Wegrzyn, M.; et al. Recombinant human erythropoietin in the treatment of acute ischemic stroke. *Stroke* **2009**, *40*, e647–e656. [CrossRef] [PubMed]

66. Whiteley, W.N.; Emberson, J.; Lees, K.R.; Blackwell, L.; Albers, G.; Bluhmki, E.; Brott, T.; Cohen, G.; Davis, S.; Donnan, G.; et al. Risk of intracerebral haemorrhage with alteplase after acute ischaemic stroke: A secondary analysis of an individual patient data meta-analysis. *Lancet Neurol.* **2016**, *15*, 925–933. [CrossRef]

67. Albers, G.W.; Goldstein, L.B.; Hess, D.C.; Wechsler, L.R.; Furie, K.L.; Gorelick, P.B.; Hurn, P.; Liebeskind, D.S.; Nogueira, R.G.; Saver, J.L.; et al. Stroke Treatment Academic Industry Roundtable (STAIR) recommendations for maximizing the use of intravenous thrombolytics and expanding treatment options with intra-arterial and neuroprotective therapies. *Stroke* **2011**, *42*, 2645–2650. [CrossRef] [PubMed]

68. Lapchak, P.A.; Zhang, J.H.; Noble-Haeusslein, L.J. RIGOR guidelines: Escalating STAIR and STEPS for effective translational research. *Transl. Stroke Res.* **2013**, *4*, 279–285. [CrossRef] [PubMed]

69. Diamandis, T.; Borlongan, C.V. One, two, three steps toward cell therapy for stroke. *Stroke* **2015**, *46*, 588–591. [CrossRef] [PubMed]

70. Rubin, M.N.; Barrett, K.M. What to do with wake-up stroke. *Neurohospitalist* **2015**, *5*, 161–172. [CrossRef] [PubMed]

71. Parsons, M.; Spratt, N.; Bivard, A.; Campbell, B.; Chung, K.; Miteff, F.; O'Brien, B.; Bladin, C.; McElduff, P.; Allen, C.; et al. A randomized trial of tenecteplase versus alteplase for acute ischemic stroke. *N. Engl. J. Med.* **2012**, *366*, 1099–1107. [CrossRef] [PubMed]

72. Henninger, N.; Fisher, M. Extending the Time Window for Endovascular and Pharmacological Reperfusion. *Transl. Stroke Res.* **2016**, *7*, 284–293. [CrossRef] [PubMed]

5

Endovascular Treatment of Stroke Caused by Carotid Artery Dissection

Grzegorz Meder [1],*, Milena Świtońska [2,3], Piotr Płeszka [2], Violetta Palacz-Duda [2], Dorota Dzianott-Pabijan [4] and Paweł Sokal [3]

[1] Department of Interventional Radiology, Jan Biziel University Hospital No. 2, Ujejskiego 75 Street, 85-168 Bydgoszcz, Poland

[2] Stroke Intervention Centre, Department of Neurosurgery and Neurology, Jan Biziel University Hospital No. 2, Ujejskiego 75 Street, 85-168 Bydgoszcz, Poland; m.switonska@cm.umk.pl (M.Ś.); pio.ple@wp.pl (P.P.); violkapduda1@tlen.pl (V.P.-D.)

[3] Department of Neurosurgery and Neurology, Faculty of Health Sciences, Nicolaus Copernicus University in Toruń, Ludwik Rydygier Collegium Medicum, Ujejskiego 75 Street, 85-168 Bydgoszcz, Poland; pawel.sokal@cm.umk.pl

[4] Neurological Rehabilitation Ward Kuyavian-Pomeranian Pulmonology Centre, Meysnera 9 Street, 85-472 Bydgoszcz, Poland; dorota.dzianott-pabijan@wp.pl

* Correspondence: grzegorz.meder@gmail.com;

Abstract: Ischemic stroke due to large vessel occlusion (LVO) is a devastating condition. Most LVOs are embolic in nature. Arterial dissection is responsible for only a small proportion of LVOs, is specific in nature and poses some challenges in treatment. We describe 3 cases where patients with stroke caused by carotid artery dissection were treated with mechanical thrombectomy and extensive stenting with good outcome. We believe that mechanical thrombectomy and stenting is a treatment of choice in these cases.

Keywords: stroke; artery dissection; endovascular treatment; stenting; mechanical thrombectomy

---

1. Introduction

Ischemic stroke due to large vessel occlusion (LVO) is a devastating condition, bearing great risk of severe disability and death [1]. Most LVOs are embolic in nature. Although only a small proportion of all LVOs arise from an arterial dissection, it accounts for approximately 20% of strokes among individuals under the age of 45 [2,3]. While some dissections can be caused by traumatic arterial injury, in most cases, dissection is considered to be idiopathic. There are some conditions that can predispose to dissection such as atherosclerosis, hypertension, Marfan syndrome, and fibromuscular dysplasia [4]. Managing stroke caused by carotid dissection can be challenging. In this report, we present a series of three cases of patients with stroke due to acute extracranial carotid artery dissection that were admitted to our stroke centre and treated with mechanical thrombectomy and extensive stenting with good outcome. We believe that mechanical thrombectomy and stenting can be a treatment of choice in these cases.

2. Case Presentation

The first patient was a 34-year old woman, with no previous drug and medical history, involved, as a passenger, in a car accident a few hours before stroke symptoms appeared. After the accident, she was an Emergency Room (ER) patient in a local hospital undergoing observation and a series of tests: trauma computed tomography (CT) scan, X-ray scans etc., which only revealed fracture of the sternum, face, and scalp bruises. After a few hours, being in a well and stable condition, she suddenly deteriorated and presented with dense left-sided weakness. She was immediately transferred to the CT suite and non-contrast CT scan of the head was performed followed by CT angiography of the neck and head. The CT scan of the head, apart the aforementioned face and scalp bruises, was normal, while the CT angiography revealed right middle cerebral artery (MCA) and Internal Cerebral Artery (ICA) occlusion with probable carotid dissection as an underlying cause. The patient was transferred to our stroke centre for endovascular treatment. During diagnostic arteriography, we confirmed dissection and thrombosis of the right carotid artery in segments C1–C2 (Figure 1A).

The first treatment goal was to remove the thrombus and open the artery. We used, a 8F short introducer sheath in the groin and then placed a long neuro sheath (6F NeuronMax, Penumbra Inc., Alameda, CA, USA) in the common carotid artery. Through the long sheath, an aspirating system (ACE68, Penumbra Inc.) was introduced into the ICA and the large thrombus was removed by aspiration only. The extent of the dissection and ICA-T occlusion were visualized (Figure 1B). With the microcatheter (Rebar 18, Medtronic, Dublin, Ireland) and J-shaped microguidewire (Hybrid 1214, Balt Extrusion, Montmorency, France), the true lumen of the dissected artery was found and catheterized to the point above the visible dissection (C3). In the next step, the ACE68 catheter was gently pushed over the Rebar microcatheter to the ICA terminus and then over the microguidewire, we pushed the Rebar microcatheter into the M2 segment of the MCA. In the next step, we used a stent-retriever (Catch V20, Balt Extrusion) and with continuous aspiration from the ACE68, we removed the clot from MCA-ICA, leaving the aspiration catheter in place. The last steps of the procedure consisted of placing three intracranial self-expanding braided stents (Leo+, Balt Extrusion) in a telescopic manner starting from the C3 ICA segment and moving caudally to the C1 segment and at the end, a braided carotid stent (Roadsaver, Terumo, Tokyo, Japan) was placed to reach the CCA (Figure 2). After placing the stents, we performed an internal massage maneuver with the microcatheter and then balloon angioplasty of the stents using a 5 mm compliant intracranial balloon (Copernic, Balt Extrusion) in the ICA C1-C3 segments, a 5 mm PTA balloon (Submarine, Medtronic) in ICA C1 and a Roadsaver stent to obtain optimal stents apposition. During the procedure, the patient was given 5000 units of heparin through intravenous (IV) administration and a weight-based bolus of eptifibatide. After the procedure, the patient remained in the angio-suite for 30 min, during which time we performed three check-runs for early stent thrombosis. The patient was then transferred to the neurologic intensive care unit for 1 day with continuous eptifibatide IV; 4 h before it was completed, she was started on oral dual antiplatelet therapy: ticagrelor 90 mg twice a day and acetylsalicylic acid (ASA) 75 mg once a day. She was in our hospital for 25 days, undergoing early neuro-rehabilitation with good clinical improvement: NIHSS 15→8 (National Institute of Health Stroke Scale). During the stay, we observed transient 1-day haematuria, which resolved without treatment. After 25 days, the patient was in stable condition modified Rankin Scale (mRS): 4/3 and transferred to the rehabilitation unit. After 3 months, she was independent, walking and had minor left-hand weakness (mRS 1). Control CT angiography showed patent stents in the right ICA and patent intracranial arteries.

The second patient was a 62-year old male, with a medical history of smoking and arterial hypertension—treated with lercanidypine and telmisartan. He was driving a truck when neurological symptoms associated with the right brain hemisphere (dense left-sided weakness) occurred, leading to a minor car accident. The patient was transferred to our hospital by a paramedic team. A CT scan performed at ER revealed occlusion of the right ICA and hyperdense right MCA. During diagnostic angiography, we confirmed right ICA occlusion, starting from the C1 segment. Using the same technique as described for the previous patient, we aspirated a large clot from the ICA, which allowed us to find a long ICA dissection (Figure 3).

After removing the clot from the ICA, we performed mechanical thrombectomy of the MCA and implanted four overlapping stents covering the dissected ICA segments (Figure 4). In this case, we also used braided intracranial stents (Leo+) and the last stent covering the CCA-ICA junction was a typical carotid laser-cut stent (Protégé, Medtronic). During the procedure, the patient was given IV of a weight-based bolus of eptifibatide and 5000 units of heparin, but we observed early clot formation at the top of the first implanted stent (C3) during the first control run. The clot was removed with an aspiration catheter (ACE68, Penumbra). After a 30-min observation with control angiographies every 10 min, the patient, without sequelae of the clot formation, was transferred to the neurology department where he underwent early rehabilitation, improving quickly (NIHSS 17→5). After 7 days, he was released to go home with no significant disability (mRS 1). Control CT angiography showed patent stents in the right ICA and patent intracranial arteries.

The third patient was a 56-year old male, with no previous medical and drug history, who suffered from a spontaneous left ICA C1 dissection with total ICA occlusion, pseudoaneurysm, and left MCA occlusion resulting in large left hemisphere syndrome, NIHSS 18 at admission. Using the technique described above, we removed the clot from the ICA and then from the MCA and stented the dissected ICA segment using 2 braided intracranial stents (Leo+, BALT) with good result (Figure 5). After 3 months of rehabilitation, the patient was discharged in stable condition, walking with minor aphasia and mild right arm weakness (mRS 2). We were unable to reach this patient for follow-up control CT angiography as he was a citizen of a foreign country and returned home after treatment.

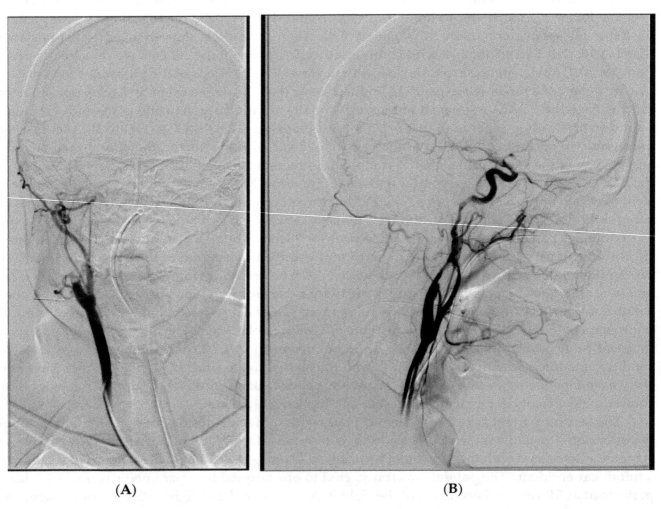

(A)   (B)

Figure 1. (A) Thrombosis and dissection of the right ICA, AP view. (B) Extent of the dissection, lateral view.

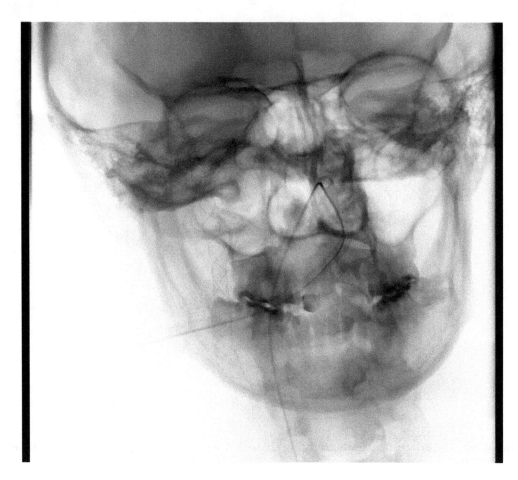

Figure 2. Stented right ICA (non DSA image).

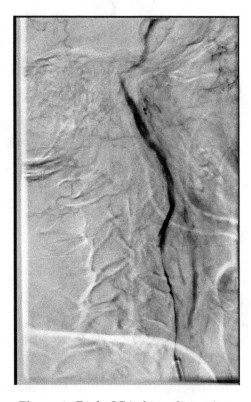

Figure 3. Right ICA, long dissection.

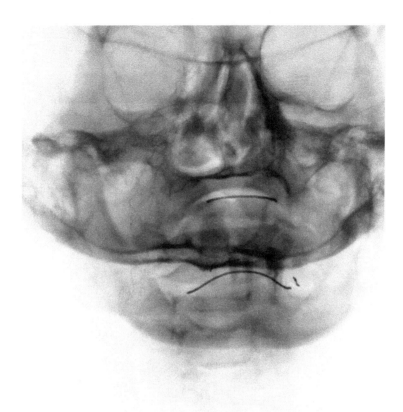

Figure 4. Four overlapping stents covering dissected ICA segments (non-subtracted image).

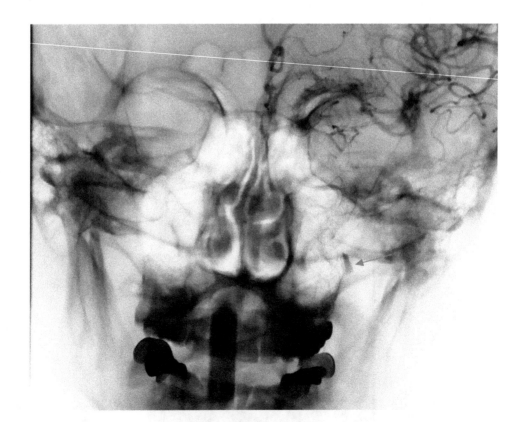

Figure 5. Stented left ICA with 2 overlapping stents covering the dissection and pseudoaneurysm with contrast medium stagnation (arrow) in late phase.

3. Discussion

Arterial dissection is characterized by the penetration of blood into the arterial wall through a tear, which develops in one or more layers of the wall. If the tear is shallow, only the intima may be dissected, which can lead to the presence of an intimal flap with or without formation of the thrombus inside the true and false vessel lumen. Deeper tears of the arterial wall may lead to a sub-adventitial dissecting aneurysm or even transection of the arterial wall and lethal bleeding [4,5].

Most dissections occur spontaneously. The second most common causative factor is head or neck trauma, especially in car accident victims. Reported trauma can sometimes be very minor or even anecdotal like sudden head turns, playing golf, jumping or chiropractic maneuvers [4,5].

Severity of the disease, anatomical features, and potential complications are well characterized by the classification proposed by Colorado University [6,7] (Table 1). Apart from lethal bleeding due to artery transection, the second most serious and common complication of artery dissection are ischemic in nature. Although artery dissection is a rather uncommon cause of stroke in the general population, it accounts for 20% of strokes in patients under the age of 45. Those strokes are caused by thrombus formation and either occlusion or narrowing of the vessel lumen. Clots originating from the dissected artery segments may also migrate distally to cerebral arteries causing secondary occlusions.

The diagnosis of dissection is based on radiologic findings in ultrasound, CT, computed tomography angiography (CTA), magnetic resonance imaging (MRI), and magnetic resonance angiography (MRA); however, digital subtraction arteriography (DSA) is still considered to be the gold standard [5]. Typical radiologic findings include: narrowed and irregular vessel lumen, tapered ICA occlusion with the carotid bulb spared, double lumen appearance, pseudonaneurysm, intimal flap, or eccentric thickening of the arterial wall. In our experience, recognizing dissection as the cause of stroke is quite easy in young patients with trauma but may be challenging in older patients with unknown medical history and total artery occlusion as the radiologic features of the artery dissection may sometimes mimic tandem occlusions or massive emboli.

Table 1. Denver dissection grading system in blunt cerebrovascular injury and associated stroke rates.

Grade	Type of Dissection	Stroke in Carotid Artery Dissection (%)	Stroke in Vertebral Artery Dissection (%)
I	Luminal irregularity or dissection with < 25% luminal narrowing	3	19
II	Intimal flap or intramural hematoma with luminal narrowing ≥ 25% or intraluminal thrombus	11	40
III	Pseudoaneurysm	33	13
IV	Total occlusion	44	33
V	Transection and free bleeding	100	N/A

There is no clear consensus regarding management of dissections. Grade V is considered to be lethal. It is widely accepted that low grade [1] dissections with no bleeding and minor or transient ischemic symptoms can be treated with 3–6 months of antithrombotic therapy with anticoagulant or antiplatelet agents [8–10]. To our understanding, as the pharmacologic treatment of higher-grade dissections carries a very low success rate, the approach in these cases should be more aggressive i.e., surgical or endovascular [11,12]. In the case of stroke symptoms with intraluminal thrombus formation such as total artery occlusion or distal emboli, the only viable option seems to be prompt endovascular treatment.

The nature of the condition must indicate the type of endovascular treatment. The first goal is the same as in typical embolic stroke—to remove the clot within the time window advised for mechanical thrombectomy [13]. After this, further (especially intracranial) progression of the dissection should be prevented, and the artery should be kept patent.

There are two main methods of retrieving a thrombus from an artery: aspiration or using stent retrievers [14]. In our opinion, it is advisable to not introduce metal devices such as stent retrievers into the dissected artery segment in order to prevent vessel walls from incurring further damage. Moreover, if the artery is completely occluded, there is no clear answer as to whether the thrombus is inside the true or false lumen. In these cases, we always use aspiration first, which seems to be less traumatic and suction power can be adjusted. While it may be debatable in the cases described here whether the thrombus was aspirated from the true or false lumen, it is important to remove it in its entirety, or as much of it as possible. Suction applied to the false vessel lumen may even be beneficial, leading to its collapse and opening of the true lumen. Revealing the true vessel lumen is of great importance as it allows for the visualization of the extent of the dissection and potential distal emboli.

In two of the described cases, patients had thrombi in the intracranial arteries. Removing such clots requires placing catheters in the true vessel lumen. Catheterization may sometimes be difficult and has to be done gently to avoid progression of the dissection. We strongly suggest using a microcatheter with a J-shaped microguidewire placed in a large lumen aspiration catheter and confirm its advance and placement by injecting contrast into the microcatheter. Passing the intracranial thrombus with the microguidewire and microcatheter allows you to use a combination of a stent retriever and aspiration, which seems to be the most efficient method [15,16]. During clot removal, we leave the aspiration catheter in place to reduce the number of passes through the dissected segment of the artery. After removing the clot from intracranial arteries, you can progress to the next step, which involves placing stents to keep the artery patent.

Final confirmation of proper microcatheter placement is mandatory before stent placement. The technique used in the cases described here consists of placing intracranial braided stents in a telescopic manner starting from the top of the dissected segment and moving caudally to cover the whole damaged portion of the artery. If there is a need for microcatheter exchange, it should be done carefully with the long microguidewire left in place first in order to prevent losing the access route. We found that the intracranial braided stents made by Balt suited our needs best due to the largest diameter available being up to 5.5 mm, and longest length being up to 75 mm; this helps to reduce the number of necessary maneuvers and stents implanted. The radial force of the stent seems to be sufficient to push the damaged intima back against the vessel wall, especially when the false vessel lumen is collapsed after aspiration. In the case of dissections starting from the internal carotid origin, the last stent we used was a carotid stent, either braided or laser cut. In the final step, we performed balloon angioplasty to achieve the best possible stent apposition. Angioplasty is performed also from the top to the bottom using intracranial remodeling balloons at first, and then high-pressure balloons in the carotid or intracranial stents placed in the C1 segment if needed.

Placing stents in the acute phase requires a prompt introduction of antiplatelet therapy to avoid early in-stent thrombosis. In the cases described here, we administered 5000 IU of heparin before the first stent was placed, and patient weight-calculated (180 mcg/kg) bolus of GP IIb/IIIa inhibitor-eptifibatide. We prefer unfractionated heparin to the low molecular weight heparin (LMWH) such as enoxaparin, since in the case of intraprocedural bleeding, the effect of unfractionated heparin can be reversed by administration of protamine sulphate. After the procedure, GP IIb/IIIa inhibitors were infused continuously (2 mcg/kg/min) for 24 h. In emergency cases of stenting such as those described in this paper, we use GP IIb/IIIa inhibitors as the first line of antiplatelet treatment—as intravenous administration of these drugs, provide almost instant platelet inhibition. Of the GP IIb/IIIa inhibitors we mostly choose eptifibatide since its effect is reversible and platelet function returns towards baseline within 4 h after stopping a continuous infusion.

Oral antiplatelets (300 mg of ASA and 180 mg of ticagrelor) were introduced 4 h before the end of the GP IIb/IIIa inhibitors' infusions. Oral dual antiplatelet therapy was continued for the next 3 months: 75 mg of ASA once a day with 90 mg ticagrelor twice a day, and after that 75 mg of ASA once a day for one year was prescribed. We have chosen a combination of ASA and ticagrelor because of their efficacy and safety profile [17]. Introducing anticoagulants and antiplatelets in patients with stroke and emergency stenting has been widely discussed, and although there are currently no clear guidelines regarding their use, recent papers show the safety of this approach [18–22].

Large extent of the brain ischemia prior to endovascular treatment (EVT) is a known predictor for both intracranial hemorrhage (ICH) and later poor clinical outcome in patients with stroke [23–25]. In our institution, we use widely accepted 10-point Alberta Stroke Program Early CT score (ASPECTS) to assess the ischemic changes on a non-contrast head CT before treatment and avoid mechanical thrombectomy (MT), in patients with ASPECTS < 6 and MT combined with stenting in patients with ASPECTS < 7 [25]. The first two described patients were treated early (less than 3 h) in the time window for mechanical thrombectomy and had high (9–10) ASPECTS before the treatment. In control CT, which is made in every patient 24 h after EVT, they developed only moderate ischemic changes in the affected MCA territories, measuring 4 cm in diameter for the first patient and 3 cm for the second one. The third patient was treated in the 5th hour from the symptoms' onset, with initial ASPECTS 7. In control CT, he developed large left MCA territory edema with slight 5 mm midline shift, both of which decreased significantly after 7 days of symptomatic treatment with mannitol and diuretics. In all cases, we achieved complete reperfusion during EVT and none of the patients developed ICH after EVT despite the introduction of antiplatelet drugs. Still, it is worth noting that caution should be taken when administering these medications to patients treated towards the end of the time window for MT, with low initial ASPECTS, incomplete reperfusion and especially in the case of trauma patients as it may trigger potential bleeding [23,26,27]. For each individual case, the expected benefits should outweigh the risk. We only noticed one event of bleeding, which occurred 3 days post-treatment as an episode of mild haematuria in the first patient and it resolved with no intervention and without sequelae. This patient had a full body trauma CT scan performed after the accident, which had been evaluated by two experienced radiologists and any active internal bleeding had been excluded. She also had another CT scan of the abdomen and pelvis after the episode of bleeding, showing the same result.

4. Conclusions and Future Directions

Mechanical thrombectomy and extensive artery stenting can be beneficial in patients with acute, high grade extracranial carotid artery dissections with artery occlusions and distal embolic complications. Medical consensus is lacking regarding ideal therapeutic strategy in those cases. Results of randomized-controlled trials like ongoing TITAN (Thrombectomy In TANdem lesion) (NCT03978988) will probably help to determine potential benefits and risk associated with acute stent placement and periprocedural antiplatelet therapy. Additionally, recent advances in vascular biology such as using microvessel-on-chip can potentially help to study in vitro the best practice regarding the use anti-coagulants and determine their optimal dose using humanized models [28,29].

Author Contributions: Conceptualization, original draft preparation: G.M. Review and editing: G.M., M.Ś., P.P., V.P.-D. and D.D.-P. Supervision, funding acquisition: G.M., P.S. All authors have read and agreed to the published version of the manuscript.

Abbreviations

CT	Computed tomography
DSA	Digital subtraction arteriography
ER	Emergency Room
GCS	Glasgow Coma Scale
mRS	modified Rankin Scale
ICA	Internal carotid artery
ICU	Intensive Care Unit
MCA	Middle cerebral artery
MRA	Magnetic resonance angiography
MRI	Magnetic resonance imaging
NIHSS	National Institute of Health Stroke Scale
ICA segments	Bouthillier classification (C1–C7)
LVO:	Large vessel occlusion
ASA	acetylsalicylic acid
MT	mechanical thrombectomy
EVT	endovascular treatment
LMWH	low molecular weight heparin
ICH	intracranial hemorrhage
ASPECTS	Alberta Stroke Program Early CT score

References

1. Rennert, R.C.; Wali, A.R.; Steinberg, J.A.; Santiago-Dieppa, D.R.; Olson, S.E.; Pannell, J.S.; Khalessi, A.A. Epidemiology, Natural History, and Clinical Presentation of Large Vessel Ischemic Stroke. *Neurosurgery* **2019**, *85* (Suppl. 1), S4–S8. [CrossRef]

2. Nagumo, K.; Nakamori, A.; Kojima, S. Spontaneous intracranial internal carotidartery dissection: 6 case reports and a review of 39 cases in the literature. *Rinsho Shinkeigaku* **2003**, *43*, 313–321.

3. Chandra, A.; Suliman, A.; Angle, N. Spontaneous dissection of the carotid andvertebral arteries: The 10-year UCSD experience. *Ann. Vasc. Surg.* **2007**, *21*, 178–185. [CrossRef]

4. Fusca, M.R.; Harrigan, M.R. Cerebrovascular dissections—A review part I: Spontaneous dissections. *Neurosurgery* **2011**, *68*, 242–257. [CrossRef] [PubMed]

5. Mehdi, E.; Aralasmak, A.; Toprak, H.; Yıldız, S.; Kurtcan, S.; Kolukisa, M.; Asıl, T.; Alkan, A. Craniocervical Dissections: Radiologic Findings, Pitfalls, Mimicking Diseases: A Pictorial Review. *Curr. Med. Imaging Rev.* **2018**, *14*, 207–222. [CrossRef] [PubMed]

6. Biffl, W.L.; Moore, E.E.; Offner, P.J.; Brega, K.E.; Franciose, R.J.; Burch, J.M. Blunt Carotid Arterial Injuries: Implications of a New Grading Scale. *J. Trauma Inj. Infect. Crit. Care* **1999**, *47*, 845–853. [CrossRef] [PubMed]

7. Biffl, W.L.; Moore, E.E.; Offner, P.J.; Burch, J.M. Blunt Carotid and Vertebral Arterial Injuries. *World J. Surg.* **2001**, *25*, 1036–1043. [CrossRef]

8. Stence, N.V.; Fenton, L.Z.; Goldenberg, N.A.; Armstrong-Wells, J.; Bernard, T.J. Craniocervical arterial dissectionin children: Diagnosis and treatment. *Curr. Treat. Options Neurol.* **2011**, *13*, 636–648. [CrossRef]

9. Brott, T.G.; Halperin, J.L.; Abbara, S.; Bacharach, J.M.; Barr, J.D.; Bush, R.L.; Cates, C.U.; Creager, M.A.; Fowler, S.B.; Friday, G.; et al. 2011 ASA/ACCF/AHA/AANN/AANS/ACR/ASNR/CNS/SAIP/SCAI/SIR/SNIS/SVM/SVS guideline on the management of patients with extracranial carotid and vertebral artery disease. *Stroke* **2011**, *42*, e420–e463.

10. Lyrer, P.; Engelter, S.T. Antithrombotic drugs for carotid artery dissection. *Cochrane Database Syst. Rev.* **2010**, *10*, CD000255. [CrossRef]

11. Lavallée, P.C.; Mazighi, M.; Saint-Maurice, J.-P.; Meseguer, E.; Abboud, H.; Klein, I.F.; Houdart, E.; Amarenco, P. Stent-Assisted Endovascular Thrombolysis Versus Intravenous Thrombolysis in Internal Carotid Artery Dissection with Tandem Internal Carotid and Middle Cerebral Artery Occlusion. *Stroke* **2007**, *38*, 2270–2274. [CrossRef]

12. Mourand, I.; Brunel, H.; Vendrell, J.-F.; Thouvenot, E.; Bonafé, A. Endovascular stent-assisted thrombolysis in acute occlusive carotid artery dissection. *Neuroradiology* **2010**, *52*, 135–140. [CrossRef] [PubMed]

13. Wahlgren, N.; Moreira, T.; Michel, P.; Steiner, T.; Jansen, O.; Cognard, C.; Mattle, H.P.; van Zwam, W.; Holmin, S.; Tatlisumak, T.; et al. Mechanical thrombectomy in acute ischemic stroke: Consensus statement by ESO-Karolinska Stroke Update 2014/2015, supported by ESO, ESMINT, ESNR and EAN. *Int. J. Stroke* **2016**, *11*, 134–147. [CrossRef]

14. Procházka, V.; Jonszta, T.; Czerny, D.; Krajca, J.; Roubec, M.; Hurtikova, E.; Urbanec, R.; Streitová, D.; Pavliska, L.; Vrtkova, A. Comparison of Mechanical Thrombectomy with Contact Aspiration, Stent Retriever, and Combined Procedures in Patients with Large-Vessel Occlusion in Acute Ischemic Stroke. *Med. Sci. Monit.* **2018**, *24*, 9342–9353. [CrossRef] [PubMed]

15. Lee, J.S.; Hong, J.M.; Lee, S.J.; Joo, I.S.; Lim, Y.C.; Kim, S.Y. The combined use of mechanical thrombectomy devices is feasible for treating acute carotid terminus occlusion. *Acta Neurochir.* **2013**, *155*, 635–641. [CrossRef]

16. Humphries, W.; Hoit, D.; Doss, V.T.; Elijovich, L.; Frei, D.; Loy, D.; Dooley, G.; Turk, A.S.; Chaudry, I.; Turner, R.; et al. Distal aspiration with retrievable stent assisted thrombectomy for the treatment of acute ischemic stroke. *J. NeuroInterventional Surg.* **2015**, *7*, 90–94. [CrossRef]

17. Wang, Y.; Chen, W.; Lin, Y.; Meng, X.; Chen, G.; Wang, Z.; Wu, J.; Wang, D.; Li, J.; Cao, Y.; et al. Ticagrelor plus aspirin versus clopidogrel plus aspirin for platelet reactivity in patients with minor stroke or transient ischaemic attack: Open label, blinded endpoint, randomised controlled phase II trial. *BMJ* **2019**, *365*, l2211. [CrossRef]

18. Stampfl, S.; Ringleb, P.A.; Mohlenbruch, M.; Hametner, C.; Herweh, C.; Pham, M.; Bosel, J.; Haehnel, S.; Bendszus, M.; Rohde, S. Emergency Cervical Internal Carotid Artery Stenting in Combination with Intracranial Thrombectomy in Acute Stroke. *Am. J. Neuroradiol.* **2014**, *35*, 741–746. [CrossRef] [PubMed]

19. Matsubara, N.; Miyachi, S.; Tsukamoto, N.; Kojima, T.; Izumi, T.; Haraguchi, K.; Asai, T.; Yamanouchi, T.; Ota, K.; Wakabayashi, T. Endovascular intervention for acute cervical carotid artery occlusion. *Acta Neurochir.* **2013**, *155*, 1115–1123. [CrossRef]

20. Papanagiotou, P.; Roth, C.; Walter, S.; Behnke, S.; Grunwald, I.Q.; Viera, J.; Politi, M.; Körner, H.; Kostopoulos, P.; Haass, A.; et al. Carotid Artery Stenting in Acute Stroke. *J. Am. Coll. Cardiol.* **2011**, *58*, 2363–2369. [CrossRef]

21. Jadhav, A.P.; Zaidat, O.; Liebeskind, D.S.; Yavagal, D.R.; Haussen, D.; Hellinger, F.R.; Jahan, R.; Jumaa, M.A.; Szeder, V.; Nogueira, R.G.; et al. Emergent Management of Tandem Lesions in Acute Ischemic Stroke. *Stroke* **2019**, *50*, 428–433. [CrossRef]

22. Zhu, F.; Anadani, M.; Labreuche, J.; Spiotta, A.; Turjman, F.; Piotin, M.; Steglich-Arnholm, H.; Holtmannspötter, M.; Taschner, C.; Eiden, S.; et al. Impact of Antiplatelet Therapy During Endovascular Therapy for Tandem Occlusions. *Stroke* **2020**, *51*, 1522–1529. [CrossRef]

23. Nawabi, J.; Kniep, H.; Schön, G.; Flottmann, F.; Leischner, H.; Kabiri, R.; Sporns, P.; Kemmling, A.; Thomalla, G.; Fiehler, J.; et al. Hemorrhage After Endovascular Recanalization in Acute Stroke: Lesion Extent, Collaterals and Degree of Ischemic Water Uptake Mediate Tissue Vulnerability. *Front. Neurol.* **2019**, *10*, 569. [CrossRef] [PubMed]

24. Dostovic, Z.; Dostovic, E.; Smajlovic, D.; Avdic, L.; Ibrahimagic, O.C. Brain Edema After Ischaemic Stroke. *Med. Arch.* **2016**, *70*, 339–341. [CrossRef] [PubMed]

25. Barber, P.A.; Demchuk, A.M.; Zhang, J.; Buchan, A.M. Validity and reliability of a quantitative computed tomography score in predicting outcome of hyperacute stroke before thrombolytic therapy. *Lancet* **2000**, *355*, 1670–1674, Erratum in **2000**, *355*, 2170. [CrossRef]

26. Ferraris, V.A.; Bernard, A.C.; Hyde, B.; Kearney, P.A. The impact of antiplatelet drugs on trauma outcomes. *J. Trauma Acute Care Surg.* **2012**, *73*, 492–497. [CrossRef]

27. Hao, Y.; Zhang, Z.; Zhang, H.; Xu, L.; Ye, Z.; Dai, Q.; Liu, X.; Xu, G. Risk of Intracranial Hemorrhage after Endovascular Treatment for Acute Ischemic Stroke: Systematic Review and Meta-Analysis. *Interv. Neurol.* **2017**, *6*, 57–64. [CrossRef]

28. Salman, M.M.; Marsh, G.; Kusters, I.; Delincé, M.; Di Caprio, G.; Upadhyayula, S.; De Nola, G.; Hunt, R.; Ohashi, K.G.; Gray, T.; et al. Design and Validation of a Human Brain Endothelial Microvessel-on-a-Chip Open Microfluidic Model Enabling Advanced Optical Imaging. *Front. Bioeng. Biotechnol.* **2020**, *8*, 1077. [CrossRef]

29. Zheng, Y.; Chen, J.; Craven, M.; Choi, N.W.; Totorica, S.; Diaz-Santana, A.; Kermani, P.; Hempstead, B.; Fischbach-Teschl, C.; López, J.A.; et al. In vitro microvessels for the study of angiogenesis and thrombosis. *Proc. Natl. Acad. Sci. USA* **2012**, *109*, 9342–9347. [CrossRef]

The Prognostic Value of High Platelet Reactivity in Ischemic Stroke Depends on the Etiology

Adam Wiśniewski [1,*], Karolina Filipska [2], Joanna Sikora [3], Robert Ślusarz [2] and Grzegorz Kozera [4]

[1] Department of Neurology, Faculty of Medicine, Nicolaus Copernicus University in Toruń, Collegium Medicum in Bydgoszcz, 85-094 Bydgoszcz, Poland
[2] Department of Neurological and Neurosurgical Nursing, Faculty of Health Sciences, Nicolaus Copernicus University in Toruń, Collegium Medicum in Bydgoszcz, 85-821 Bydgoszcz, Poland; karolinafilipskakf@gmail.com (K.F.); robert_slu_cmumk@wp.pl (R.Ś.)
[3] Experimental Biotechnology Research and Teaching Team, Department of Transplantology and General Surgery, Nicolaus Copernicus University in Toruń, Collegium Medicum in Bydgoszcz, 85-094 Bydgoszcz, Poland; joanna.sikora@cm.umk.pl
[4] Medical Simulation Centre, Medical University of Gdańsk, Faculty of Medicine, 80-210 Gdańsk, Poland; gkozera1@wp.pl
* Correspondence: adam.lek@wp.pl

Abstract: Background: Reduced aspirin response may result in a worse prognosis and a poor clinical outcome in ischemic stroke. The aim of this prospective pilot study was to assess the relationship between platelet reactivity and early and late prognosis, and the clinical and functional status in ischemic stroke, with the role of stroke etiology. Methods: The study involved 69 subjects with ischemic stroke, divided into large and small vessel etiological subgroups. Platelet function testing was performed with two aggregometric methods—impedance and optical—while the clinical condition was assessed using the National Institute of Health Stroke Scale (NIHSS) and the functional status was assessed using the modified Rankin Scale (mRS) on the first and eighth day (early prognosis) and the 90th day of stroke (late prognosis). Results: The initial platelet reactivity was found to be higher in patients with severe neurological deficits on the 90th day after stroke, than in the group with mild neurological deficits (median, respectively, 40 area under the curve (AUC) units vs. 25 AUC units, $p = 0.033$). In the large vessel disease group, a significant correlation between the platelet reactivity and the functional status on the first day of stroke was found (correlation coefficient (R) = 0.4526; $p = 0.0451$), the platelet reactivity was higher in the subgroup with a severe clinical condition compared to a mild clinical condition on the first day of stroke ($p = 0.0372$), and patients resistant to acetylsalicylic acid (aspirin) had a significantly greater possibility of a severe neurological deficit on the first day of stroke compared to those who were sensitive to aspirin (odds ratio (OR) = 14.00, 95% confidence interval (CI) 1.25–156.12, $p = 0.0322$). Conclusion: High on-treatment platelet reactivity in ischemic stroke was associated with a worse late prognosis regardless of the etiology. We demonstrated a significant relationship between high platelet reactivity and worse early prognosis and poor clinical and functional condition in the large vessel etiologic subgroup. However, due to the pilot nature of this study, its results should be interpreted with caution and further validation on a larger cohort is required.

Keywords: ischemic stroke; platelet reactivity; aspirin resistance; large vessel disease; carotid stenosis; clinical outcome; prognosis

1. Introduction

Stroke is a leading cause of disability and death worldwide and is associated with a worse quality of life [1]. Antiplatelet therapy is used to reduce the risk of recurrent ischemic stroke [2]. Acetylsalicylic acid (aspirin) is a primary antiplatelet agent; however, its effect can vary in different patients [3]. In some patients, a reduced aspirin response may be observed, resulting in a failure to inhibit the platelet reactivity [4]. Platelet function testing can evaluate the effectiveness of aspirin in decreasing platelet aggregation and activation. High on-treatment platelet reactivity or biochemical aspirin resistance is a multifactorial, negative feature that is associated with insufficient antiplatelet therapy [5].

One of the better-understood causes of cerebral ischemia is the pathology of large pre-cranial vessels, most often the internal carotid artery, which accounts for approximately 20–30% of all causes of stroke [6]. Our previous papers demonstrated the hyperaggregation and hyperactivation of platelets in this etiological subtype of ischemic stroke [7,8]. Furthermore, we hypothesize that it may be related to aspirin resistance and affect the clinical condition and prognosis due to the reduced inhibition of platelets. In the next step, we estimate the role of high on-treatment platelet reactivity for the clinical evaluation and prognosis of stroke patients.

Previous reports regarding the relationship between high platelet reactivity and clinical deterioration did not present clear conclusions [9–12]. The researchers did not focus on the potential role of stroke etiology for significant correlations in this field. The main objective of this study was to determine the relationship between platelet reactivity in the acute phase of ischemic strokes in patients treated with acetylsalicylic acid and the clinical and functional condition of patients, as well as early and late prognosis, with a particular emphasis on cerebral ischemic etiopathogenesis.

2. Materials and Methods

2.1. Study Population

The perspective, single-center, observational study was conducted at the Department of Neurology at the University Hospital No. 1 in Bydgoszcz. We consecutively enrolled 69 patients between February 2016 and December 2017 who underwent ischemic stroke according to the updated definition of stroke by the American Heart Association/American Stroke Association [13]. All subjects received a standard dose (150 mg) of acetylsalicylic acid based on the current guidelines. We divided the enrolled subjects into two subgroups considering the etiology of ischemic strokes. For the large vessel disease subgroup, we included patients with at least 50% of a carotid artery stenosis on the site correlated with clinical symptoms that were confirmed in an ultrasound examination [14]. The second etiological subgroup, small vessel disease, consisted of subjects with clinical and radiological features related to small vessel disease. We included patients with classic lacunar syndromes (pure motor or sensory stroke or ataxic hemiparesis) and typical neuroimaging markers (small subcortical infarcts <2 cm, hyperintensities in the white matter, lacunes < 15 mm, prominent perivascular spaces, microbleeds, and brain atrophy), where acute ischemic infarcts in neuroimaging were related to clinical symptoms of stroke [15]. The exclusion criteria were: a subject's inability to make an informed signature (speech disorders, or quantitative or qualitative disturbances of consciousness), an embolic background of ischemic stroke, a previous history of stroke, the chronic use of acetylsalicylic acid before stroke onset, gastrointestinal or urinary bleeding within the last 2 years, low platelet count <100,000/μL, anemia (hemoglobin <9 g/dL), or low hematocrit <35%, "silent" infarcts (infarcts in neuroimaging that are not related to clinical symptoms of stroke).

2.2. Clinical Outcome

Both the clinical status and functional status were assessed within 24 h after admission (first day) to the hospital, on the eighth day of hospitalization (early prognosis), and on the 90th (+/− 5 days) day (late prognosis) after the stroke onset. The clinical status and functional status were assessed using standardized research tools, the National Institute of Health Stroke Scale (NIHSS) and modified Rankin Scale (mRS), respectively. When analyzing the severity of the neurological deficit, two subgroups of patients with stroke were distinguished: a subgroup with a mild neurological deficit (0–5 points on the NIHSS) and a subgroup with moderate and severe neurological deficits (≥6 points on the NIHSS). Regarding the functional status of the patients, two subgroups of stroke patients were distinguished: a favorable prognosis (on the mRS 0–2 points) and an unfavorable prognosis (on the mRS 3–5 points). A comparison of the clinical and functional conditions in both etiological subgroups of the subjects is presented in Table 1.

Table 1. A comparison of the anthropometric data, platelet reactivity, clinical, and functional status in patients with stroke in both etiological subgroups.

Parameter	Large Vessel Disease $n = 20$	Small Vessel Disease $n = 49$	p-Value
Age median (range) *	67 (45–85)	68 (40–89)	0.7761
Male N, (%) **	14 (70%)	21 (42.9%)	0.0408
Platelet reactivity: optical aggregometry (AUC) median (range) *	17.1 (0–208.6)	20.4 (0–154.2)	0.7147
Platelet reactivity: impedance aggregometry (AUC) median (range) *	42 (9–101)	27.5 (6–108)	0.0622
NIHSS 1 day median (range) *	5 (2–17)	5 (1–17)	0.6770
NIHSS 8 day median (range) *	2 (0–10)	2 (0–10)	0.8324
NIHSS 90 day median (range) *	1 (0–8)	2 (0–10)	0.6625
mRS 1 day median (range) *	4 (1–5)	4 (1–5)	0.7304
mRS 8 day median (range) *	1 (0–5)	2 (0–4)	0.4999
mRS 90 day median (range) *	1 (0–4)	2 (0–4)	0.5740

* Mann–Whitney U test, ** Chi-squared calculation. AUC, area under the curve; NIHSS, National Institute of Health Stroke Scale; mRS, modified Rankin scale.

2.3. Ethics Statement

Written informed consent, after revision of the study protocol, was obtained from each participant. This study was approved by the Bioethics Committee of Nicolaus Copernicus University in Torun at Collegium Medicum of Ludwik Rydygier in Bydgoszcz (KB number 73/2016).

2.4. Platelet Function Testing

Aspirin-induced platelet function testing was measured using two methods: optical aggregometry and impedance aggregometry. Blood samples were collected from the participants within 24 h after the stroke onset. To standardize and to unify the time-points of measurements, most cases were performed between 18 and 24 h after the stroke onset, at the same time of day (10–12 AM). The optical aggregometry or light transmission aggregometry (LTA) was performed with an aggregometer (Chrono-Log Corp., Havertown, PA, USA) and the results were expressed as area under the curve (AUC) units. Values over 115 AUC units were defined as high on-treatment platelet reactivity or aspirin resistance. We performed impedance aggregometry using the Multiplate® platelet function analyzer (Roche Diagnostics, France) and its results were expressed as AUC units. For the aspirin-resistant group, we enrolled subjects with values over 40 AUC units. The procedures for performing platelet function testing were similar as described in the previous studies [16,17]. Of our 69 subjects, 43 underwent optical aggregometry measurements, and all 69 subjects underwent impedance aggregometry assessment.

2.5. Statistical Analysis

STATISTICA 13.1 (Dell Inc., Round Rock, TX, USA) was used to perform all statistical evaluations. The non-parametric Mann–Whitney U test was used to compare continuous variables. Categorical variables were compared with a Chi-squared test. Spearman's rank test was used to evaluate the correlations between the variables. The influence of platelet reactivity levels on stroke severity was performed with logistic regression analysis. In the present study, the statistical significance was defined as $p < 0.05$.

3. Results

3.1. All Subjects

There was no correlation between the platelet reactivity, assessed by Multiplate® and LTA methods, and the severity of the neurological deficit assessed using the NIHSS and functional status of the patients assessed on the mRS in the whole study group (Table 2). The comparison of the severity of neurological deficit (NIHSS) in patients with stroke assessed on the first, eighth, and 90th day after the stroke onset did not show significant differences between the subgroups of patients resistant and sensitive to aspirin (on the first day $p = 0.8663$, on the eighth day $p = 0.9234$, and on the 90th day $p = 0.8225$). There were no differences between the above groups regarding the functional status (mRS) of patients (on the first day $p = 0.9808$, on the eighth day $p = 0.4610$, and on the 90th day $p = 0.5892$).

In the present study, we found that the initial platelet reactivity assessed by Multiplate® was higher in patients with moderate/severe neurological deficits compared to a mild deficit on the 90th day after the stroke onset (median, respectively, 40 AUC units vs. 25 AUC units, $p = 0.033$) (Figure 1).

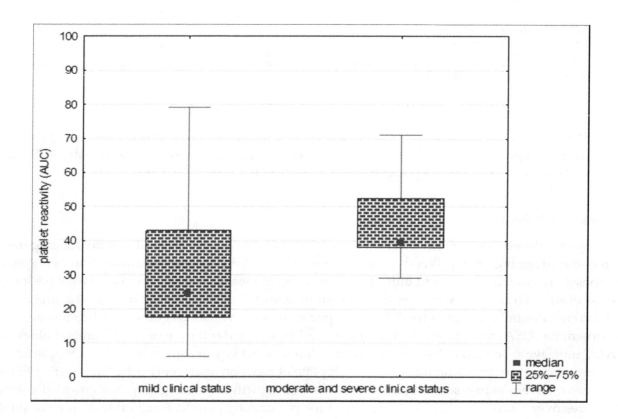

Figure 1. Comparison of platelet reactivity by Multiplate® (in area under the curve (AUC) units) in subgroups of patients with mild and moderate/severe neurological deficits on the 90th day in the general population of stroke patients.

However, there were no differences in the platelet reactivity between the groups distinguished on the basis of the severity of the deficit on the first and eighth day of stroke (on the first day $p = 0.6599$; on the eighth day $p = 0.3271$). The platelet reactivity assessed by Multiplate® did not differ between patients with a favorable and unfavorable prognosis on the first ($p = 0.6455$), eighth ($p = 0.6744$), and 90th day of the disease ($p = 0.7414$). The analysis of the relationship between the platelet reactivity in the LTA method and the clinical and functional status of stroke patients in the whole group of subjects showed no significant relationships ($p > 0.05$).

Logistic regression analysis showed that in the whole group of patients with stroke, aspirin-resistant subjects were 5.5 times more likely to have a severe neurological deficit on the 90th day of stroke than patients who were sensitive to aspirin; however, these differences did not reach statistical significance (odds ratio (OR) = 5.52, 95% confidence interval (CI) 0.54–56.86; $p = 0.1506$).

3.2. Two Etiological Subgroups

In the subgroups of patients with the pathology of large and small vessel disease, there were no statistically significant differences in the clinical and functional status of the stroke patients (NIHSS and mRS) (Table 1). In the subgroup of patients with large vessel disease, a significant correlation was found between the platelet reactivity assessed by Multiplate® and the functional status (mRS) on the first day of stroke (correlation coefficient (R) = 0.4526; $p = 0.0451$) (Figure 2, Table 2).

Table 2. Correlations of the clinical and functional conditions and platelet reactivity in both methods on individual days of stroke in the general population and in the subgroup of patients with large vessel disease.

| | General Population | | | | Large Vessel Disease | | | |
| | Multiplate® | | LTA | | Multiplate® | | LTA | |
	R	p	R	p	R	p	R	p
NIHSS 1 day	0.0713	0.5603	0.0010	0.9948	0.4908	0.0728	0.0010	0.9947
NIHSS 8 days	0.0473	0.6996	0.1472	0.3462	0.2636	0.2614	0.1472	0.3462
NIHSS 90 days	0.0781	0.5233	0.0859	0.5838	0.2801	0.2017	0.0859	0.5837
mRS 1 day	0.0273	0.8240	0.0170	0.9139	0.4526	0.0451	0.01698	0.9139
mRS 8 days	0.1233	0.3128	0.0781	0.6186	0.4068	0.0750	0.0781	0.6186
mRS 90 days	0.0968	0.4288	0.1099	0.4829	0.3676	0.1108	0.1099	0.4826

Spearman's rank correlation. R, correlation coefficient; LTA, light transmission aggregometry; NIHSS, National Institute of Health Stroke Scale; mRS, modified Rankin scale.

Assessing the relationship between the aspirin resistance groups and the severity of clinical deficit in patients with large vessel disease, we found that the aspirin-resistant patients did not differ in the NIHSS scores from aspirin-sensitive patients (on the first day $p = 0.06$, on the eighth day $p = 0.1167$, and on the 90th day $p = 0.0986$). Assessing the relationship with the functional status in patients with large vessel disease, we found that patients with aspirin resistance achieved a higher median of points on mRS on the eighth day of the disease than patients sensitive to aspirin ($p = 0.0352$) (Figure 3).

There were no differences in the mRS scores on the first and 90th day of stroke (respectively, $p = 0.0523$ for the first day, $p = 0.0631$ for the 90th day). In the subgroup of patients with the pathology of small vessels there were no significant differences in the severity of the clinical deficit and the functional status between the groups distinguished on the basis of the presence or absence of aspirin resistance ($p > 0.05$).

Comparing the platelet reactivity in patients with moderate/severe (NIHSS ≥6 points) and mild neurological deficits (NIHHS <6 points), we found that in the subgroup of patients with the pathology of large vessels, the median of platelet reactivity in the Multiplate® method was higher than in the subgroup of patients with severe neurological deficit compared to mild deficit on the first day of the disease (respectively, median 58.5 vs. 23.5 AUC units; $p = 0.0372$) (Figure 4); this did not differ on the eighth day ($p = 0.0762$), on the 90th day ($p = 0.0982$), or on particular days in the subgroup of patients with the pathology of small vessels ($p > 0.05$).

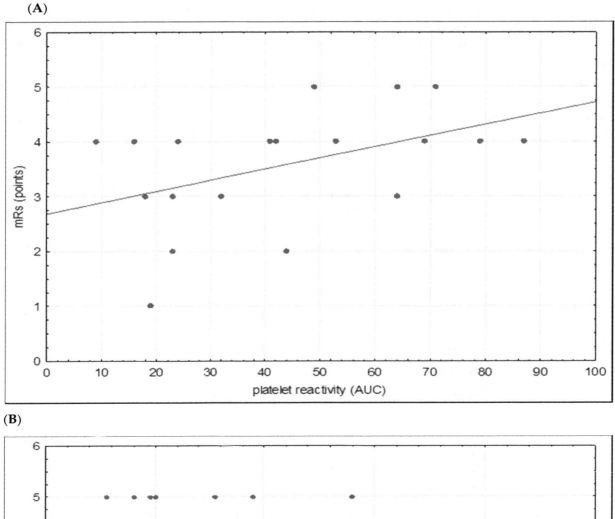

Figure 2. Correlation of platelet reactivity assessed by Multiplate® (in area under the curve (AUC) units) and functional status (modified Rankin scale (mRS) on the first day of stroke) in the subgroup of patients with large vessel disease (**A**) and small vessel disease (**B**).

Comparing the platelet reactivity in patients with favorable and unfavorable prognosis, the median of platelet reactivity in Multiplate® method did not differ between the above-mentioned groups both on the first, eighth, and 90th day of stroke in both subgroups ($p > 0.05$).

Logistic regression analysis showed that in the subgroup with large vessel disease, aspirin-resistant subjects had a 14 times greater probability of a severe neurological deficit on the first day of stroke than subjects sensitive to aspirin (OR = 14.00, 95% CI 1.25–156.12, $p = 0.0322$).

(A)

(B)

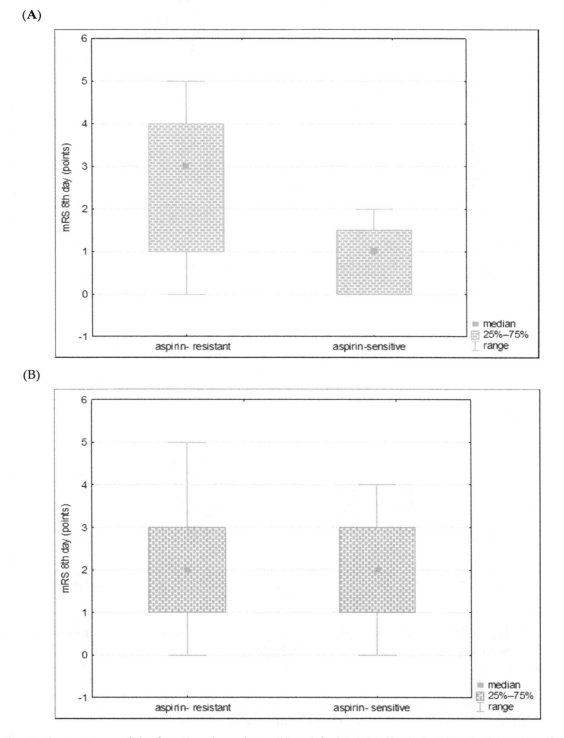

Figure 3. Comparison of the functional conditions (modified Rankin Scale (mRS)) on the eighth day of stroke in aspirin-resistant and aspirin-sensitive subjects in large vessel disease subgroup (**A**) and small vessel disease subgroup (**B**).

(A)

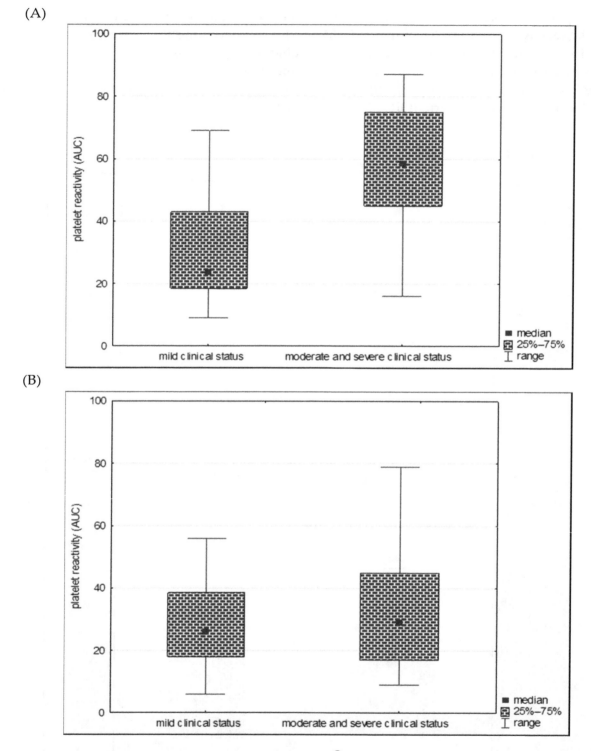

(B)

Figure 4. Comparison of platelet reactivity by Multiplate® (in AUC units) in the subgroup of patients with mild and moderate/severe neurological deficits on the first day of stroke in large vessel disease subgroup (**A**) and small vessel disease subgroup (**B**).

4. Discussion

In the present study, we demonstrated a significant role of ischemic stroke etiology for the prognostic value of high on-treatment platelet reactivity. We underline that the association between aspirin resistance and poor early clinical and functional conditions in ischemic stroke depends on the etiological subtype of the stroke. In the large vessel disease subgroup, we found a higher platelet reactivity in patients with severe neurological deficits on the first day of stroke, and that aspirin-resistant patients have a significantly higher probability of a severe clinical condition compared to aspirin-sensitive patients.

The division of patients according to the etiopathogenesis of stroke revealed a significant effect of platelet reactivity on the early functional condition. There was an average, though significant, correlation between platelet reactivity and functional status assessed on mRS on the first day of stroke, and patients resistant to aspirin had higher scores on the mRS (worse prognosis) on the eighth day of stroke than patients who were sensitive to aspirin. Both were present only in the large vessel disease subgroup. No similar results were demonstrated in the whole study population or in the small vessel disease subgroup.

These novel findings emphasize the great impact of stroke etiology on the association of high on-treatment platelet reactivity and poor early prognosis. However, it is difficult to refer the results of this research with other publications due to the heterogenous populations of the studied groups and different methodologies, and the lack of references in the literature on the impact of stroke etiopathogenesis on the relationship of platelet function testing with the prognosis of stroke subjects. Other authors did not assess the effect of stroke etiopathogenesis on the relationship of platelet reactivity with clinical and functional conditions.

In this study, there was no correlation between the platelet reactivity and the clinical condition in the whole group of subjects using the NIHSS on the first, eighth, and 90th day of stroke. In addition, the division into aspirin-resistant and -sensitive patients did not significantly differentiate the clinical status on particular days of the disease. Only the division of patients with mild to moderate/severe neurological deficits (according to the NIHSS score) revealed a significant effect on a higher initial platelet reactivity (within 24 h after onset) on the more severe clinical conditions, but this relationship was recorded only on the 90th day of stroke. Numerous authors showed that the aspirin-resistant group was characterized by a more severe early clinical condition, assessed on the NIHSS on the first day, than the group sensitive to aspirin [9–12]. Cheng et al. [12] indicated a significant correlation (R = 0.56) between platelet reactivity and the severity of neurological deficits assessed in the NIHSS. These results led to the conclusion that excessive platelet reactivity and aspirin resistance are associated with a worse clinical condition of patients in the acute phase of stroke. A different observation was demonstrated by Kim et al. [18] and Lai et al. [19], whose studies did not show the effect of platelet reactivity on the severity of the clinical condition assessed on the first day using the NIHSS. Similarly, Englyst et al. [20] did not find significant differences in the clinical status assessed on the NIHSS on the third day of stroke between the groups of patients resistant and sensitive to aspirin. The few literature reports on the long-term clinical conditions assessed on the 30th and 90th days of stroke showed contradictory results. Yip et al. [21] reported that aspirin-resistant patients were characterized by a worse clinical condition (NIHSS) both on the 30th and 90th days than patients sensitive to aspirin, while Lai et al. [19] did not find differences in the clinical condition (NIHSS) between these groups on the 90th day. We hypothesize that the contradictory conclusions from the presented studies may have resulted from omitting the important role of stroke etiology, as demonstrated in the current study.

The impact of platelet reactivity on the functional status of stroke patients is also debatable. Lai et al. [19] suggested a lack of relationship between platelet reactivity and early prognosis, as they did not reveal significant differences on the first day of stroke on mRS in the groups of patients sensitive and resistant to aspirin. On the other hand, Englyst et al. [20] showed a worse functional status of patients evaluated on mRS on the third day of stroke in aspirin-resistant patients compared to the aspirin-sensitive group (mRS median, respectively, 4 vs. 2, $p = 0.013$). Similar conclusions were reached by Sobol et al. [22] (mRS median 3 vs. 2, $p = 0.02$) assessing the functional status of patients on the 10th day of stroke. In our study, in the whole study population, there was no effect of platelet reactivity on the early prognosis—the functional status—on the first and eighth day of stroke or significant differences in the functional status of patients resistant and sensitive to aspirin. The differences in the results of this study from the data presented by other authors may be a result of including all etiological types of stroke (e.g., embolic) and other methodologies (Englyst et al., hemostatic thromboelastography; Sobol et al., Platelet Function Assay (PFA-100)). In addition, according to the results of Amy et al. [23] and Wilterdink et al. [24], aspirin administration before ischemic stroke onset results in a better prognosis of patients evaluated on mRS. Englyst et al. [20] assessed only patients treated with aspirin (for at least three days) before the incident. In the study by Sobol et al. [22], there is no information on whether patients with stroke had previously taken aspirin or only from the first day of stroke. In the only paper regarding late prognosis, Lai et al. [19] showed that on the 90th day of stroke, in the group with aspirin resistance, subjects with a worse functional status were more often reported, rated on mRS at 3–5 points, than in the group sensitive to aspirin ($p = 0.037$). However, the current study did not show any significant effects of platelet reactivity on the late functional status (even considering the etiopathogenesis of stroke). It is worth noting that Lai et al. evaluated the platelet reactivity with the PFA-100 method and recruited patients with stroke who received a dose of 100 mg of aspirin at least five days before platelet reactivity testing, which may have resulted in different functional outcomes than in this study.

The present study and previous reports, despite various methodologies and inclusion and exclusion criteria of the study population, underline that high on-treatment platelet reactivity may have a negative impact on early and late prognosis and a significant association with poor clinical and functional outcomes in stroke subjects. The novelty demonstrated in this research emphasizes that stroke etiology may be a key factor for the above dependencies.

According to the results obtained in this study, carotid artery stenosis appears to be an essential platelet activating factor. Tsai et al. [25], who assessed platelet function using flow cytometry, also demonstrated significantly higher platelet aggregation in patients with large vessel pathology compared to small vessel pathology. Importantly, the study was conducted on a similar population of patients with cerebral ischemia to this study (i.e., they excluded patients with stroke due to the embolic background. Similar results were presented by Zheng et al. [11], Kinsella et al. [26], and Dawson et al. [27], who demonstrated that platelet reactivity assessed by different methods is significantly elevated in patients with carotid artery stenosis. Kinsella et al. [28], using the PFA-100, reported that surgical treatment (e.g., stenting) in stroke subjects due to a carotid artery stenosis was associated with a significant reduction of platelet activation. These results were consistent with our current findings, highlighting the role of large vessel disease etiology for ischemic stroke in increasing platelet reactivity. These results indicate that platelet function monitoring may be useful for stroke subjects due to carotid artery stenosis. Additionally, platelet-function-guided individualized antiplatelet therapy can be essential to optimize clinical outcomes and to improve the functional status.

Unfortunately, both the American and European guidelines for the treatment and prevention of stroke do not distinguish between antiplatelet therapy and stroke pathomechanisms. Regardless of whether it is lacunar stroke or stroke due to a pathology of large extracranial vessels, aspirin administration is recommended for all patients with thrombotic stroke [2]. The current guidelines do not address the issue of aspirin resistance. It seems that this may be due to the lack of large, randomized clinical trials that could be used to develop clear guidelines.

As stroke in large extracranial pathology accounts for a fairly significant proportion of all strokes, and the results of current and previous studies highlight the significant impact of carotid artery pathology on platelet reactivity relationships with worse clinical conditions and prognoses, we recommend routinely determining platelet reactivity and detecting aspirin resistance, especially in cases of recurrent ischemic events. The authors believe that this would allow for personalized antiplatelet treatment based on platelet function testing, whose effectiveness for this group of patients is a priority.

The authors are aware that this study has several limitations. The evaluation of platelet function was performed only once and at different times during the first 24 h after the onset of stroke and at different times after the first dose of acetylsalicylic acid. It could have contributed to the variations in the measurements of platelet function. A single measurement with poorly validated methods in light of the marked variability of platelet reactivity that was previously demonstrated, may not be sufficient to properly assess the effect of high on-treatment platelet reactivity on the clinical condition and prognosis in ischemic stroke. More work is essential to sequentially determine platelet reactivity on successive days. Another limitation is that biochemical resistance does not always correspond with clinical resistance. The sample size in the study was small and imbalanced between the two etiological subgroups. The lack of recruitment of patients with severe stroke (especially those with impaired consciousness), due to the inability to obtain informed consent, constitutes a huge limitation of the study. Despite using stringent inclusion and exclusion criteria, in the face of low rates of in-hospital atrial fibrillation detection, there is a possibility that a small percentage of subjects may have had another etiology of stroke, such as embolism.

5. Conclusions

This pilot study demonstrated that high on-treatment platelet reactivity is associated with a worse late prognosis in ischemic stroke. In patients with large vessel disease, high platelet reactivity is associated with a worse early prognosis and clinical and functional condition of patients in the acute phase of stroke. The role of etiology demonstrated in this paper is novelty. However, due to the pilot nature of this study, the obtained results should be interpreted with caution. Further research, performed on larger sample size, is essential to validate and confirm our findings and to determine the optimal and personalized antiplatelet therapy.

Author Contributions: Conceptualization, A.W.; methodology, A.W., G.K., and J.S.; software, J.S.; validation, G.K.; formal analysis, A.W., K.F., and G.K.; investigation, A.W.; resources, J.S.; data curation, J.S..; writing—original draft preparation, A.W. and K.F.; writing—review and editing, A.W.; visualization, A.W.; supervision, G.K. and R.Ś.; project administration, A.W. and G.K. All authors have read and agreed to the published version of the manuscript.

References

1. Naghavi, M.; Wang, H.; Lozano, R.; Davis, A.; Liang, X.; Zhou, M.; Vollset, S.E.; Ozgoren, A.A.; Abdalla, S.; Abd-Allah, F.; et al. Global, regional, and national age-sex specific all-cause and cause-specific mortality for 240 causes of death, 1990–2013: A systematic analysis for the Global Burden of Disease Study 2013. *Lancet* **2015**, *385*, 117–171.

2. Powers, W.J.; Rabinstein, A.A.; Ackerson, T.; Adeove, O.M.; Bambakidis, N.C.; Becker, K.; Biller, J.; Brwon, M.; Demaerschalk, B.M.; Hoh, B.; et al. 2018 Guidelines for the Early Management of Patients with Acute Ischemic Stroke: A Guideline for Healthcare Professionals from the American Heart Association/American Stroke Association. *Stroke* **2018**, *49*, e46–e110. [CrossRef] [PubMed]

3. Rondina, M.T.; Weyrich, A.S.; Zimmerman, G.A. Platelets as cellular effectors of inflammation in vascular diseases. *Circ. Res.* **2013**, *112*, 1506–1519. [CrossRef] [PubMed]

4. Linden, M.D.; Jackson, D.E. Platelets: Pleiotropic roles in atherogenesis and atherothrombosis. *Int. J. Biochem. Cell Biol.* **2010**, *42*, 1762–1766. [CrossRef] [PubMed]

5. Paniccia, R.; Priora, R.; Liotta, A.A.; Agatina, A. Platelet function tests: A comparative review. *Vasc. Health Risk Manag.* **2015**, *11*, 133–148. [CrossRef]

6. Marulanda-Londono, E.; Chaturvedi, S. Stroke due to large vessel atherosclerosis. *Neurol. Clin. Pract.* **2016**, *6*, 252–258. [CrossRef]

7. Wiśniewski, A.; Sikora, J.; Filipska, K.; Kozera, G. Assessment of the relationship between platelet reactivity, vascular risk factors and gender in cerebral ischaemia patients. *Neurol. Neurochir. Pol.* **2019**, *53*, 258–264. [CrossRef]

8. Wiśniewski, A.; Sikora, J.; Sławińska, A.; Filipska, K.; Karczmarska-Wódzka, A.; Serafin, Z.; Kozera, G. High On-Treatment Platelet Reactivity Affects the Extent of Ischemic Lesions in Stroke Patients Due to Large-Vessel Disease. *J. Clin. Med.* **2020**, *9*, 251. [CrossRef]

9. Oh, M.S.; Yu, K.H.; Lee, J.H.; Jung, S.; Kim, C.; Jang, M.U.; Lee, J.; Lee, B.C. Aspirin resistance is associated with increased stroke severity and infarct volume. *Neurology* **2016**, *86*, 1808–1817. [CrossRef]

10. Agayeva, N.; Topcuoglu, M.A.; Arsava, E.M. The Interplay between Stroke Severity, Antiplatelet Use, and Aspirin Resistance in Ischemic Stroke. *J. Stroke Cerebrovasc. Dis.* **2016**, *25*, 397–403. [CrossRef]

11. Zheng, A.S.; Churilov, L.; Colley, R.E.; Goh, C.; Davis, S.M.; Yan, B. Association of aspirin resistance with increased stroke severity and infarct size. *JAMA Neurol.* **2013**, *70*, 208–213. [CrossRef] [PubMed]

12. Cheng, X.; Xie, N.C.; Hu, H.L.; Chen, C.; Lian, Y.J. Biochemical aspirin resistance is associated with increased stroke severity and infarct volumes in ischemic stroke patients. *Oncotarget* **2017**, *8*, 77086–77095. [CrossRef] [PubMed]

13. Sacco, R.L.; Kasner, S.E.; Broderick, J.P.; Caplan, L.R.; Connors, J.J.; Culebras, A.; Elkind, M.S.; George, M.G.; Hamdan, A.D.; Higashida, R.T.; et al. An updated definition of stroke for the 21st century: A statement for healthcare professionals from the American Heart Association/American Stroke Association. *Stroke* **2013**, *44*, 2064–2089. [CrossRef] [PubMed]

14. Wojczal, J.; Tomczyk, T.; Luchowski, P. Standards in neurosonology. *J. Ultrason.* **2016**, *16*, 44–45. [CrossRef] [PubMed]

15. Wardlaw, J.M.; Smith, E.E.; Biessels, G.J.; Cordonnier, C.; Fazekas, F.; Frayne, R.; Lindley, R.I.; O'Brien, J.T.; Barkhof, F.; Benavente, O.R.; et al. Neuroimaging standards for research into small vessel disease and its contribution to ageing and neurodegeneration. *Lancet Neurol.* **2013**, *12*, 822–838. [CrossRef]

16. Sibbing, D.; Braun, S.; Jawansky, S.; Vogt, W.; Mehilli, J.; Schömig, A.; Kastrati, A.; von Beckerath, N. Assessment of ADP-induced platelet aggregation with light transmission aggregometry and multiplate electrode platelet aggregometry before and after clopidogrel treatment. *Thromb. Haemost.* **2008**, *99*, 121–126.

17. Tóth, O.; Calatzis, A.; Penz, S.; Losonczy, H.; Siess, W. Multiple electrode aggregometry: A new device to measure platelet aggregation in whole blood. *Thromb. Haemost.* **2006**, *96*, 781–788.

18. Kim, J.T.; Heo, S.H.; Lee, J.S.; Choi, M.J.; Choi, K.H.; Nam, T.S.; Lee, S.H.; Park, M.S.; Kim, B.C.; Kim, M.K.; et al. Aspirin resistance in the acute stages of acute ischemic stroke is associated with the development of new ischemic lesions. *PLoS ONE* **2015**, *10*, e0120743. [CrossRef]

19. Lai, P.T.; Chen, S.Y.; Lee, Y.S.; Ho, Y.P.; Chiang, Y.Y.; Hsu, H.Y. Relationship between acute stroke outcome, aspirin resistance, and humoral factors. *J. Chin. Med. Assoc.* **2012**, *75*, 513–518. [CrossRef]

20. Englyst, N.A.; Horsfield, G.; Kwan, J.; Byrne, C.D. Aspirin resistance is more common in lacunar strokes than embolic strokes and is related to stroke severity. *J. Cereb. Blood Flow Metab.* **2008**, *28*, 1196–1203. [CrossRef]

21. Yip, H.K.; Liou, C.W.; Chang, H.W.; Lan, M.Y.; Liu, J.S.; Chen, M.C. Link between platelet activity and outcomes after an ischemic stroke. *Cerebrovasc. Dis.* **2005**, *20*, 120–128. [CrossRef] [PubMed]

22. Sobol, A.B.; Mochecka, A.; Selmaj, K.; Loba, J. Is there a relationship between aspirin responsiveness and clinical aspects of ischemic stroke? *Adv. Clin. Exp. Med.* **2009**, *18*, 473–479.

23. Amy, Y.X.; Keezer, M.R.; Zhu, B.; Wolfson, C.; Côté, R. Pre-stroke use of antihypertensives, antiplatelets, or statins and early ischemic stroke outcomes. *Cerebrovasc. Dis.* **2009**, *27*, 398–402.

24. Wilterdink, J.L.; Bendixen, B.; Adams, H.P., Jr.; Woolson, R.F.; Clarke, W.R.; Hansen, M.D. Effect of prior aspirin use on stroke severity in the trial of Org 10172 in acute stroke treatment (TOAST). *Stroke* **2001**, *32*, 2836–2840. [CrossRef] [PubMed]

25. Tsai, N.W.; Chang, W.N.; Shaw, C.F.; Jan, C.R.; Chang, H.W.; Huang, C.R.; Chen, S.D.; Chuang, Y.C.; Lee, L.H.; Wang, H.C.; et al. Levels and value of platelet activation markers in different subtypes of acute non-cardio-embolic ischemic stroke. *Thromb. Res.* **2009**, *124*, 213–218. [CrossRef] [PubMed]

26. Kinsella, J.A.; Tobin, W.O.; Hamilton, G.; McCabe, D.J. Platelet activation, function, and reactivity in atherosclerotic carotid artery stenosis: A systematic review of the literature. *Int. J. Stroke* **2013**, *8*, 451–464. [CrossRef]

27. Dawson, J.; Quinn, T.; Lees, K.R.; Walters, M.R. Microembolic signals and aspirin resistance in patients with carotid stenosis. *Cardiovasc. Ther.* **2012**, *30*, 234–239. [CrossRef]

28. Kinsella, J.A.; Tobin, W.A.; Tierney, S. Assessment of 'on-treatment platelet reactivity' and relationship with cerebral micro-embolic signals in asymptomatic and symptomatic carotid stenosis. *J. Neurol. Sci.* **2017**, *376*, 133–139. [CrossRef]

7

Predicting Stroke Outcomes Using Ankle-Brachial Index and Inter-Ankle Blood Pressure Difference

Minho Han [1], Young Dae Kim [1,2], Jin Kyo Choi [1], Junghye Choi [1], Jimin Ha [1], Eunjeong Park [3], Jinkwon Kim [4], Tae-Jin Song [5], Ji Hoe Heo [1,2] and Hyo Suk Nam [1,2,*]

[1] Department of Neurology, Yonsei University College of Medicine, Seoul 03722, Korea; umsthol18@yuhs.ac (M.H.); neuro05@yuhs.ac (Y.D.K.); JKSNAIL85@yuhs.ac (J.K.C.); hye07@yuhs.ac (J.C.); jiminha@yuhs.ac (J.H.); jhheo@yuhs.ac (J.H.H.)

[2] Integrative Research Center for Cerebrovascular and Cardiovascular Diseases, Seoul 03722, Korea

[3] Cardiovascular Research Institute, Yonsei University College of Medicine, Seoul 03722, Korea; EUNJEONG-PARK@yuhs.ac

[4] Department of Neurology, Yongin Severance Hospital, Yonsei University College of Medicine, Yongin-si 16995, Korea; ANTITHROMBUS@yuhs.ac

[5] Department of Neurology, Seoul Hospital, Ewha Womans University College of Medicine, Seoul 07804, Korea; knstar@ewha.ac.kr

* Correspondence: hsnam@yuhs.ac

Abstract: Background: This study investigated the association of high ankle-brachial index difference (ABID) and systolic inter-ankle blood pressure difference (IAND) with short- and long-term outcomes in acute ischemic stroke patients without peripheral artery disease (PAD). Methods: Consecutive patients with acute ischemic stroke who underwent ankle-brachial index (ABI) measurement were enrolled. ABID was calculated as |right ABI-left ABI|. IAND and systolic inter-arm blood pressure difference (IAD) were calculated as |right systolic blood pressure – left systolic blood pressure|. Poor functional outcome was defined as modified Rankin Scale score ≥ 3 at 3 months. Major adverse cardiovascular events (MACEs) were defined as stroke recurrence, myocardial infarction, or death. Results: A total of 2901 patients were enrolled and followed up for a median of 3.1 (interquartile range, 1.6–4.7) years. Among them, 2643 (84.9%) patients did not have PAD. In the logistic regression analysis, ABID ≥ 0.15 and IAND ≥ 15 mmHg were independently associated with poor functional outcome (odds ratio (OR), 1.970, 95% confidence interval (CI), 1.175-3.302; OR, 1.665, 95% CI, 1.188-2.334, respectively). In Cox regression analysis, ABID ≥ 0.15 and IAND ≥ 15 mmHg were independently associated with MACEs (hazard ratio (HR), 1.514, 95% CI, 1.058-2.166; HR, 1.343, 95% CI, 1.051-1.716, respectively) and all-cause mortality (HR, 1.524, 95% CI, 1.039-2.235; HR, 1.516, 95% CI, 1.164-1.973, respectively) in patients without PAD. Conclusion: High ABID and IAND are associated with poor short-term outcomes, long-term MACE occurrence, and all-cause mortality in acute ischemic stroke without PAD.

Keywords: ankle-brachial index difference; inter-ankle blood pressure difference; stroke; peripheral artery disease; outcome

1. Introduction

Blood pressure (BP) ratios and differences between the four limbs can be simultaneously obtained and calculated with ankle-brachial index (ABI) measurement [1]. Among the ratios and differences, ABI difference (ABID), systolic inter-ankle blood pressure difference (IAND), and systolic inter-arm BP difference (IAD) have been reported to be useful in predicting the prognosis in patients with cardiovascular disease, high-risk populations, and the general population [2,3].

Lower extremity peripheral artery disease (PAD) is defined by a low ABI, calculated by dividing the ankle systolic BP by the arm systolic BP. ABI has high specificity and sensitivity for the diagnosis of PAD [4], and ABI may also provide information beyond PAD. A previous study showed that ABID ≥ 0.15 was an independent risk factor for overall mortality in patients undergoing hemodialysis [5]. However, the prognostic value of ABID in patients with ischemic stroke remains uncertain.

IAD is strongly associated with increased cardiovascular and all-cause mortality [6]. Previous studies showed that IAND provided additional information to estimate stroke incidence and cardiovascular mortality beyond IAD [1,3]. To the best of our knowledge, no study has reported the prognostic impact of IAND on the outcomes of patients with acute ischemic stroke.

A previous study showed that the prevalence of PAD in patients with ischemic stroke was 32% and the rate of asymptomatic PAD in patients with stroke was 68% [7]. Another study showed that stroke patients with asymptomatic PAD had an increased risk of recurrent vascular events, including stroke [8]. Therefore, the prognostic significance needs to be separately assessed in ischemic stroke patients without PAD.

In this regard, we hypothesized that ABID and IAND are associated with poor short-term functional outcomes, major adverse cardiovascular events (MACEs), and all-cause mortality in patients with acute ischemic stroke. Whether the prognostic values of these parameters are valid in acute ischemic stroke patients without PAD was also investigated.

2. Materials and Methods

2.1. Patients and Evaluation

A hospital-based, retrospective observational study using prospectively collected stroke registry data was conducted. The Yonsei Stroke Registry collected the data of patients with acute cerebral infarction or transient ischemic attack (TIA) who presented to the emergency department within 7 days of symptom onset between January 1, 2007 and June 30, 2013 [9]. Acute cerebral infarction was defined as sudden onset of acute neurological deficits of presumed vascular etiology lasting 24 h or evidence of acute infarction on brain computed tomography (CT) or magnetic resonance imaging (MRI). TIA was diagnosed when a patient had transient (<24 h) neurologic dysfunction of vascular origin and did not show acute lesions on CT or MRI. Among these candidates, only patients with available four-limb BPs measured by ABI examination and a cerebral angiographic evaluation using either CT angiography, MR angiography, or digital subtraction angiography performed during the admission period were included. Patients were treated by standard treatment protocols based on the guidelines for acute ischemic stroke [10–13]. Stroke classifications were determined during weekly conferences. Based on a consensus of three stroke neurologists, stroke subtypes were classified according to the Trial of ORG 10172 in Acute Stroke Treatment (TOAST) classification [14].

2.2. Demographic Characteristics and Risk Factors

We collected data on baseline characteristics, including sex, age, and neurological deficit (National Institutes of Health Stroke Scale (NIHSS) score) upon admission; presence of risk factors; and laboratory data (glucose, high-density lipoprotein (HDL), and low-density lipoprotein (LDL)). Hypertension was defined as resting systolic blood pressure (SBP) of ≥140 mmHg or diastolic blood pressure (DBP) of ≥90 mmHg after repeated measurements during hospitalization or currently taking antihypertensive medication. Diabetes mellitus was defined as fasting plasma glucose levels of ≥7 mmol/L or taking an oral hypoglycemic agent or insulin. Current smoking was defined as having smoked a cigarette within 1 year prior to admission. Congestive heart failure was determined from the history of heart failure diagnosis, treatment with loop diuretics, and ejection fraction of ≤35% on echocardiography. Coronary artery disease (CAD) was diagnosed when a patient had a previous history of CAD (acute myocardial infarction, unstable angina, coronary artery bypass graft, or percutaneous coronary artery stent/angioplasty) or the presence of significant stenosis (≥50%) in any of the three main coronary arteries on multi-slice CT coronary angiography upon admission. Cerebral artery atherosclerosis (CAA) was defined as occlusion or significant stenosis (≥50%) of any intracranial or extracranial cerebral artery. PAD was determined if a patient had an ABI of <0.9 or a history of angiographically confirmed PAD.

2.3. ABI and Brachial-Ankle Pulse Wave Velocity Measurement

ABI and brachial-ankle pulse wave velocity (baPWV) were measured in the supine position using an automatic device (VP-1000; Colin Co., Ltd., Komaki, Japan), which has been validated previously [6,15]. This device automatically and simultaneously measures four-limb pulse wave forms and BP using the oscillometric method. Right ABI was calculated by the ratio of the right ankle SBP divided by the higher SBP of the arms. Left ABI was calculated by the ratio of the left ankle SBP divided by the higher SBP of the arms. ABID was calculated as |right ABI-left ABI|. IAND was extracted as BPs from both legs and calculated as |right ankle SBP-left ankle SBP|. IAD was extracted as BPs from arms and calculated as |right brachial SBP-left brachial SBP|. BaPWV on each side was automatically calculated as the transmission distance divided by the transmission time and expressed in centimeters per second. Transmission distance from the arm to each ankle was automatically calculated according to the patient's height. Transmission time was defined as the time interval between the initial increase of brachial and tibial waveforms. The higher values of baPWV on both sides were used for analysis.

2.4. Follow-Up and Outcome Measures

Patients were followed up in the outpatient clinic or by a structured telephone interview at 3 months and yearly after discharge. Short-term functional outcomes at 3 months were determined by a structured interview using the modified Rankin Scale (mRS). Poor outcome was defined as an mRS of ≥3. Deaths among participants from January 1, 2007 to December 31, 2013, were confirmed by matching the information in the death records and identification numbers assigned to the participants at birth [16]. We obtained data for the date and causes of death from the Korean National Statistical Office, which were identified based on death certificates. MACEs were defined as any stroke recurrence, myocardial infarction occurrence, or death.

2.5. Statistical Analysis

SPSS for Windows (version 23, SPSS, Chicago, IL, USA) was used for the statistical analysis. Intergroup statistical analyses were performed to compare the demographic characteristics and risk factors in the whole study population. The statistical significance of intergroup differences was assessed using the χ^2 or Fisher's exact test for categorical variables and independent two-sample t-test or Mann–Whitney U-test for continuous variables. Data were expressed as means ± standard deviations or medians (interquartile ranges (IQRs)) for continuous variables and numbers (%) for categorical variables. Cutoff values for IAND and IAD were based on those used in the previous study [3]. In elderly people, IAND of ≥15 mmHg and IAD of ≥15 mmHg were cutoff values that could predict mortality [3]. The cutoff value of ABID of ≥0.15 mmHg was based on a study wherein ABID predicted the mortality of patients with chronic hemodialysis [5]. Multivariable logistic regression analysis was performed after adjusting for sex, age, cardiovascular risk factors (hypertension, diabetes mellitus, hypercholesterolemia, current smoking, congestive heart failure, CAD, CAA, and PAD), and variables that exhibited a p value of <0.05 in the univariate analysis, to investigate the association of ABID, IAND, or IAD with short-term functional outcomes. Survival curves were generated according to the Kaplan–Meier method and compared using the log-rank test. Multivariable Cox proportional hazard regression was performed to determine independent factors associated with survival after an ischemic stroke. Subgroup analysis was also performed to confirm that the associations between short- and long-term outcomes and BP differences were valid in patients without PAD. We analyzed the diastolic IAND and diastolic IAD separately as supplemental data. All P values were two-tailed, and differences were considered significant at $p < 0.05$.

2.6. Standard Protocol Approval, Registration, and Patient Consent

The Institutional Review Board of Severance Hospital, Yonsei University Health System, approved this study and waived the need for informed consent because of the retrospective design and observational nature of this study (approval date: 2020-01-16; approval number: 4-2019-1196).

2.7. Data availability Statement

De-identified participant data are available upon reasonable request.

3. Results

3.1. Patient Demographic and Clinical Characteristics

A total of 3822 patients with acute ischemic stroke or TIA were recruited during the study period. After exclusions (follow-up loss ($n = 154$), no ABI measurements ($n = 729$), hemodialysis of one arm ($n = 16$), and TIA ($n = 22$)), 2901 patients were finally enrolled in this study (Figure 1).

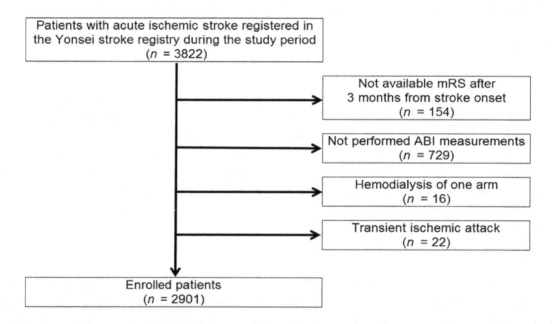

Figure 1. Flowchart of participants according to inclusion and exclusion criteria. ABI, ankle brachial index; mRS; modified Rankin Scale score.

A total of 258 (8.9%) patients had PAD. The mean age was 65.4 ± 12.2 years, and 61.8% were men. Among them, 582 (20.1%) had poor outcomes (Table 1). Compared with patients with good outcomes, those with poor outcomes were older, were more likely to be women, had more severe initial stroke severity, were less likely to be current smokers, and were more likely to have CAA, PAD, and a stroke subtype of large artery atherosclerosis (all p values <0.05). For four-limb BP profiles, both ankle SBP and ABI were lower in patients with poor outcomes than in those with good outcomes (all p values <0.001). All BP differences including ABID, IAND, and IAD were higher in patients with poor outcomes than in those with good outcomes (all p values <0.001). Compared with the included patients, excluded patients were older, were more likely to be women, had higher NIHSS score, were more likely to have congestive heart failure, and were less likely to be current smokers or have CAD (Supplementary Table S1).

Table 1. Patient demographic and clinical characteristics.

	Total (n = 2901)	Good Outcomes (mRS of 0-2; n = 2319)	Poor Outcomes (mRS of 3-6; n = 582)	p Value
Age, y	65.4 ± 12.2	64.0 ± 12.0	71.0 ± 11.4	<0.001
Men	1793 (61.8)	1489 (64.2)	304 (52.2)	<0.001
NIHSS score at admission	3.0 (1.0, 6.0)	2.0 (1.0, 4.0)	8.0 (4.0, 15.0)	<0.001
Risk factors				
Hypertension	2164 (74.6)	1712 (73.8)	452 (77.7)	0.057
Diabetes mellitus	920 (31.7)	728 (31.4)	192 (33.0)	0.459
Hypercholesterolemia	622 (21.4)	486 (21.0)	136 (23.4)	0.205
Current smoking	717 (24.7)	622 (26.8)	95 (16.3)	<0.001
Congestive heart failure	119 (4.1)	92 (4.0)	27 (4.6)	0.465
Coronary artery disease	686 (23.6)	549 (23.7)	137 (23.5)	0.946
Cerebral artery atherosclerosis	1727 (59.5)	1292 (55.7)	435 (74.7)	<0.001
Peripheral artery disease	258 (8.9)	152 (6.6)	106 (18.2)	<0.001
Laboratory findings				
Glucose, mg/dL	143.5 ± 63.9	142.7 ± 63.2	1468 ± 66.0	0.168
HDL, mg/dL	42.8 ± 11.0	42.6 ± 10.8	43.4 ± 11.6	0.127
LDL, mg/dL	114.5 ± 38.6	114.7 ± 37.5	113.8 ± 42.5	0.651
Stroke subtype				
LAA	587 (20.2)	440 (19.0)	147 (25.3)	<0.001
CE	754 (26.0)	600 (25.9)	154 (26.5)	
SVO	261 (9.0)	232 (10.0)	29 (5.0)	
OC	72 (2.5)	58 (2.5)	14 (2.4)	
UE	1227 (42.3)	989 (42.6)	238 (40.9)	
Arm BP, mmHg				
Right SBP	146.3 ± 23.5	146.7 ± 23.2	145.1 ± 24.6	0.147
Left SBP	145.3 ± 23.8	145.6 ± 23.6	144.0 ± 24.6	0.129
IAD	4.90 ± 6.51	4.71 ± 6.45	5.77 ± 7.15	0.001
Ankle BP, mmHg				
Right SBP	164.5 ± 31.3	166.3 ± 30.1	157.7 ± 35.1	<0.001
Left SBP	163.6 ± 31.3	165.2 ± 30.4	157.2 ± 34.6	<0.001
IAND	9.23 ± 11.94	8.42 ± 10.82	12.65 ± 15.87	<0.001
ABI				
Right ABI	1.111 ± 0.132	1.122 ± 0.118	1.071 ± 0.170	<0.001
Left ABI	1.105 ± 0.130	1.114 ± 0.118	1.069 ± 0.171	<0.001
ABID	0.063 ± 0.083	0.058 ± 0.077	0.086 ± 0.104	<0.001
Right ABI >1.30	58 (2.0)	44 (1.9)	14 (2.4)	0.434
Left ABI >1.30	44 (1.5)	31 (1.3)	13 (2.2)	0.113
Both ABI >1.30	18 (0.6)	14 (0.6)	4 (0.7)	0.818

Data are expressed as means ± standard deviations, medians [interquartile ranges], or numbers (%). ABI, ankle brachial index; ABID, ankle brachial index difference; BP, blood pressure; CE, cardioembolism; DBP, diastolic blood pressure; HDL, high density lipoprotein; IAD, systolic inter-arm blood pressure difference; IAND, systolic inter-ankle blood pressure difference; LAA, large artery atherosclerosis; LDL, low density lipoprotein; mRS, modified Rankin Scale; NIHSS, National Institutes of Health Stroke Scale; OC, other cause; SBP, systolic blood pressure; SVO, small vessel occlusion; and UE, undetermined etiology.

In all study patients, 236 (8.1%) patients showed ABID ≥0.15, 450 (15.5%) had IAND ≥15 mmHg, and 116 (4.0%) had IAD ≥15 mmHg. Among atherosclerotic diseases, CAA and PAD were independent determinants of ABID ≥0.15 (CAA: odds ratio (OR), 1.718, 95% confidence interval (CI), 1.211-2.437; PAD: OR, 22.124, 95% CI, 15.844-30.894) and IAND ≥15 mmHg (CAA: OR, 1.646, 95% CI, 1.281-2.114; PAD: OR, 13.328, 95% CI, 9.876-17.987). However, only PAD was an independent determinant of IAD ≥15 mmHg (PAD: OR, 3.044, 95% CI, 1.890-4.904) (Table 2).

Table 2. Determinants of IAD ≥15 mmHg, IAND ≥15 mmHg, and ABID ≥0.15.

	ABID ≥0.15		IAND ≥15 mmHg		IAD ≥15 mmHg	
	OR (95% CI)	*p* value *	OR (95% CI)	*p* value *	OR (95% CI)	*p* value *
CAD	1.290 (0.954-1.745)	0.098	0.957 (0.752-1.217)	0.718	0.912 (0.580-1.434)	0.689
CAA	1.718 (1.211-2.437)	0.002	1.646 (1.281-2.114)	<0.001	1.451 (0.926-2.274)	0.104
PAD	22.124 (15.844-30.894)	<0.001	13.328 (9.876-17.987)	<0.001	3.044 (1.890-4.904)	<0.001

Data were derived from the multivariable logistic regression analysis. ABID, ankle brachial index difference; CAD, coronary artery disease; CAA, cerebral artery atherosclerosis; CI, confidence interval; IAD, systolic inter-arm blood pressure difference; IAND, systolic inter-ankle blood pressure difference; NIHSS, National Institutes of Health Stroke Scale; OR, odds ratio; and PAD, peripheral artery disease. *adjusted for sex, age, NIHSS score at admission, hypertension, diabetes mellitus, hypercholesterolemia, current smoking, congestive heart failure, and stroke subtype.

ABID ≥0.15 and IAND ≥15 mmHg were more likely to have ABI >1.30 (all *p* values <0.001), but not IAD ≥15 mmHg (Table 3). BaPWVs were well correlated with ABID, IAND, and IAD (with ABID, $r = 0.139$, $p < 0.001$; with IAND, $r = 0.207$, $p < 0.001$; and with IAD, $r = 0.121$, $p < 0.001$) (Supplementary Table S2).

Table 3. Relationship between IAD, IAND, ABID, and ABI >1.30.

	Right ABI >1.30		Left ABI >1.30		Both ABI >1.30	
	n (%)	*p* value	*n* (%)	*p* value	*n* (%)	*p* value
ABID						
ABID <0.15	45 (1.7)	0.001	30 (1.1)	<0.001	18 (0.7)	0.392
ABID ≥0.15	13 (5.5)		14 (5.9)		0 (0.0)	
IAND						
IAND <15 mmHg	36 (1.5)	<0.001	27 (1.1)	<0.001	16 (0.7)	1.000
IAND ≥15 mmHg	22 (4.9)		17 (3.8)		2 (0.4)	
IAD						
IAD <15 mmHg	55 (2.0)	0.503	42 (1.5)	0.695	17 (0.6)	0.521
IAD ≥15 mmHg	3 (2.6)		2 (1.7)		1 (0.9)	

ABI, ankle brachial index; ABID, ankle brachial index difference; IAD, systolic inter-arm blood pressure difference; and IAND, systolic inter-ankle blood pressure difference.

3.2. Poor Functional Outcome

All patients with ($n = 2901$) and without PAD ($n = 2643$) were separately analyzed. In all study patients, poor outcome was independently associated with ABID (OR, 5.289, 95% CI, 1.723-16.236) and cutoff of ABID ≥0.15 (OR, 1.920, 95% CI, 1.361-2.708). Poor outcome was also independently associated with IAND (OR, 1.015, 95% CI, 1.007-1.023) and cutoff of IAND ≥15 mmHg (OR, 1.818, 95% CI, 1.389-2.381). In patients without PAD, the cutoff of ABID ≥0.15 was independently associated with poor outcomes (OR, 1.970, 95% CI, 1.175-3.302). IAND and cutoff of IAND ≥15 mmHg were also independently associated with poor outcomes (IAND: OR, 1.025, 95% CI, 1.009-1.041; IAND ≥15 mmHg: OR, 1.665, 95% CI, 1.188-2.334). Conversely, IAD ≥15 mmHg was associated with poor outcomes in the whole population (OR, 1.623, 95% CI, 1.011-2.605) but was not associated with poor outcomes in patients without PAD (Table 4).

Table 4. Predictors of poor outcome at 3 months.

	All Patients (*n* = 2901)		Patients without PAD (*n* = 2643)	
	OR (95% CI)	*p* value*	OR (95% CI)	*p* value*
ABI				
ABID	5.289 (1.723-16.236)	0.004	5.774 (0.948-35.151)	0.057
ABID ≥0.15	1.920 (1.361-2.708)	<0.001	1.970 (1.175-3.302)	0.010
Ankle BP, mmHg				
IAND	1.015 (1.007-1.023)	<0.001	1.025 (1.009-1.041)	0.002
IAND ≥15 mmHg	1.818 (1.389-2.381)	<0.001	1.665 (1.188-2.334)	0.003
Arm BP, mmHg				
IAD	1.009 (0.995-1.024)	0.190	1.009 (0.991-1.027)	0.329
IAD ≥15 mmHg	1.623 (1.011-2.605)	0.045	1.337 (0.758-2.360)	0.316

Data were derived from the multivariable logistic regression analysis. ABI, ankle brachial index; ABID, ankle brachial index difference; BP, blood pressure; CI, confidence interval; IAD, systolic inter-arm blood pressure difference; IAND, systolic inter-ankle blood pressure difference; NIHSS, National Institutes of Health Stroke Scale; OR, odds ratio; and PAD, peripheral artery disease. *adjusted for sex, age, NIHSS score at admission, hypertension, diabetes mellitus, hypercholesterolemia, current smoking, congestive heart failure, coronary artery disease, cerebral artery atherosclerosis, and stroke subtype.

3.3. All-Cause Mortality and MACEs

Study patients were followed up for a median of 3.1 (IQR, 1.6–4.7) years. A total of 622 patients had MACEs (21.4%) including 496 all-cause deaths (17.1%) during the study period. In Kaplan–Meier survival curves (Figure 2), higher all-cause mortality and MACEs (log-rank test; $p < 0.001$) were found in patients with ABID ≥0.15 or IAND ≥15 mmHg (log-rank test; all $p < 0.001$). Higher all-cause mortality (log-rank test; $p = 0.007$) and MACEs (log-rank test; $p = 0.008$) were also found in patients with IAD ≥15 mmHg.

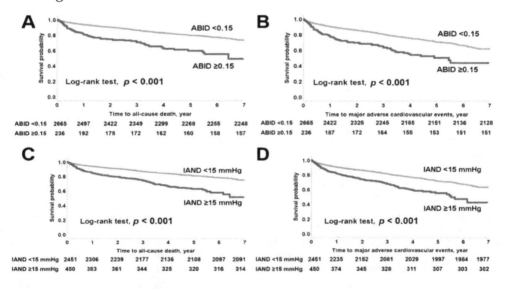

Figure 2. Kaplan–Meier survival analysis. (**A**) All-cause mortality; (**B**) major adverse cardiovascular event according to ABID ≥0.15. (**C**) All-cause mortality; (**D**) major adverse cardiovascular event according to IAND ≥15 mmHg. ABID; ankle-brachial index difference; IAND, systolic inter-ankle blood pressure difference.

In multivariable Cox regression analysis, ABID and ABID ≥0.15 were independently associated with all-cause mortality (ABID: hazard ratio (HR), 6.221, 95% CI, 2.973-13.018; ABID ≥0.15: HR, 1.567, 95% CI, 1.223-2.009) and MACEs (ABID: HR, 3.926, 95% CI, 1.906-8.087; ABID ≥0.15: HR, 1.416, 95% CI, 1.117-1.794). IAND and IAND ≥15 mmHg were also independently associated with all-cause mortality

(IAND: HR, 1.013, 95% CI, 1.007-1.019; IAND ≥15 mmHg: HR, 1.616, 95% CI, 1.317-1.982) and MACEs (IAND: HR, 1.010, 95% CI, 1.005-1.015; IAND ≥15 mmHg: HR, 1.380, 95% CI, 1.139-1.672).

In patients without PAD, ABID and ABID ≥0.15 were independently associated with all-cause mortality (ABID: HR, 9.221, 95% CI, 3.013-28.220; ABID ≥0.15: HR, 1.524, 95% CI, 1.039-2.235) and MACEs (ABID: HR, 6.605, 95% CI, 2.281-19.124; ABID ≥0.15: HR, 1.514, 95% CI, 1.058-2.166). IAND and IAND ≥15 mmHg were also independently associated with all-cause mortality (IAND: HR, 1.017, 95% CI, 1.004-1.030; IAND ≥15 mmHg: HR, 1.516, 95% CI, 1.164-1.973) and MACEs (IAND: HR, 1.015, 95% CI, 1.004-1.027; IAND ≥15 mmHg: HR, 1.343, 95% CI, 1.051-1.716). Meanwhile, IAD was associated only with the long-term occurrence of MACEs in all patients (HR, 1.010, 95% CI, 1.001-1.019), but not in those without PAD (HR, 1.006, 95% CI, 0.993-1.018, $p = 0.374$) (Table 5).

Table 5. Predictors of long-term outcome.

| | All Patients ($n = 2901$) | | | |
| | All-Cause Mortality | | MACE | |
	HR (95% CI)	p value*	HR (95% CI)	p value*
ABI				
ABID	6.221 (2.973-13.018)	<0.001	3.926 (1.906-8.087)	<0.001
ABID ≥0.15	1.567 (1.223-2.009)	<0.001	1.416 (1.117-1.794)	0.004
Ankle BP, mmHg				
IAND	1.013 (1.007-1.019)	<0.001	1.010 (1.005-1.015)	<0.001
IAND ≥15 mmHg	1.616 (1.317-1.982)	<0.001	1.380 (1.139-1.672)	0.001
Arm BP, mmHg				
IAD	1.009 (0.999-1.019)	0.068	1.010 (1.001-1.019)	0.027
IAD ≥15 mmHg	1.176 (0.810-1.708)	0.395	1.151 (0.820-1.617)	0.417
	Patients without PAD ($n = 2643$)			
	All-Cause Mortality		MACE	
	HR (95% CI)	p value*	HR (95% CI)	p value*
ABI				
ABID	9.221 (3.013-28.220)	<0.001	6.605 (2.281-19.124)	0.001
ABID ≥0.15	1.524 (1.039-2.235)	0.031	1.514 (1.058-2.166)	0.023
Ankle BP, mmHg				
IAND	1.017 (1.004-1.030)	0.010	1.015 (1.004-1.027)	0.010
IAND ≥15 mmHg	1.516 (1.164-1.973)	0.002	1.343 (1.051-1.716)	0.019
Arm BP, mmHg				
IAD	1.007 (0.993-1.021)	0.333	1.006 (0.993-1.018)	0.374
IAD ≥15 mmHg	1.075 (0.681-1.697)	0.755	1.032 (0.682-1.563)	0.881

Data were derived from the cox proportional hazards regression analysis. ABI, ankle brachial index; ABID, ankle brachial index difference; BP, blood pressure; CI, confidence interval; HR, hazard ratio; IAD, systolic inter-arm blood pressure difference; IAND, systolic inter-ankle blood pressure difference; MACE, major adverse cardiovascular event; NIHSS, National Institutes of Health Stroke Scale; and PAD, peripheral artery disease. *adjusted for sex, age, NIHSS score at admission, hypertension, diabetes mellitus, hypercholesterolemia, current smoking, congestive heart failure, coronary artery disease, cerebral artery atherosclerosis, and stroke subtype.

4. Discussion

We demonstrated that higher ABID and IAND were independently associated with poor short-term functional outcomes, long-term MACE occurrence, and all-cause mortality in patients with acute ischemic stroke. In particular, higher ABID and IAND had prognostic effects even in patients without PAD. Meanwhile, IAD was associated with poor short-term outcomes and MACEs in all patients, but not in those without PAD. These findings suggest that higher ABID and IAND have prognostic value for both poor short- and long-term outcomes of acute ischemic stroke and are more sensitive than IAD for predicting outcomes in acute ischemic stroke patients without PAD.

Primarily, increased ABID and IAND are attributable to the presence of PAD [17]. PAD affects approximately 200 million people worldwide and is the third most common cause of atherosclerotic cardiovascular death after CAD and stroke [18]. Traditional cardiovascular risk factors (smoking, hypertension, diabetes mellitus, and hypercholesterolemia) and advanced aging are important determinants of PAD. Therefore, patients with PAD often have concomitant atherosclerosis on the cerebral and coronary artery. In the Reduction of Atherothrombosis for Continued Health registry involving 44 countries worldwide, 39% of patients with PAD had CAD, 10% had cerebral artery disease, and 13% had both [19]. Accumulated systemic atherosclerosis worsens stroke prognosis [20]. Among the atherosclerotic burdens, ABID and IAND were associated with CAA and PAD. In contrast, IAD was only associated with PAD. It can be assumed that stroke patients with large ABID and IAND are more likely to have additional cerebral atherosclerotic burden and may have a poorer prognosis.

To the best of our knowledge, no study has previously evaluated ABID as a prognosis predictor in patients with acute ischemic stroke. ABI measurement is a well-established method to identify patients with PAD. Low ABI is commonly defined as ABI <0.9 and provides good sensitivity (80%) and excellent specificity (95%) to detect PAD [4]. ABI is also associated with poor initial stroke severity [21] and predicts poor prognosis and mortality in patients with stroke [2]. However, several previous studies have shown that low ABI was not sensitive enough to detect asymptomatic PAD in the general population [22]. To detect PAD and predict stroke prognosis accurately, novel parameters besides ABI should be developed. We found that ABID and IAND were independent and strong predictors of MACEs and all-cause mortality in patients with acute ischemic stroke. Interestingly, ABID and IAND remained to be significantly associated with poor short- and long-term outcomes in patients without PAD. This finding suggests that ABID and IAND may provide additional information for patients with subclinical or mild PAD. The strength of ABID might be related to the consideration of IAND and arm BP simultaneously. In addition, ABID and IAND can be obtained and easily calculated during ABI measurement in routine clinical practice.

In patients with stroke, IAD has been demonstrated to be associated with recurrent stroke [23], poor prognosis [24], and mortality [6]. However, some patients undergo dialysis with one arm because of end-stage renal disease, making it difficult to measure IAD. In addition, IAD (and ABI) may be "pseudonormal" when a patient has severe stenosis in both arms and in one leg. In contrast, IAND can be calculated without BP measurement in the arm and provide consistent data [3]. Several studies showed the increased usefulness of IAND and ABI relative to IAD. One study showed that IAND could better predict both overall and cardiovascular mortality than IAD in elderly patients [3]. ABI exhibits better association with cardiovascular outcomes than IAD in patients with type 2 diabetes [25]. However, no study has reported the comparison between IAND and IAD in patients with acute ischemic stroke.

Because lower limbs are more prone to be affected by PAD than upper limbs, IAND could be a better predictor of PAD than IAD [26]. High IAND was associated with increased left ventricular mass index [27] and arterial stiffness [28] and also predicted mortality in the elderly people [3]. Similarly, large ABID provided the prognostic value for mortality in patients undergoing chronic hemodialysis [5]. These findings suggest that the cardiovascular risk was higher in patients with lower extremity PAD than in those with upper extremity PAD [29]. Therefore, the circulatory burden assumed from the heart to the ankles may be greater than that from the heart to the arms.

Endothelial dysfunction [26], calcification burden [30], and arterial stiffness [27] are more frequent in the lower extremities than in the upper extremities. The degree of endothelial dysfunction in leg circulation is related to PAD severity. Endothelial dysfunction of leg circulation may occur before the impairment of forearm circulation in PAD [26]. Our data showed that high ABID and IAND were more likely to have ABI >1.30 than IAD. High ABI (i.e., ABI >1.30) is generally believed to occur because of medial arterial calcification and may be a marker for vascular stiffness [4]. High ABI was associated with an increase in both overall and cardiovascular mortality in patients with chronic kidney disease undergoing hemodialysis [31] and in the general population [32]. PWV and ABI are both atherosclerotic markers. ABI reflects stenosis or peripheral artery obstruction, whereas PWV represents arterial stiffness [5]. ABID, IAND, and IAD was positively correlated with baPWV.

The correlation coefficient was highest in IAND, followed by ABID and IAD. In patients undergoing hemodialysis, high PWV and low ABI are significantly associated with mortality [33]. Therefore, ABID and IAND could be more influenced by endothelial dysfunction, systemic atherosclerosis, calcification burden, and arterial stiffness than IAD, which may be related to more frequent PAD in the lower extremities [25,26,28,29].

This study has several limitations. First, radiological studies to detect atherosclerosis in the lower extremities were not routinely performed. A correlation study between apparent atherosclerosis and IAND or ABID might be helpful for better understanding [4,17]. Second, multiple, automatic, and simultaneous assessments are recommended for accurate BP difference measurement rather than single, manual, and sequential evaluation methods [34]. We used an automatic and simultaneous measurement device, but BP difference was investigated only once during the ABI measurement, and additional follow-up data were limited. Third, BP differences in this study focused on SBP, rather than DBP. Additional analysis was performed with DBP data, which found that the prognostic effect of DBP was not different from that of SBP (Supplementary Tables S3 and S4). Fourth, our findings may not be generalized to other populations or cohorts because our study population is limited to Korean patients. Fifth, the stroke standard treatment guidelines were updated and changed several times during the study period. Lastly, a total of 921 patients were excluded from the analysis. Among them, patients who did not undergo ABI measurements were mostly excluded. Therefore, the possibility of selection bias exists because of the retrospective study design; however, consecutive patients were included, and a relatively large sample size was analyzed.

5. Conclusions

This study suggests that high ABID and IAND are associated with poor short-term outcomes, long-term MACE occurrence, and all-cause mortality in patients with acute ischemic stroke. In addition, ABID and IAND predict post-stroke outcomes, even in patients without PAD. Therefore, ABID and IAND can be simple and reliable methods for identifying patients with an increased risk of poor short- and long-term outcomes in acute ischemic stroke.

Author Contributions: Conceptualization, M.H. and H.S.N.; methodology, M.H. and H.S.N.; formal analysis, M.H.; investigation, M.H. and H.S.N.; writing—original draft preparation, M.H. and H.S.N.; writing—review and editing, M.H., J.K., T.-J.S. and H.S.N.; data curation, M.H., J.K.C., J.C., J.H. and E.P.; supervision, Y.D.K., J.H.H. and H.S.N.; funding acquisition, H.S.N. All authors have read and agreed to the published version of the manuscript.

Acknowledgments: We thank Kangsik Seo, MT, for his small consideration in the course of writing the paper.

References

1. Guo, H.; Sun, F.; Dong, L.; Chang, H.; Gu, X.; Zhang, H.; Sheng, L.; Tian, Y. The Association of Four-Limb Blood Pressure with History of Stroke in Chinese Adults: A Cross-Sectional Study. *PLoS ONE* **2015**, *10*, e0139925. [CrossRef] [PubMed]
2. Milionis, H.; Vemmou, A.; Ntaios, G.; Makaritsis, K.; Koroboki, E.; Papavasileiou, V.; Savvari, P.; Spengos, K.; Elisaf, M.; Vemmos, K. Ankle-brachial index long-term outcome after first-ever ischaemic stroke. *Eur. J. Neurol.* **2013**, *20*, 1471–1478. [CrossRef] [PubMed]
3. Sheng, C.S.; Liu, M.; Zeng, W.F.; Huang, Q.F.; Li, Y.; Wang, J.G. Four-limb blood pressure as predictors of mortality in elderly Chinese. *Hypertension* **2013**, *61*, 1155–1160. [CrossRef] [PubMed]

4.   Aboyans, V.; Criqui, M.H.; Abraham, P.; Allison, M.A.; Creager, M.A.; Diehm, C.; Fowkes, F.G.; Hiatt, W.R.; Jonsson, B.; Lacroix, P.; et al. Measurement and interpretation of the ankle-brachial index: A scientific statement from the American Heart Association. *Circulation* **2012**, *126*, 2890–2909. [CrossRef] [PubMed]

5.   Lin, C.Y.; Leu, J.G.; Fang, Y.W.; Tsai, M.H. Association of interleg difference of ankle brachial index with overall and cardiovascular mortality in chronic hemodialysis patients. *Ren. Fail.* **2015**, *37*, 88–95. [CrossRef] [PubMed]

6.   Kim, J.; Song, T.J.; Song, D.; Lee, H.S.; Nam, C.M.; Nam, H.S.; Kim, Y.D.; Heo, J.H. Interarm blood pressure difference and mortality in patients with acute ischemic stroke. *Neurology* **2013**, *80*, 1457–1464. [CrossRef]

7.   Huttner, H.B.; Kohrmann, M.; Mauer, C.; Lucking, H.; Kloska, S.; Doerfler, A.; Schwab, S.; Schellinger, P.D. The prevalence of peripheral arteriopathy is higher in ischaemic stroke as compared with transient ischaemic attack and intracerebral haemorrhage. *Int. J. Stroke* **2010**, *5*, 278–283. [CrossRef]

8.   Sen, S.; Lynch, D.R., Jr.; Kaltsas, E.; Simmons, J.; Tan, W.A.; Kim, J.; Beck, J.; Rosamond, W. Association of asymptomatic peripheral arterial disease with vascular events in patients with stroke or transient ischemic attack. *Stroke* **2009**, *40*, 3472–3477. [CrossRef]

9.   Han, M.; Kim, Y.D.; Park, H.J.; Hwang, I.G.; Choi, J.; Ha, J.; Heo, J.H.; Nam, H.S. Prediction of functional outcome using the novel asymmetric middle cerebral artery index in cryptogenic stroke patients. *PLoS ONE* **2019**, *14*, e0208918. [CrossRef]

10. Sacco, R.L.; Adams, R.; Albers, G.; Alberts, M.J.; Benavente, O.; Furie, K.; Goldstein, L.B.; Gorelick, P.; Halperin, J.; Harbaugh, R.; et al. Guidelines for prevention of stroke in patients with ischemic stroke or transient ischemic attack: A statement for healthcare professionals from the American Heart Association/American Stroke Association Council on Stroke: Co-sponsored by the Council on Cardiovascular Radiology and Intervention: The American Academy of Neurology affirms the value of this guideline. *Stroke* **2006**, *37*, 577–617. [CrossRef]

11. Adams, R.J.; Albers, G.; Alberts, M.J.; Benavente, O.; Furie, K.; Goldstein, L.B.; Gorelick, P.; Halperin, J.; Harbaugh, R.; Johnston, S.C.; et al. Update to the AHA/ASA recommendations for the prevention of stroke in patients with stroke and transient ischemic attack. *Stroke* **2008**, *39*, 1647–1652. [CrossRef] [PubMed]

12. Furie, K.L.; Kasner, S.E.; Adams, R.J.; Albers, G.W.; Bush, R.L.; Fagan, S.C.; Halperin, J.L.; Johnston, S.C.; Katzan, I.; Kernan, W.N.; et al. Guidelines for the prevention of stroke in patients with stroke or transient ischemic attack: A guideline for healthcare professionals from the american heart association/american stroke association. *Stroke* **2011**, *42*, 227–276. [CrossRef] [PubMed]

13. Jauch, E.C.; Saver, J.L.; Adams, H.P., Jr.; Bruno, A.; Connors, J.J.; Demaerschalk, B.M.; Khatri, P.; McMullan, P.W., Jr.; Qureshi, A.I.; Rosenfield, K.; et al. Guidelines for the early management of patients with acute ischemic stroke: A guideline for healthcare professionals from the American Heart Association/American Stroke Association. *Stroke* **2013**, *44*, 870–947. [CrossRef] [PubMed]

14. Adams, H.P., Jr.; Bendixen, B.H.; Kappelle, L.J.; Biller, J.; Love, B.B.; Gordon, D.L.; Marsh, E.E., 3rd. Classification of subtype of acute ischemic stroke. Definitions for use in a multicenter clinical trial. TOAST. Trial of Org 10172 in Acute Stroke Treatment. *Stroke* **1993**, *24*, 35–41. [CrossRef]

15. Han, M.; Kim, Y.D.; Park, H.J.; Hwang, I.G.; Choi, J.; Ha, J.; Heo, J.H.; Nam, H.S. Brachial-ankle pulse wave velocity for predicting functional outcomes in patients with cryptogenic stroke. *J. Clin. Neurosci.* **2019**, *69*, 214–219. [CrossRef]

16. Nam, H.S.; Kim, H.C.; Kim, Y.D.; Lee, H.S.; Kim, J.; Lee, D.H.; Heo, J.H. Long-term mortality in patients with stroke of undetermined etiology. *Stroke* **2012**, *43*, 2948–2956. [CrossRef]

17. Herraiz-Adillo, A.; Soriano-Cano, A.; Martinez-Hortelano, J.A.; Garrido-Miguel, M.; Mariana-Herraiz, J.A.; Martinez-Vizcaino, V.; Notario-Pacheco, B. Simultaneous inter-arm and inter-leg systolic blood pressure differences to diagnose peripheral artery disease: A diagnostic accuracy study. *Blood Press.* **2018**, *27*, 121–122. [CrossRef]

18. Fowkes, F.G.; Rudan, D.; Rudan, I.; Aboyans, V.; Denenberg, J.O.; McDermott, M.M.; Norman, P.E.; Sampson, U.K.; Williams, L.J.; Mensah, G.A.; et al. Comparison of global estimates of prevalence and risk factors for peripheral artery disease in 2000 and 2010: A systematic review and analysis. *Lancet* **2013**, *382*, 1329–1340. [CrossRef]

19. Bhatt, D.L.; Steg, P.G.; Ohman, E.M.; Hirsch, A.T.; Ikeda, Y.; Mas, J.L.; Goto, S.; Liau, C.S.; Richard, A.J.; Rother, J.; et al. International prevalence, recognition, and treatment of cardiovascular risk factors in outpatients with atherothrombosis. *JAMA* **2006**, *295*, 180–189. [CrossRef]

20. Hoshino, T.; Sissani, L.; Labreuche, J.; Ducrocq, G.; Lavallee, P.C.; Meseguer, E.; Guidoux, C.; Cabrejo, L.; Hobeanu, C.; Gongora-Rivera, F.; et al. Prevalence of systemic atherosclerosis burdens and overlapping stroke etiologies and their associations with long-term vascular prognosis in stroke with intracranial atherosclerotic disease. *JAMA Neurol.* **2018**, *75*, 203–211. [CrossRef]

21. Lee, D.H.; Kim, J.; Lee, H.S.; Cha, M.J.; Kim, Y.D.; Nam, H.S.; Nam, C.M.; Heo, J.H. Low ankle-brachial index is a predictive factor for initial severity of acute ischaemic stroke. *Eur. J. Neurol.* **2012**, *19*, 892–898. [CrossRef] [PubMed]

22. Zhang, Z.; Ma, J.; Tao, X.; Zhou, Y.; Liu, X.; Su, H. The prevalence and influence factors of inter-ankle systolic blood pressure difference in community population. *PLoS ONE* **2013**, *8*, e70777. [CrossRef] [PubMed]

23. Chang, Y.; Kim, J.; Kim, Y.J.; Song, T.J. Inter-arm blood pressure difference is associated with recurrent stroke in non-cardioembolic stroke patients. *Sci. Rep.* **2019**, *9*, 12758. [CrossRef] [PubMed]

24. Chang, Y.; Kim, J.; Kim, M.H.; Kim, Y.J.; Song, T.J. Interarm Blood Pressure Difference is Associated with Early Neurological Deterioration, Poor Short-Term Functional Outcome, and Mortality in Noncardioembolic Stroke Patients. *J. Clin. Neurol.* **2018**, *14*, 555–565. [CrossRef]

25. Yan, B.P.; Zhang, Y.; Kong, A.P.; Luk, A.O.; Ozaki, R.; Yeung, R.; Tong, P.C.; Chan, W.B.; Tsang, C.C.; Lau, K.P.; et al. Borderline ankle-brachial index is associated with increased prevalence of micro- and macrovascular complications in type 2 diabetes: A cross-sectional analysis of 12,772 patients from the Joint Asia Diabetes Evaluation Program. *Diab. Vasc. Dis. Res.* **2015**, *12*, 334–341. [CrossRef]

26. Sanada, H.; Higashi, Y.; Goto, C.; Chayama, K.; Yoshizumi, M.; Sueda, T. Vascular function in patients with lower extremity peripheral arterial disease: A comparison of functions in upper and lower extremities. *Atherosclerosis* **2005**, *178*, 179–185. [CrossRef]

27. Su, H.M.; Lin, T.H.; Hsu, P.C.; Lee, W.H.; Chu, C.Y.; Chen, S.C.; Lee, C.S.; Voon, W.C.; Lai, W.T.; Sheu, S.H. Association of interankle systolic blood pressure difference with peripheral vascular disease and left ventricular mass index. *Am. J. Hypertens.* **2014**, *27*, 32–37. [CrossRef]

28. Su, H.M.; Lin, T.H.; Hsu, P.C.; Lee, W.H.; Chu, C.Y.; Chen, S.C.; Lee, C.S.; Voon, W.C.; Lai, W.T.; Sheu, S.H. Association of bilateral brachial-ankle pulse wave velocity difference with peripheral vascular disease and left ventricular mass index. *PLoS ONE* **2014**, *9*, e88331. [CrossRef]

29. Lin, L.Y.; Hwu, C.M.; Chu, C.H.; Won, J.G.S.; Chen, H.S.; Chang, L.H. The ankle brachial index exhibits better association with cardiovascular outcomes than interarm systolic blood pressure difference in patients with type 2 diabetes. *Medicine (Baltimore)* **2019**, *98*, e15556. [CrossRef]

30. Aboyans, V.; Ho, E.; Denenberg, J.O.; Ho, L.A.; Natarajan, L.; Criqui, M.H. The association between elevated ankle systolic pressures and peripheral occlusive arterial disease in diabetic and nondiabetic subjects. *J. Vasc. Surg.* **2008**, *48*, 1197–1203. [CrossRef]

31. Chen, S.C.; Chang, J.M.; Hwang, S.J.; Tsai, J.C.; Liu, W.C.; Wang, C.S.; Lin, T.H.; Su, H.M.; Chen, H.C. Ankle brachial index as a predictor for mortality in patients with chronic kidney disease and undergoing haemodialysis. *Nephrology (Carlton)* **2010**, *15*, 294–299. [CrossRef] [PubMed]

32. Resnick, H.E.; Lindsay, R.S.; McDermott, M.M.; Devereux, R.B.; Jones, K.L.; Fabsitz, R.R.; Howard, B.V. Relationship of high and low ankle brachial index to all-cause and cardiovascular disease mortality: The Strong Heart Study. *Circulation* **2004**, *109*, 733–739. [CrossRef]

33. Chen, S.C.; Chang, J.M.; Tsai, Y.C.; Tsai, J.C.; Su, H.M.; Hwang, S.J.; Chen, H.C. Association of interleg BP difference with overall and cardiovascular mortality in hemodialysis. *Clin. J. Am. Soc. Nephrol.* **2012**, *7*, 1646–1653. [CrossRef] [PubMed]

34. Verberk, W.J.; Kessels, A.G.; Thien, T. Blood pressure measurement method and inter-arm differences: A meta-analysis. *Am. J. Hypertens.* **2011**, *24*, 1201–1208. [CrossRef] [PubMed]

8

Potential Utility of Neurosonology in Paroxysmal Atrial Fibrillation Detection in Patients with Cryptogenic Stroke

Chrissoula Liantinioti [1], Lina Palaiodimou [1], Konstantinos Tympas [2], John Parissis [2],
Aikaterini Theodorou [1], Ignatios Ikonomidis [2], Maria Chondrogianni [1], Christina Zompola [1],
Sokratis Triantafyllou [1], Andromachi Roussopoulou [1], Odysseas Kargiotis [3], Aspasia Serdari [4],
Anastasios Bonakis [1], Konstantinos Vadikolias [4], Konstantinos Voumvourakis [1],
Leonidas Stefanis [1,5], Gerasimos Filippatos [2] and Georgios Tsivgoulis [1,*]

[1] Second Department of Neurology, "Attikon" University Hospital, School of Medicine,
National and Kapodistrian University of Athens, 12462 Athens, Greece; chrissa21@hotmail.com (C.L.);
lina_palaiodimou@yahoo.gr (L.P.); katetheo24@gmail.com (A.T.); mariachondrogianni@hotmail.gr (M.C.);
chriszompola@yahoo.gr (C.Z.); socrates_tr@hotmail.com (S.T.); an.rousso@yahoo.gr (A.R.);
bonakistasos@yahoo.com (A.B.); cvoumvou@otenet.gr (K.V.); lstefanis@bioacademy.gr (L.S.)
[2] Second Department of Cardiology, "Attikon" University Hospital, Medical School,
National and Kapodistrian University of Athens, 12462 Athens, Greece; kostas.tympas@yahoo.gr (K.T.);
jparissis@yahoo.com (J.P.); ignoik@gmail.com (I.I.); geros@otenet.gr (G.F.)
[3] Stroke Unit, Metropolitan Hospital, 18547 Piraeus, Greece; kargiody@gmail.com
[4] Department of Neurology, University Hospital of Alexandroupolis, Democritus University of Thrace,
School of Medicine, 68100 Alexandroupolis, Greece; aserdari@yahoo.com (A.S.);
vadikosm@yahoo.com (K.V.)
[5] First Department of Neurology, Eginition Hospital, National and Kapodistrian University of Athens,
School of Medicine, 11528 Athens, Greece
* Correspondence: tsivgoulisgiorg@yahoo.gr

Abstract: Background: Occult paroxysmal atrial fibrillation (PAF) is a common and potential treatable cause of cryptogenic stroke (CS). We sought to prospectively identify independent predictors of atrial fibrillation (AF) detection in patients with CS and sinus rhythm on baseline electrocardiogram (ECG), without prior AF history. We had hypothesized that cardiac arrhythmia detection during neurosonology examinations (Carotid Duplex (CDU) and Transcranial Doppler (TCD)) may be associated with higher likelihood of AF detection. Methods: Consecutive CS patients were prospectively evaluated over a six-year period. Demographics, clinical and imaging characteristics of cerebral ischemia were documented. The presence of arrhythmia during spectral waveform analysis of CDU/TCD was recorded. Left atrial enlargement was documented during echocardiography using standard definitions. The outcome event of interest included PAF detection on outpatient 24-h Holter ECG recordings. Statistical analyses were performed using univariate and multivariate logistic regression models. Results: A total of 373 patients with CS were evaluated (mean age 60 ± 11 years, 67% men, median NIHSS-score 4 points). The rate of PAF detection of any duration on Holter ECG recordings was 11% (95% CI 8%–14%). The following three variables were independently associated with the likelihood of AF detection on 24-h Holter-ECG recordings in both multivariate analyses adjusting for potential confounders: age (OR per 10-year increase: 1.68; 95% CI: 1.19–2.37; $p = 0.003$), moderate or severe left atrial enlargement (OR: 4.81; 95% CI: 1.77–13.03; $p = 0.002$) and arrhythmia detection during neurosonology evaluations (OR: 3.09; 95% CI: 1.47–6.48; $p = 0.003$). Conclusion: Our findings underline the potential utility of neurosonology in improving the detection rate of PAF in patients with CS.

Keywords: cryptogenic stroke; atrial fibrillation; neurosonology; Holter monitoring; transcranial Doppler; cervical duplex

---

1. Introduction

The etiology of acute cerebral ischemia (ACI) remains undetermined in more than one-third of all ischemic stroke (IS) patients upon discharge [1,2]. According to Trial of ORG 10172 in Acute Stroke Treatment (TOAST) classification, an IS is classified as cryptogenic stroke (CS) when no cause can be identified after the baseline diagnostic workup [3]. A well-defined etiopathogenic mechanism is cardioembolism, which actually accounts for 17% to 30% of all IS, with more than half of cardioembolic strokes being attributed to atrial fibrillation (AF) [4–6]. However, paroxysmal AF (PAF) is frequently undetected, due to episodic and asymptomatic nature and short duration [7]. It is therefore evident that a proportion of strokes labeled as CS are cardioembolic in origin because of occult PAF [8].

The detection of PAF is of utmost importance in order to provide the most suitable treatment for stroke secondary prevention. Antiplatelet treatment, advocated by current guideline recommendations for patients with CS [9], is known to provide inadequate protection from future cardioembolic events in patients with AF [10]. On the contrary, it has been estimated that the administration of anticoagulant therapy reduces the annual IS recurrence risk by 8.4% compared with antiplatelet therapy in IS patients with AF [11]. Both ESO/AHA guidelines recommend at least 24-h Holter monitoring in patients with CS to detect PAF [9,12].

Neurovascular imaging is also essential for accurate delineation of the stroke mechanism and the development of acute stroke therapies [13]. Carotid duplex ultrasound (CDU) and transcranial doppler ultrasound (TCD) are ancillary diagnostic tests in support of the etiological workup of IS and the evaluation of neurovascular status [14,15]. Both neurosonological modalities can be performed at the bedside in the very early stages of IS and are relatively inexpensive and noninvasive. Additionally, they allow monitoring and provide actual hemodynamic information. Thus, CDU and TCD may detect heart rhythm alterations in real-time during spectral waveform analysis [16,17] and provide complementary information to 24-h Holter-ECG recordings.

In view of former considerations, we sought to identify independent predictors of AF detection in patients with CS and sinus rhythm on baseline cardiac evaluation (electrocardiogram (ECG) and 24-h Holter-ECG recordings), without prior AF history. More specifically, we had hypothesized that cardiac arrhythmia detected during neurosonology evaluation (CDU and TCD) may be associated with higher likelihood of AF detection.

2. Methods

Consecutive patients with CS, no prior AF history and sinus rhythm on the baseline ECG and the 24-h Holter-ECG recordings were prospectively evaluated at a tertiary care stroke center ("Attikon" University Hospital, National and Kapodistrian University of Athens, Athens, Greece) over a six-year period. CS was defined according to TOAST criteria [3], following an extensive diagnostic workup of all patients presenting with symptoms of ischemic stroke (IS) or transient ischemic attack (TIA). More specifically, all patients underwent the following laboratory and imaging examinations: brain CT-scan or MRI-scan, full blood count, biochemical blood analysis (cholesterol and glucose values included), ECG, cardiac ultrasound, 24-h Holter heart-rhythm monitoring, CDU and TCD. Additional information regarding the diagnostic workup of CS patients in our center has been previously described [18,19].

Stroke severity at hospital admission was documented using National Institute of Health Stroke Scale (NIHSS) score [20] by certified vascular neurologists [18,19]. Baseline characteristics including demographics, vascular risk factors, admission NIHSS-scores, neuroimaging and neurosonology findings, echocardiographic measurements, and number of 24-h Holter monitoring evaluations were recorded. Radiologists blinded to the patients' clinical data analyzed neuroimaging examinations and cerebral infarctions were subsequently categorized according to their location as either cortical or non-cortical including subcortical, brainstem and cerebellar location [21].

CDU and TCD examinations were performed by a certified neurosonologist (GT) with a Refurbished Philips® CX50 portable ultrasound machine, using L12-3 and S5-1 ultrasound transducer probes respectively. Neurosonology examinations were performed in each patient within 48 h from hospital admission. Irregular duration of the intervals between consecutive peak-systolic velocities during spectral waveform analysis of extra- or intra-cranial arteries in at least three complexes indicated the presence of cardiac arrhythmia and this finding was prospectively documented. (Figure 1) [16,17]. Echocardiogram was performed by certified cardiologists and left atrial (LA) diameter was measured using standardized methodology as previously described [22]. LA enlargement was classified into mild, moderate or severe, according to the guidelines of the American Society of Echocardiography (ASE) [23].

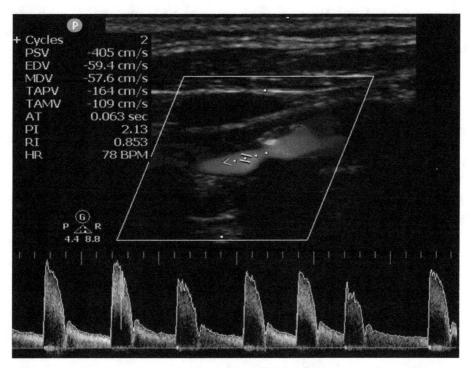

Figure 1. Detection of cardiac arrhythmia during spectral waveform analysis of external carotid artery in cervical duplex ultrasound.

Twenty-four-hour Holter ECG was performed using a 12-channel Holter monitoring Mortara H12+™ instrument. The inpatient recordings were completed within 96 h from hospital admission. It should be emphasized that sinus rhythm on baseline 24-h Holter ECG was a prerequisite for patients' inclusion in our study and for the diagnosis of CS [3]. During the follow-up period that varied between three to 60 months, CS patients underwent ≥1 outpatient 24-h Holter ECG recordings, based on the presence of premature atrial contractions on the baseline 24-h Holter ECG and that decision was not related to the neurosonology findings. The primary outcome event of interest included PAF detection of any duration as previously described [18]. Two blinded investigators using dedicated analysis software analyzed all ECG recordings [18]. Total time in AF was calculated as the sum of each individual AF episode for patients with multiple episodes during monitoring. The secondary outcome of interest included the current definition of PAF according to ACC/AHA/ESC guidelines, which applies to AF episodes without a reversible cause lasting >30 s [24].

The study protocol was approved by the ethics committee of our hospital and signed informed consent was obtained from the patient or legal representative before enrollment in all cases.

Statistical Analyses

Continuous variables are presented as mean ± SD (normal distribution) and as median with interquartile range (skewed distribution). Categorical variables are presented as percentages with their corresponding 95% Confidence Intervals (95% CI). Statistical comparisons between two groups were performed using χ^2 test, or in case of small expected frequencies, Fisher's exact test. Continuous variables were compared by the use of the unpaired t-test or Mann–Whitney U test, as indicated. Univariable and multivariable binary logistic regression models were used to evaluate associations between baseline characteristics (demographics, vascular risk factors, stroke severity, neuroimaging and neurosonology findings, echocardiographic measurements, and number of 24-h Holter monitoring evaluations) with the likelihood of detecting AF on Holter monitoring in patients with CS before and after adjusting for potential confounders. A cut-off of $p < 0.1$ was used to select variables for inclusion in multivariable analyses that were conducted using backward stepwise selection procedure. To confirm the robustness of multivariable models, we repeated all multivariable analyses using a forward selection procedure. Associations are presented as odds ratios (OR) with corresponding 95% confidence intervals (CI). Statistical significance was achieved if the p value was ≤ 0.05 in multivariable logistic regression analyses. The Statistical Package for Social Science (SPSS Inc., Armonk, NY, USA; version 23.0 for Windows) was used for statistical analyses.

3. Results

A total of 373 patients with CS (mean age 60 ± 11 years, 67% men, median NIHSS score on admission: four, IQR: 3–10) underwent 24-h Holter-ECG evaluations during the six-year study period. The baseline characteristics of the study population are presented in Table 1. The mean CHA2DS2-VASC score and the mean number of outpatient 24-h Holter-ECG recordings were 3.8 ± 1.3 and 1.5 ± 1.5 respectively. Moderate or severe left atrial enlargement were present in 6% of the study population, while in 20% we detected cardiac arrhythmia during neurosonology evaluations.

Table 1. Baseline characteristics of the study population ($n = 373$).

Variable	Overall
Age, years (mean ± SD)	60 ± 11
Female sex (%)	122 (33%)
NIHSS-Score, points (median, IQR)	4 (3–10)
Hypertension (%)	230 (62%)
Diabetes (%)	82 (22%)
Hyperlipidemia (%)	215 (58%)
Current Smoking (%)	158 (22.5%)
Coronary Artery Disease (%)	58 (16%)
Excessive Alcohol Intake (%)	37 (10%)
Previous History of TIA or Stroke (%)	74 (20%)
Heart Failure (%)	17 (5%)
Peripheral Arterial Disease (%)	15 (4%)
Vascular Disease (%)	70 (19%)
CHA2DS2-VASc Score, Points (mean ± SD)	3.8 ± 1.3
Left Atrial Enlargement (%)	155 (42%)
Mild	133 (36%)
Moderate	17 (5%)
Severe	5 (1%)
Cortical Location of Infarction (%)	76 (20%)
Cardiac Arrhythmia Detected during Neurosonology Evaluation (%)	66 (18%)
Number of 24-h Holter Recordings (mean ± SD)	1.5 ± 1.5
1	254 (68%)
2	85 (23%)
≥3	34 (9%)

IQR: interquartile range, TIA: transient ischemic attack.

AF of any duration was documented on outpatient 24-h Holter-ECG recordings in 40 patients with CS (11%, 95% CI: 8–14%). The mean duration of AF was 4940 ± 1043 s, while in 12 patients (30% of AF patients) AF duration was ≤30 s. The detection rate of AF ≥30 s was 8% (95% CI: 5–11%) in our cohort. AF detection rates differed significantly ($p < 0.001$) according to the degree of left atrial enlargement (Table 2). More specifically, the rates of AF detection were 7%, 12%, and 36% in patients with no, mild, moderate, or severe left atrial enlargement respectively (p for linear trend <0.001). AF detection rates also differed significantly ($p = 0.048$) according to the number of 24-h Holter-ECG recordings (Table 3). More specifically, the rates of AF detection were 8%, 14%, and 21% in patients with 1, 2, and ≥3 Holter recordings respectively (p for linear trend 0.014).

Table 2. Prevalence of atrial fibrillation detection on 24-h Holter monitoring stratified by degree of left atrial enlargement.

Left Atrial Enlargement	Atrial Fibrillation (−)	Atrial Fibrillation (+)	p-Value *	p-Value for Linear Trend **
None (%)	93%	7%		
Mild (%)	88%	12%	<0.001	<0.001
Moderate or Severe (%)	64%	36%		

* Pearson chi-square: 17.952 (df = 2); ** Linear by linear association: 12.887 (df = 1).

Table 3. Prevalence of atrial fibrillation detection on 24-h Holter monitoring stratified by the number of 24-h Holter-ECG recordings.

Number of 24-h Holter ECG Recordings	Atrial Fibrillation (−)	Atrial Fibrillation (+)	p Value *	p-Value for Linear Trend **
1 (%)	92%	8%		
2 (%)	86%	14%	0.048	0.014
≥3 (%)	79%	21%		

* Pearson chi-square: 6.079 (df = 2); ** Linear by linear association: 6.057 (df = 1).

Further evaluation regarding the cardiac structure was also conducted in a subset of our patients. Fifty-three percent of our patients (199/373) had undergone transesophageal echocardiogram (TEE). Cardiac CT and/or cardiac MRI were performed in three cases only, since these two investigations were not readily available in our hospital. All TEE, cardiac CT, and cardiac MRI investigations did not disclose any cardiogenic source of embolization in our cohort.

The univariable and multivariable associations of baseline characteristics with the likelihood of AF detection on 24-h Holter-ECG recordings are presented in Table 4. The following variables were associated with AF detection on initial univariable analyses using a p value of <0.1 as threshold for inclusion in multivariable models: age (OR per 10-year increase: 1.81; 95%CI: 1.31–2.50; $p < 0.001$), heart failure (OR: 2.74; 95% CI: 0.85–8.83; $p = 0.093$), CHA2DS2-VASC score (OR per 1-point increase: 1.53; 95% CI: 1.20–1.941; $p = 0.001$), ≥3 Holter recordings (OR: 2.40; 95% CI: 0.97–5.95; $p = 0.058$), moderate or severe left atrial enlargement (OR: 5.70; 95% CI: 2.22–14.61; $p < 0.001$), and cardiac arrhythmia detection during neurosonology evaluations (OR: 3.77; 95% CI: 1.87–7.60; $p < 0.001$). The following three variables were independently ($p < 0.05$) associated with the likelihood of AF detection on 24-h Holter-ECG recordings in multivariable logistic regression analyses conducted by backward selection procedure: age (OR per 10-year increase: 1.68; 95% CI: 1.19–2.37; $p = 0.003$), moderate or severe left atrial enlargement (OR: 4.81; 95% CI: 1.77–13.03; $p = 0.002$), and cardiac arrhythmia detection during neurosonology evaluations (OR: 3.09; 95%CI: 1.47–6.48; $p = 0.003$). We repeated the multivariable analyses using the forward selection procedure and obtained identical results. The independent associations of age (OR per 10-year increase: 1.68; 95% CI: 1.19–2.37; $p = 0.003$), moderate or severe left atrial enlargement (OR: 4.81; 95%CI: 1.77–13.03; $p = 0.002$) and cardiac arrhythmia detection during neurosonology evaluations (OR: 3.09; 95% CI: 1.47–6.48; p = 0.003) with the likelihood of AF detection persisted also on multivariable logistic regression analyses conducted by the forward selection procedure.

Table 4. Univariable and multivariable logistic regression analyses depicting the associations of baseline characteristics with the likelihood of atrial fibrillation detection during 24-h Holter monitoring.

Variable	Univariable Logistic Regression Analysis		Multivariable Logistic Regression Analysis	
	Odds Ratio (95%CI)	p *	Odds Ratio (95%CI)	p
Age (per 10-year increase)	1.81 (1.31–2.50)	<0.001	1.68 (1.19–2.37)	0.003
Female Sex	1.43 (0.73–2.80)	0.300		
NIHSS-Score at Admission (per 1-point increase)	0.97 (0.91–1.03)	0.295		
Hypertension	1.51 (0.74–3.08)	0.254		
Diabetes Mellitus	1.40 (0.67–2.94)	0.374		
Hyperlipidemia	1.60 (0.80–3.21)	0.185		
Previous History of TIA or Stroke	1.20 (0.54–2.64)	0.655		
Coronary Artery Disease	1.17 (0.49–2.80)	0.719		
Congestive Heart Failure	2.74 (0.85–8.83)	0.093	2.74 (0.85–8.83)	0.165
Current Smoking	1.22 (0.63–2.35)	0.558		
Excessive Alcohol Intake	1.34 (0.49–3.67)	0.565		
Peripheral Arterial Disease	1.30 (0.28–5.96)	0.739		
Vascular Disease	1.09 (0.48–2.49)	0.833		
CHA2DS2-VASc Score (per 1-point increase)	1.53 (1.20–1.94)	0.001	1.15 (0.80–1.66)	0.451
≥3 (24-h) Holter Evaluations	2.40 (0.97–5.95)	0.058	1.62 (0.58–4.52)	0.354
Cortical Location of Infarction	1.35 (0.63–2.90)	0.444		
Cardiac Arrhythmia Detected during Neurosonology Evaluation	3.77 (1.87–7.60)	<0.001	3.09 (1.47–6.48)	0.003
Moderate or Severe Left Atrial Enlargement	5.70 (2.22–14.61)	<0.001	4.81 (1.77–13.03)	0.002

* cutoff of p < 0.1 was used for selection of candidate variables for inclusion in multivariable logistic regression models.

4. Discussion

Our prospective single-center cohort study showed that detection of PAF in patients with CS is independently associated with increasing age, LA enlargement, and cardiac arrhythmia detection during neurosonology evaluations. In addition, the detection rates of AF of any duration and AF ≥ 30 s on outpatient 24-h Holter-ECG recordings were 11% and 8% respectively in our cohort.

There is mounting literature suggesting that newly diagnosed AF is identified in ≈5% of patients with stroke in the inpatient setting [25], while the rate of PAF detection in CS patients varies between 5–20%, according to different studies and prolonged Holter-ECG monitoring [26–28]. Repetition of 24-h Holter recording can detect AF at a higher rate, as it was also demonstrated in the present study, but it still carries lower diagnostic yield compared to continuous arrhythmia monitoring [29]. The detection of occult PAF has important therapeutic implications in CS patients, as anticoagulation is the optimal treatment for secondary stroke prevention in AF-associated stroke and can substantially reduce recurrent stroke and systemic embolism compared to antiplatelet therapy [30–34]. Furthermore, secondary prevention in CS includes oral anticoagulation when AF is detected, regardless of AF pattern (paroxysmal or chronic). Notably, the benefit of oral anticoagulation therapy in secondary stroke prevention in patients with AF has been established both for chronic and intermittent AF [35].

Another important finding is that AF duration was ≤30 s in 30% of the patients recognized with AF in outpatient Holter monitoring in our study, while the current American College of Cardiology/American Heart Association definition of PAF requires >30 s as a threshold for AF diagnosis [24]. However, AF of any duration should be considered clinically relevant in patients with CS, as recognized bursts of PAF may be markers of longer periods of AF that occur outside of the monitoring period. Interestingly, prior studies in CS patients have used a variety of time thresholds, ranging from 0 s to 5 minutes, reflecting the lack of consensus regarding AF duration yield [36–38].

Our study also disclosed an association between advancing age and detection of PAF in patients with CS, which persisted on multivariable analysis. This finding is consistent with other cohort studies, which demonstrated that older age was an independent predictor of occult PAF in CS patients [39,40].

AF detection on 24-h Holter monitoring is also associated with LA enlargement. According to our study, the rates of AF detection were 7%, 12% and 36% in patients with no, mild, moderate or severe left atrial enlargement respectively and that association was statistically significant. However, the metric used for indicating LA in our study was the LA diameter, whereas LA volume indexed to the subjects' body surface area, which represents a three-dimensional size of the LA is thought to be a superior metric of LA dimension in terms of predicting cardiovascular outcomes [41]. A recent study outlined the association of higher LA volume index with cardioembolic stroke and the rate of AF detection in patients with embolic stroke of undetermined source (ESUS), who completed four-week outpatient cardiac event monitoring [42]. ESUS is a subtype of CS and is used to describe non-lacunar CS in which embolism is a likely underlying mechanism [43]. However, ESUS constitutes a heterogenous group of patients, in whom other embolic mechanisms (patent foramen ovale, aortic plaque, non-stenosing unstable carotid plaque, cardiac valve disorders, coagulation disorders in patients with occult cancer) might be responsible for stroke, except for occult AF. Those underlying mechanisms mandate different management than oral anticoagulation, thus clinical utility of ESUS is debatable [44]. Consequently, our findings lend support to the recent concept that LA diameter measurement may help stratify ESUS patients with the greater benefit from anticoagulation due to underlying occult AF [44].

The potential diagnostic utility of neurosonology examinations (CDU and TCD) in the early detection of PAF in patients with CS is also supported by our results. Specifically, it was shown that cardiac arrhythmia detection during spectral waveform analysis in CDU/TCD evaluations was associated with the likelihood of AF detection on outpatient 24-h Holter-ECG recordings. A plausible explanation for this association may be related to the psychological stress induced by the TCD and CDU examinations to the patients that in turn may provoke episodes of arrhythmia, thus increasing the neurosonology rates of arrhythmia detection [45,46]. Being inexpensive, readily available, performed by-the-bed in the early stages of IS, even before the first 24-h Holter recording has been completed, CDU/TCD examination can be a useful tool for delineating stroke etiology in a multifactorial approach; both evaluating extracranial/intracranial vascular stenosis or occlusion and detecting cardiac arrhythmias in real-time [15–17]. One limiting factor is that, although neurosonology examinations can detect arrhythmias, it is not possible to differentiate them among the many different types and provide a certain diagnosis of AF. Abnormal neurosonology examination can represent AF as simple extra-systolic beats and consequently the specificity of this examination as a predictor of AF appears low. However, AF appears to account for a substantial proportion of rhythm abnormalities [47]. Even if the cardiac arrhythmia detected by neurosonology examinations is finally diagnosed as paroxysmal supraventricular tachycardia (PSVT) in ECG studies, this is also clinically relevant information, as PSVT patients have higher prevalence rate of AF [48]. Consequently, arrhythmia detection by CDU/TCD can be used as a potential marker that may assist in the identification of CS patients that should undergo prolonged cardiac monitoring using implantable cardiac monitors. If the present findings are externally validated, the echocardiographic and neurosonology findings may be included in current risk stratification scores (e.g., HAVOC) and other schemata for AF detection in CS [49,50].

Certain limitations of the present study need to be acknowledged. First, the sample size of the present single center study was moderate ($n = 373$). Second, there was no core laboratory analysis of CDU/TCD recordings for arrhythmia detection and no central adjudication of neuroimaging parameters. However, considering that investigators evaluating neuroimaging and neurosonology studies were blinded to the AF status of each patient, it is unlikely that this may have led to significant bias. Third, ECG detection of AF in CS patients was assessed by repetitive short-term (24-h) external monitoring devices in an outpatient setting and such an intermittent monitoring strategy has lower sensitivity and lower negative predictive value than continuous arrhythmia monitoring. Moreover, patients were not under continuous ECG monitoring during hospitalization, since the policy of our institution did not allow prolonged cardiac monitoring with repeated 24-h Holter-ECG recordings or cardiac telemetry or implantable cardiac monitoring during hospitalization. Fourth, the optimal duration of CDU/TCD recording for arrhythmia detection was not assessed in our study. It may be postulated that a more prolonged recording, for example continuous 1-h TCD monitoring using a headframe in search of arrhythmia and microembolic signals as well, could have identified more episodes of rhythm abnormalities, making the correlation with AF detection on ECG recordings even stronger. Finally, data about other possible confounders, such as secondary prevention therapies or patients' body mass index (BMI) were not collected.

5. Conclusions

In conclusion, to the best of our knowledge, this is the first study demonstrating an independent association between arrhythmia detection during neurosonology examinations in the early stages of IS and the detection of AF on outpatient 24-h Holter-ECG recordings in CS patients. Our findings appear to expand the utility of CDU/TCD studies in determining stroke etiology. However, our study was not designed to evaluate the diagnostic utility of neurosonology in comparison to outpatient prolonged cardiac monitoring. Further external validation of the present findings in larger cohorts of patients with more extensive duration of cardiac monitoring is required.

Author Contributions: Study concept and design: C.L., G.T.; Acquisition of Data: C.L., L.P., K.T., J.P., A.T., I.I., M.C., C.Z., S.T., A.R., G.T.; Analysis and interpretation: C.L., L.P., A.T., G.T.; Critical revision of the manuscript for important intellectual content: C.L., L.P., K.T., J.P., A.T., I.I., M.C., C.Z., S.T., A.R., O.K., A.S., A.B., K.V. (Konstantinos Vadikolias), K.V. (Konstantinos Voumvourakis), L.S., G.F., G.T.

References

1. Schulz, U.G.; Rothwell, P.M. Differences in vascular risk factors between etiological subtypes of ischemic stroke: Importance of population based studies. *Stroke* **2003**, *34*, 2050–2059. [CrossRef] [PubMed]
2. Tsivgoulis, G.; Patousi, A.; Pikilidou, M.; Birbilis, T.; Katsanos, A.H.; Mantatzis, M.; Asimis, A.; Papanas, N.; Skendros, P.; Terzoudi, A.; et al. Stroke incidence and outcomes in Northeastern Greece: The Evros stroke registry. *Stroke* **2018**, *49*, 288–295. [CrossRef] [PubMed]
3. Adams, H.P., Jr.; Bendixen, B.H.; Kappelle, L.J.; Biller, J.; Love, B.B.; Gordon, D.L.; Marsh, E.E., 3rd. Classification of subtype of acute ischemic stroke. Definitions for use in a multicenter clinical trial. TOAST. Trial of Org 10172 in Acute Stroke Treatment. *Stroke* **1993**, *24*, 35–41. [CrossRef] [PubMed]
4. Murtagh, B.; Smalling, R.W. Cardioembolic stroke. *Curr. Atheroscler.* **2006**, *8*, 310–316. [CrossRef]
5. Khoo, C.W.; Lip, G.Y. Clinical outcomes of acute stroke patients with atrial fibrillation. *Expert. Rev. Cardiovasc. Ther.* **2009**, *7*, 371–374. [CrossRef]
6. Arboix, A.; Vericat, M.C.; Pujades, R.; Massons, J.; García-Eroles, L.; Oliveres, M. Cardioembolic infarction in the Sagrat Cor-Alianza Hospital of Barcelona Stroke Registry. *Acta Neurol. Scand.* **1997**, *96*, 407–412. [CrossRef]
7. Lip, G.Y.; Hee, F.L. Paroxysmal atrial fibrillation. *QJM* **2001**, *94*, 665–678. [CrossRef]

8. Kishore, A.; Vail, A.; Majid, A.; Dawson, J.; Lees, K.R.; Tyrrell, P.J.; Smith, C.J. Detection of atrial fibrillation after ischemic stroke or transient ischemic attack: A systematic review and meta-analysis. *Stroke* **2014**, *45*, 520–526. [CrossRef]

9. Kernan, W.N.; Ovbiagele, B.; Black, H.R.; Bravata, D.M.; Chimowitz, M.I.; Ezekowitz, M.D.; Fang, M.C.; Fisher, M.; Furie, K.L.; Heck, D.V. Guidelines for the prevention of stroke in patients with stroke and transient ischemic attack: A guideline for healthcare professionals from the American Heart Association/American Stroke Association. *Stroke* **2014**, *45*, 2160–2236. [CrossRef]

10. EAFT (European Atrial Fibrillation Trial) Study Group. Secondary prevention in non-rheumatic atrial fibrillation after transient ischaemic attack or minor stroke. *Lancet* **1993**, *342*, 1255–1262. [CrossRef]

11. Hart, R.G.; Benavente, O.; McBride, R.; Pearce, L.A. Antithrombotic therapy to prevent stroke in patients with atrial fibrillation: A meta-analysis. *Ann. Intern. Med.* **1999**, *131*, 492–501. [CrossRef] [PubMed]

12. European Stroke Organisation (ESO); Executive Committee; ESO Writing Committee. Guidelines for management of ischaemic stroke and transient ischaemic attack 2008. *Cerebrovasc Dis.* **2008**, *25*, 457–507. [CrossRef] [PubMed]

13. Masdeu, J.C.; Irimia, P.; Asenbaum, S.; Bogousslavsky, J.; Brainin, M.; Chabriat, H.; Herholz, K.; Markus, H.S.; Martínez-Vila, E.; Niederkorn, K.; et al. EFNS guideline on neuroimaging in acute stroke. Report of an EFNS task force. *Eur. J. Neurol.* **2006**, *13*, 1271–1283. [CrossRef] [PubMed]

14. Qureshi, A.I.; Alexandrov, A.V.; Tegeler, C.H.; Hobson, R.W.; Dennis Baker, J.; Hopkins, L.N.; American Society of Neuroimaging; Society of Vascular and Interventional Neurology. Guidelines for screening of extracranial carotid artery disease: A statement for healthcare professionals from the multidisciplinary practice guidelines committee of the American Society of Neuroimaging; cosponsored by the Society of Vascular and Interventional Neurology. *J. Neurol.* **2007**, *17*, 19–47.

15. Alexandrov, A.V.; Sloan, M.A.; Wong, L.K.; Douville, C.; Razumovsky, A.Y.; Koroshetz, W.J.; Kaps, M.; Tegeler, C.H.; American Society of Neuroimaging Practice Guidelines Committee. Practice standards for transcranial Doppler ultrasound: Part I–test performance. *J. Neurol.* **2007**, *17*, 11–18.

16. Tsivgoulis, G.; Alexandrov, A.V.; Sloan, M.A. Advances in transcranial doppler ultrasonography. *Curr. Neurol. Neurosci. Rep.* **2009**, *9*, 46–54. [CrossRef]

17. Alexandrov, A.V.; Sloan, M.A.; Tegeler, C.H.; Newell, D.N.; Lumsden, A.; Garami, Z.; Levy, C.R.; Wong, L.K.; Douville, C.; Kaps, M.; et al. Practice standards for transcranial Doppler (TCD) ultrasound. Part II. Clinical indications and expected outcomes. *J. Neurol.* **2012**, *22*, 215–224.

18. Liantinioti, C.; Tympas, K.; Katsanos, A.H.; Parissis, J.; Chondrogianni, M.; Zompola, C.; Papadimitropoulos, G.; Ioakeimidis, M.; Triantafyllou, S.; Roussopoulou, A.; et al. Duration of paroxysmal atrial fibrillation in cryptogenic stroke is not associated with stroke severity and early outcomes. *J. Neurol. Sci.* **2017**, *376*, 191–195. [CrossRef]

19. Katsanos, A.H.; Bhole, R.; Frogoudaki, A.; Giannopoulos, S.; Goyal, N.; Vrettou, A.R.; Ikonomidis, I.; Paraskevaidis, I.; Pappas, K.; Parissis, J.; et al. The value of transesophageal echocardiography for embolic strokes of undetermined source. *Neurology* **2016**, *87*, 988–995. [CrossRef]

20. National Institute of Health, National Institute of Neurological Disorders and Stroke. Stroke Scale. Available online: https://www.ninds.nih.gov/sites/default/files/NIH_Stroke_Scale_Booklet.pdf (accessed on 3 September 2019).

21. Tsivgoulis, G.; Kargiotis, O.; Katsanos, A.H.; Patousi, A.; Mavridis, D.; Tsokani, S.; Pikilidou, M.; Birbilis, T.; Mantatzis, M.; Zompola, C.; et al. Incidence, characteristics and outcomes in patients with embolic stroke of undetermined source: A population-based study. *J. Neurol. Sci.* **2019**, *401*, 5–11. [CrossRef]

22. Ikonomidis, I.; Frogoudaki, A.; Vrettou, A.R.; Andreou, I.; Palaiodimou, L.; Katogiannis, K.; Liantinioti, C.; Vlastos, D.; Zervas, P.; Varoudi, M.; et al. Impaired Arterial Elastic Properties and Endothelial Glycocalyx in Patients with Embolic Stroke of Undetermined Source. *Thromb. Haemost.* **2019**. [Epub ahead of print]. [CrossRef] [PubMed]

23. Lang, R.M.; Bierig, M.; Devereux, R.B.; Flachskampf, F.A.; Foster, E.; Pellikka, P.A.; Picard, M.H.; Roman, M.J.; Seward, J.; Shanewise, J.S.; et al. Recommendations for chamber quantification: A report from the American Society of Echocardiography's Guidelines and Standards Committee and the Chamber Quantification Writing Group, developed in conjunction with the European Association of Echocardiography, a branch of the European Society of Cardiology. *J. Am. Soc. Echocardiogr.* **2005**, *18*, 1440–1463. [PubMed]

24. Heart, R.S.; Zipes, D.P.; Camm, A.J.; Borggrefe, M.; Buxton, A.E.; Chaitman, B.; Fromer, M.; Gregoratos, G.; Klein, G.; Moss, A.J.; et al. ACC/AHA/ESC 2006 Guidelines for the Management of Patients with Atrial Fibrillation: A report of the American College of Cardiology/American Heart Association Task Force on Practice Guidelines and the European Society of Cardiology Committee for Practice Guidelines (Writing Committee to Revise the 2001 Guidelines for the Management of Patients With Atrial Fibrillation): Developed in collaboration with the European Heart Rhythm Association and the Heart Rhythm Society. *Circulation* **2006**, *114*, e257–e354.

25. Liao, J.; Khalid, Z.; Scallan, C.; Morillo, C.; O'Donnell, M. Noninvasive cardiac monitoring for detecting paroxysmal atrial fibrillation or flutter after acute ischemic stroke: A systematic review. *Stroke* **2007**, *38*, 2935–2940. [CrossRef]

26. Sanna, T.; Diener, H.C.; Passman, R.S.; Di Lazzaro, V.; Bernstein, R.A.; Morillo, C.A.; Rymer, M.M.; Thijs, V.; Rogers, T.; Beckers, F.; et al. Cryptogenic Stroke and underlying Atrial Fibrillation. *N. Engl. J. Med.* **2014**, *370*, 2478–2486. [CrossRef]

27. Flint, A.C.; Banki, N.M.; Ren, X.; Rao, V.A.; Go, A.S. Detection of paroxysmal atrial fibrillation by 30-day event monitoring in cryptogenic ischemic stroke: The Stroke and Monitoring for PAF in Real Time (SMART) Registry. *Stroke* **2012**, *43*, 2788–2790. [CrossRef]

28. Seet, R.C.; Friedman, P.A.; Rabinstein, A.A. Prolonged rhythm monitoring for the detection of occult paroxysmal atrial fibrillation in ischemic stroke of unknown cause. *Circulation* **2011**, *26*, 477–486. [CrossRef]

29. Choe, W.C.; Passman, R.S.; Brachmann, J.; Morillo, C.A.; Sanna, T.; Bernstein, R.A.; Di Lazzaro, V.; Diener, H.C.; Rymer, M.M.; Beckers, F.; et al. A Comparison of Atrial Fibrillation Monitoring Strategies After Cryptogenic Stroke (from the Cryptogenic Stroke and Underlying AF Trial). *Am. J. Cardiol.* **2015**, *116*, 889–893. [CrossRef]

30. Hylek, E.M.; Go, A.S.; Chang, Y.; Jensvold, N.G.; Henault, L.E.; Selby, J.V.; Singer, D.E. Effect of intensity of oral anticoagulation on stroke severity and mortality in atrial fibrillation. *N. Engl. J. Med.* **2003**, *349*, 1019–1026. [CrossRef]

31. Evans, A.; Perez, I.; Yu, G.; Kalra, L. Secondary stroke prevention in atrial fibrillation: Lessons from clinical practice. *Stroke* **2000**, *31*, 2106–2111. [CrossRef]

32. Nieuwlaat, R.; Prins, M.H.; Le Heuzey, J.Y.; Vardas, P.E.; Aliot, E.; Santini, M.; Cobbe, S.M.; Widdershoven, J.W.; Baur, L.H.; Lévy, S.; et al. Prognosis, disease progression, and treatment of atrial fibrillation patients during 1 year: Follow-up of the Euro Heart Survey on atrial fibrillation. *Eur. Heart J.* **2008**, *29*, 1181–1189. [CrossRef] [PubMed]

33. Puccio, D.; Novo, G.; Baiamonte, V.; Nuccio, A.; Fazio, G.; Corrado, E.; Coppola, G.; Muratori, I.; Vernuccio, L.; Novo, S. Atrial fibrillation and mild cognitive impairment: What correlation? *Minerva Cardioangiol.* **2009**, *57*, 143–150. [PubMed]

34. Coppola, G.; Manno, G.; Mignano, A.; Luparelli, M.; Zarcone, A.; Novo, G.; Corrado, E. Management of Direct Oral Anticoagulants in Patients with Atrial Fibrillation Undergoing Cardioversion. *Medicina* **2019**, *55*, 660. [CrossRef] [PubMed]

35. Van Walraven, C.; Hart, R.G.; Singer, D.E.; Laupacis, A.; Connolly, S.; Petersen, P.; Koudstaal, P.J.; Chang, Y.; Hellemons, B. Oral anticoagulants vs aspirin in nonvalvular atrial fibrillation: An individual patient meta-analysis. *JAM* **2002**, *288*, 2441–2448. [CrossRef]

36. Elijovich, L.; Josephson, S.A.; Fung, G.L.; Smith, W.S. Intermittent atrial fibrillation may account for a large proportion of otherwise cryptogenic stroke: A study of 30-day cardiac event monitors. *J. Stroke Cerebrovasc. Dis.* **2009**, *18*, 185–189. [CrossRef]

37. Ziegler, P.D.; Glotzer, T.V.; Daoud, E.G.; Wyse, D.G.; Singer, D.E.; Ezekowitz, M.D.; Koehler, J.L.; Hilker, C.E. Incidence of newly detected atrial arrhythmias via implant-able devices in patients with a history of thromboembolic events. *Stroke* **2010**, *41*, 256–260. [CrossRef]

38. Gaillard, N.; Deltour, S.; Vilotijevic, B.; Hornych, A.; Crozier, S.; Leger, A.; Frank, R.; Samson, Y. Detection of paroxysmal atrial fibrillation with transtelephonic EKG in TIA or stroke patients. *Neurology* **2010**, *74*, 1666–1670. [CrossRef]

39. Alhadramy, O.; Jeerakathil, T.J.; Majumdar, S.R.; Najjar, E.; Choy, J.; Saqqur, M. Prevalence and predictors of paroxysmal atrial fibrillation on Holter monitor in patients with stroke or transient ischemic attack. *Stroke* **2010**, *41*, 2596–2600. [CrossRef]

40. Favilla, C.G.; Ingala, E.; Jara, J.; Fessler, E.; Cucchiara, B.; Messé, S.R.; Mullen, M.T.; Prasad, A.; Siegler, J.; Hutchinson, M.D.; et al. Predictors of finding occult atrial fibrillation after cryptogenic stroke. *Stroke* **2015**, *46*, 1210–1215. [CrossRef]

41. Tsang, T.S.; Abhayaratna, W.P.; Barnes, M.E.; Miyasaka, Y.; Gersh, B.J.; Bailey, K.R.; Cha, S.S.; Seward, J.B. Prediction of cardiovascular outcomes with left atrial size: Is volume superior to area or diameter? *J. Am. Coll. Cardiol.* **2006**, *47*, 1018–1023. [CrossRef]

42. Jordan, K.; Yaghi, S.; Poppas, A.; Chang, A.D.; Mac Grory, B.; Cutting, S.; Burton, T.; Jayaraman, M.; Tsivgoulis, G.; Sabeh, M.K.; et al. Left Atrial Volume Index Is Associated With Cardioembolic Stroke and Atrial Fibrillation Detection After Embolic Stroke of Undetermined Source. *Stroke* **2019**, *50*, 1997–2001. [CrossRef] [PubMed]

43. Hart, R.G.; Diener, H.C.; Coutts, S.B.; Easton, J.D.; Granger, C.B.; O'Donnell, M.J.; Sacco, R.L.; Connolly, S.J.; Cryptogenic Stroke/ESUS International Working Group. Embolic strokes of undetermined source: The case for a new clinical construct. *Lancet Neurol.* **2014**, *13*, 429–438. [CrossRef]

44. Tsivgoulis, G.; Katsanos, A.H.; Köhrmann, M.; Caso, V.; Lemmens, R.; Tsioufis, K.; Paraskevas, G.P.; Bornstein, N.M.; Schellinger, P.D.; Alexandrov, A.V.; et al. Embolic strokes of undetermined source: Theoretical construct or useful clinical tool? *Ther. Adv. Neurol. Disord.* **2019**, *12*, 1756286419851381. [CrossRef] [PubMed]

45. Hansson, A.; Madsen-Härdig, B.; Olsson, S.B. Arrhythmia-provoking factors and symptoms at the onset of paroxysmal atrial fibrillation: A study based on interviews with 100 patients seeking hospital assistance. *BMC Cardiovasc. Disord.* **2004**, *4*, 13. [CrossRef] [PubMed]

46. Severino, P.; Mariani, M.V.; Maraone, A.; Piro, A.; Ceccacci, A.; Tarsitani, L.; Maestrini, V.; Mancone, M.; Lavalle, C.; Pasquini, M.; et al. Triggers for Atrial Fibrillation: The Role of Anxiety. *Cardiol. Res. Pract.* **2019**, *2019*, 1208505. [CrossRef] [PubMed]

47. Khurshid, S.; Choi, S.H.; Weng, L.C.; Wang, E.Y.; Trinquart, L.; Benjamin, E.J.; Ellinor, P.T.; Lubitz, S. Frequency of Cardiac Rhythm Abnormalities in a Half Million Adults. *Circ. Arrhythm. Electrophysiol.* **2018**, *11*, e006273. [CrossRef]

48. Hamer, M.E.; Wilkinson, W.E.; Clair, W.K.; Page, R.L.; McCarthy, E.A.; Pritchett, E.L. Incidence of symptomatic atrial fibrillation in patients with paroxysmal supraventricular tachycardia. *J. Am. Coll. Cardiol.* **1995**, *25*, 984–988. [CrossRef]

49. Kwong, C.; Ling, A.Y.; Crawford, M.H.; Zhao, S.X.; Shah, N.H. A Clinical Score for Predicting Atrial Fibrillation in Patients with Cryptogenic Stroke or Transient Ischemic Attack. *Cardiology* **2017**, *138*, 133–140. [CrossRef]

50. Lip, G.Y.; Nieuwlaat, R.; Pisters, R.; Lane, D.A.; Crijns, H.J. Refining clinical risk stratification for predicting stroke and thromboembolism in atrial fibrillation using a novel risk factor-based approach: The euro heart survey on atrial fibrillation. *Chest* **2010**, *137*, 263–272. [CrossRef]

Improving the Clinical Outcome in Stroke Patients Receiving Thrombolytic or Endovascular Treatment in Korea

9

Young Dae Kim [1], Ji Hoe Heo [1], Joonsang Yoo [1,2], Hyungjong Park [1,2], Byung Moon Kim [3],
Oh Young Bang [4], Hyeon Chang Kim [5], Euna Han [6], Dong Joon Kim [3], JoonNyung Heo [1],
Minyoung Kim [1], Jin Kyo Choi [1], Kyung-Yul Lee [7], Hye Sun Lee [8], Dong Hoon Shin [9],
Hye-Yeon Choi [10], Sung-Il Sohn [2], Jeong-Ho Hong [2], Jang-Hyun Baek [11,12], Gyu Sik Kim [13],
Woo-Keun Seo [4], Jong-Won Chung [4], Seo Hyun Kim [14], Tae-Jin Song [15], Sang Won Han [16],
Joong Hyun Park [16], Jinkwon Kim [7,17], Yo Han Jung [18], Han-Jin Cho [19], Seong Hwan Ahn [20],
Sung Ik Lee [21], Kwon-Duk Seo [13,21] and Hyo Suk Nam [1,*]

1   Department of Neurology, Yonsei University College of Medicine, Seoul 03722, Korea;
    neuro05@yuhs.ac (Y.D.K.); jhheo@yuhs.ac (J.H.H.); JSYOO@yuhs.ac (J.Y.); hjpark209042@gmail.com (H.P.);
    jnheo@jnheo.com (J.H.); bestmykim@gmail.com (M.K.); JKSNAIL85@yuhs.ac (J.K.C.)
2   Department of Neurology, Brain Research Institute, Keimyung University School of Medicine, Daegu 41931,
    Korea; sungil.sohn@gmail.com (S.-I.S.); neurohong79@gmail.com (J.-H.H.)
3   Department of Radiology, Yonsei University College of Medicine, Seoul 03722, Korea;
    BMOON21@yuhs.ac (B.M.K.); DJKIMMD@yuhs.ac (D.J.K.)
4   Department of Neurology, Samsung Medical Center, Sungkyunkwan University School of Medicine,
    Seoul 06351, Korea; ohyoung.bang@samsung.com (O.Y.B.); mcastenosis@gmail.com (W.-K.S.);
    neurocjw@gmail.com (J.-W.C.)
5   Department of Preventive Medicine, Yonsei University College of Medicine, Seoul 03722, Korea;
    hckim@yuhs.ac
6   College of Pharmacy, Yonsei Institute for Pharmaceutical Research, Yonsei University, Incheon 21983, Korea;
    eunahan@yonsei.ac.kr
7   Department of Neurology, Gangnam Severance Hospital, Severance Institute for Vascular and Metabolic
    Research, Yonsei University College of Medicine, Seoul 06273, Korea; KYLEE@yuhs.ac (K.-Y.L.);
    antithrombus@gmail.com (J.K.)
8   Department of Research Affairs, Biostatistics Collaboration Unit, Yonsei University College of Medicine,
    Seoul 06273, Korea; HSLEE1@yuhs.ac
9   Department of Neurology, Gachon University Gil Medical Center, Incheon 21565, Korea;
    sphincter@naver.com
10 Department of Neurology, Kyung Hee University Hospital at Gangdong, Kyung Hee University School of
    Medicine, Seoul 05278, Korea; hyechoi@gmail.com
11 Department of Neurology, National Medical Center, Seoul 04564, Korea; janghyun.baek@gmail.com
12 Department of Neurology, Kangbuk Samsung Hospital, Sungkyunkwan University School of Medicine,
    Seoul 03181, Korea
13 Department of Neurology, National Health Insurance Service Ilsan Hospital, Ilsan 10444, Korea;
    gskim@nhimc.or.kr (G.S.K.); seobin7@naver.com (K.-D.S.)
14 Department of Neurology, Yonsei University Wonju College of Medicine, Wonju 26426, Korea;
    s-hkim@yonsei.ac.kr
15 Department of Neurology, Seoul Hospital, Ewha Womans University College of Medicine, Seoul 07804,
    Korea; knstar@hanmail.net
16 Department of Neurology, Sanggye Paik Hospital, Inje University College of Medicine, Seoul 01757, Korea;
    sah1puyo@gmail.com (S.W.H.); truelove1@hanmail.net (J.H.P.)
17 Department of Neurology, CHA Bundang Medical Center, CHA University, Seongnam 13496, Korea
18 Department of Neurology, Changwon Fatima Hospital, Changwon 51394, Korea; eyasyohan@gmail.com
19 Department of Neurology, Pusan National University School of Medicine, Busan 49241, Korea;
    chohj75@gmail.com
20 Department of Neurology, Chosun University School of Medicine, Gwangju 61453, Korea;
    shahn@Chosun.ac.kr

21 Department of Neurology, Sanbon Hospital, Wonkwang University School of Medicine, Sanbon 15865, Korea; neurologist@hanmail.net
* Correspondence: hsnam@yuhs.ac

Abstract: We investigated whether there was an annual change in outcomes in patients who received the thrombolytic therapy or endovascular treatment (EVT) in Korea. This analysis was performed using data from a nationwide multicenter registry for exploring the selection criteria of patients who would benefit from reperfusion therapies in Korea. We compared the annual changes in the modified Rankin scale (mRS) at discharge and after 90 days and the achievement of successful recanalization from 2012 to 2017. We also investigated the determinants of favorable functional outcomes. Among 1230 included patients, the improvement of functional outcome at discharge after reperfusion therapy was noted as the calendar year increased ($p < 0.001$). The proportion of patients who were discharged to home significantly increased (from 45.6% in 2012 to 58.5% in 2017) ($p < 0.001$). The successful recanalization rate increased over time from 78.6% in 2012 to 85.1% in 2017 ($p = 0.006$). Time from door to initiation of reperfusion therapy decreased over the years ($p < 0.05$). These secular trends of improvements were also observed in 1203 patients with available mRS data at 90 days ($p < 0.05$). Functional outcome was associated with the calendar year, age, initial stroke severity, diabetes, preadmission disability, intervals from door to reperfusion therapy, and achievement of successful recanalization. This study demonstrated the secular trends of improvement in functional outcome and successful recanalization rate in patients who received reperfusion therapy in Korea.

Keywords: reperfusion; therapy; ischemic stroke; outcome

1. Introduction

Stroke is one of the diseases with the highest burden worldwide. Although the age-standardized risk of stroke or case fatality has been improving, there is still an increase in the absolute number of stroke or stroke-related death [1]. The Global Burden of Disease Study demonstrated that the burden of cerebrovascular disease increased over several decades and ranked second in the highest burden of diseases in 2015 [2].

Intravenous tissue plasminogen activator (IV t-PA) therapy and endovascular treatment (EVT) are established treatments for eligible patients with acute ischemic stroke [3,4]. Although these modalities can lead to successful recanalization, which is a strong determinant of a good outcome [5], many patients who received reperfusion therapy did not achieve a favorable outcome [6]. Over the past decades, there has been an improvement in the stroke care program, imaging techniques, treatment devices, and experience in EVT. As a result, overall outcome of reperfusion therapy for acute ischemic stroke could be improved at a national level [7]. In Korea, there have been improvements in the care system for acute stroke patients, including easy and rapid accessibility to medical services, establishment of stroke units or centers, and acute stroke codes for reperfusion therapy [8–10]. Considering these secular trends in the stroke care system, clinical and radiologic outcomes after reperfusion therapy might have changed in Korea.

We investigated whether there was an annual change in outcomes in patients who received IV t-PA therapy or EVT in Korea. We also determined which factors had played a role in these changes using the nationwide thrombolytic and EVT registry.

2. Materials and Methods

2.1. Patients Inclusion

The study population was derived from the Selection Criteria in Endovascular Thrombectomy and thrombolytic therapy (SECRET) registry (Clinicaltrials.gov NCT02964052, https://clinicaltrials.gov/ct2/show/NCT02964052?term=NCT02964052&rank=1). The SECRET registry is a nationwide multicenter registry for exploring the selection criteria of patients who would benefit from reperfusion therapies. The SECRET registry was started on May 2016. This registry consisted of four parts: (1) clinical information, (2) information on reperfusion therapy, (3) comorbidities, and (4) imaging data.

The clinical information section includes the demographics, vascular risk factors, previous medication status, laboratory findings, and neurologic status or premorbidity before stroke. In the reperfusion therapy section, the information on time parameters, angiographic findings before and after treatment, devices used during the procedure, periprocedural complications, and concomitant thrombolytic agents used was collected. The modified Rankin scale (mRS) at discharge and after 90 days, along with mortality within 6 months, was determined in each patient during the follow-up. If a patient died, we also assessed the cause of death.

For the comorbidities section, we determined the presence of the component of the Charlson comorbidity index (CCI) for each patient. In the stroke population, we used a modified version of the CCI, which consisted of 19 diseases, including myocardial infarction, congestive heart failure, peripheral vascular disease, previous stroke, atrial fibrillation, dementia, depression, chronic pulmonary disease, ulcer disease, mild liver disease, moderate or severe renal disease, connective tissue disease or rheumatic disease, anemia, diabetes, acquired immune deficiency syndrome, cancer, leukemia, lymphoma, and metastatic cancer [11].

The imaging data section included the occlusion site, infarction core, collateral status, and thrombus characteristics on thin-section computed tomography (CT). The imaging findings were ascertained by the imaging adjudication committee (6 stroke neurologists and 4 neuroradiologists). The audit was conducted every two weeks, and the data management center verified the completeness and accuracy of the data. For this study, we used the demographics, vascular risk factors, underlying vascular diseases, time parameters, occlusion site, angiographic findings before and after treatment, and functional outcome variables.

This registry included 1026 patients who had been registered retrospectively from 15 hospitals between January 2012 and December 2015 and 333 patients who had been registered prospectively from 13 hospitals between November 2016 and December 2017. For prospectively-enrolled patients, written informed consent was obtained from patients or the next of kin. This registry was approved by the institutional review board in each participating hospital.

2.2. Reperfusion Therapy

IV t-PA and EVT was used in patients who met the criteria based on current guidelines. IV t-PA (Actilyse; Boehringer-Ingelheim, Ingelheim, Germany) was used in patients who had a stroke within 4.5 h from symptom onset and met the criteria based on current guidelines with a standard dose (0.9 mg/kg) [12,13]. If patients had large vessel occlusion on initial angiographic studies and could be treated within 8 h from symptom onset, EVT was considered. The EVT was performed primarily using mechanical devices rather than chemical agents. Among the mechanical devices, Solitaire stent retriever (Medtronic Neurovascular, Iirvine, CA, USA), Trevo retriever (Stryker Neurovascular, Fremont, CA, USA), or Penumbra reperfusion catheter (Penumbra, Alameda, CA, USA) was available in Korea and used based on target vessel site, tortuosity, or neurointerventionalist's preference. Intra-arterial thrombolysis with urokinase (Green Cross, Seoul, Korea) or glycoprotein IIb/IIIa antagonists was used as an adjuvant therapy in certain cases including those with re-occlusion or distal embolization.

If the onset of symptom was unclear, EVT was performed based on imaging findings and physician's discretion. Brain magnetic resonance imaging and magnetic resonance angiography were performed 24 h after reperfusion therapy. When brain MRI could not be performed, brain CT and/or CT angiography was performed. During hospitalization, each patient was treated on the basis of current stroke guidelines [14,15].

2.3. Outcome Measures

In this study, functional outcome was assessed with mRS at discharge and after 90 days. Favorable functional was defined as having mRS score of 0–2 and excellent functional outcomes was defined as mRS score of 0–1. In terms of radiologic outcomes, successful recanalization was determined using digital subtraction angiography (DSA), CT angiography (CTA), or magnetic resonance angiography (MRA). In this study, successful recanalization was defined as thrombolysis in cerebral infarction grade of 2b or 3 on final DSA among patients with EVT [16]. In patients who received IV t-PA only, successful recanalization was defined as arterial occlusive lesion (AOL) scoring of 3 on CTA or MRA performed within 24 h. Symptomatic intracerebral hemorrhage was defined as having any type of hemorrhage causing neurologic deterioration with National Institutes of Health Stroke Scale (NIHSS) score ≥ 4 or leading to death or surgery within 7 days of stroke onset based on the criteria in the European Cooperative Acute Stroke Study (ECASS) III trial [12].

2.4. Statistical Analysis

When we compared the baseline characteristics according to the calendar year, Student's independent t-test was used to compare age, time interval, and laboratory findings, and Pearson's χ^2 test or Fisher's exact test was used in the analysis of categorical data. Wilcoxon rank sum test was used to compare baseline NIHSS scores. Because the number of patients who received reperfusion therapy in December 2016 and registered in the SECRET registry was small, these patients were merged into the patient group treated in 2017 for this analysis. When we investigated the trends of outcomes by year, linear-by-linear or Jonckheere-Terpstra test was used for the analysis. To determine the independent predictors of outcomes, logistic regression or ordinal regression analysis was used. A multivariable analysis was performed using all variables with a p-value < 0.1 in the univariable analysis. All p-values were two-sided, and a p-value < 0.05 was considered statistically significant. All statistical analysis was performed using Windows SPSS package (version 23.0, IBM Corp., Armonk, NY, USA) and R version 3.2.1 (R Foundation for Statistical Computing, Vienna, Austria, http://www.R-project.org).

3. Results

3.1. Baseline Characteristics

Between January 2012 and December 2017, a total of 1359 patients who received reperfusion therapy with either IV t-PA therapy or EVT were registered. First, we excluded 38 patients who received intra-arterial chemical thrombolytic treatment as primary therapeutic modality. Then, we also excluded 86 patients who had in-hospital ischemic stroke, and nine patients who were transferred to the study hospital from other local hospitals ("drip-and-ship" case) because there were insufficient data on time parameters such as the intervals from stroke onset to first hospital arrival, CT, or IV t-PA. Finally, 1226 patients were included in this analysis (Figure 1).

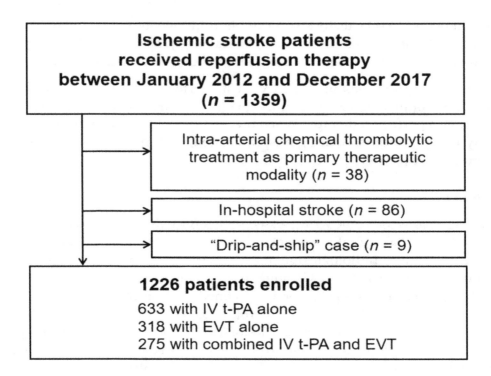

Figure 1. Flow diagram for the selection of patients in this study. IV, intravenous; t-PA, tissue plasminogen activator; EVT, endovascular.

Baseline characteristics of patients are presented in Table 1. The mean age was 68.9 ± 11.6 years, and 724 patients (58.9%) were male. The most common risk factor was hypertension (70.9%), followed by atrial fibrillation or atrial flutter (48.3%). The median NIHSS score was 12 (interquartile range [IQR], 7–17). Six-hundred and thirty-three (51.6%) patients received IV t-PA treatment alone, 318 (25.9%) patients received EVT alone, and the remaining 275 (22.4%) received combined IV t-PA and EVT. The number of patients who received IV t-PA and registered in SECRET registry was larger than those registered after EVT with/without IV t-PA, except in 2017. We could determine the location of large artery occlusion in 851 of 1021 patients who underwent angiographic studies before reperfusion therapy. The most common occlusion site was the middle cerebral artery (MCA) (56.1%, n = 477), followed by the internal carotid artery (ICA) (27.1%, n = 231), vertebrobasilar (VBA) artery (12.1%, n = 103), and others (4.7%, n = 40). During study period, thrombectomy devices including Solitaire, Trevo, and Penumbra system were available in Korea. Among 593 patients treated with EVT, Solitaire was most frequently selected in 433 (73%), followed by Penumbra system (n = 69, 11.6%), and Trevo (n = 69, 11.6%).

Table 1. Baseline characteristics of the included patients by year.

	Total	Calendar Year					p-Value for Trends
		2012 (n = 103)	2013 (n = 231)	2014 (n = 284)	2015 (n = 302)	2017 (n = 306)	
Age	68.9 ± 11.6	68.7 ± 10.3	68.8 ± 11.2	68.8 ± 11.7	70.0 ± 11.3	67.9 ± 12.6	0.941
Male sex	723 (59.0)	58 (56.3)	142 (61.5)	162 (57.0)	168 (55.6)	193 (63.1)	0.328
Hypertension	869 (70.9)	79 (76.7)	168 (72.7)	193 (68.0)	213 (70.5)	216 (70.6)	0.437
Diabetes	499 (40.7)	53 (51.5)	101 (43.7)	110 (38.7)	108 (35.8)	127 (41.5)	0.187
Hyperlipidemia	408 (33.3)	33 (32.0)	60 (26.0)	98 (34.5)	87 (28.8)	130 (42.5)	0.001
Current smoking	273 (22.3)	22 (21.4)	52 (22.5)	70 (24.6)	64 (21.2)	65 (21.2)	0.630
Coronary disease	212 (17.3)	21 (20.4)	31 (13.4)	55 (19.4)	52 (17.2)	53 (17.3)	0.903
Valvular heart disease	47 (3.8)	4 (3.9)	3 (1.3)	10 (3.5)	20 (6.6)	10 (3.3)	0.408
Mechanical valvular disease	18 (1.5)	4 (3.9)	2 (0.9)	3 (1.1)	4 (1.3)	5 (1.6)	0.714
Mitral stenosis	29 (2.4)	0 (0.0)	1 (0.4)	7 (2.5)	16 (5.3)	5 (1.6)	0.182
Atrial fibrillation or atrial flutter	592 (48.3)	55 (53.4)	112 (48.5)	144 (50.7)	159 (52.6)	122 (39.9)	0.008
Congestive heart failure	68 (5.5)	5 (4.9)	16 (6.9)	18 (6.3)	16 (5.3)	13 (4.2)	0.265
Peripheral arterial occlusive diseases	22 (1.8)	3 (2.9)	8 (3.5)	4 (1.4)	2 (2.2)	5 (1.6)	0.141
Previous stroke	246 (20.1)	26 (25.2)	42 (18.2)	60 (21.1)	55 (18.2)	63 (20.3)	0.754
Preadmission disability	50 (4.1)	8 (7.8)	10 (4.3)	16 (5.6)	8 (2.6)	8 (2.6)	0.020
Location site (n = 1021)							0.170
ICA	231 (22.6)	26 (34.7)	35 (19.7)	53 (24.5)	54 (21.7)	63 (20.8)	
MCA	477 (46.7)	24 (32.0)	81 (45.5)	110 (50.9)	125 (50.2)	137 (45.2)	
VBA	103 (10.1)	11 (14.7)	20 (11.2)	23 (10.6)	18 (7.2)	31 (10.2)	
Others	40 (3.9)	2 (2.7)	10 (5.6)	7 (3.2)	7 (2.8)	14 (4.6)	
No Occlusion	170 (16.7)	12 (16.0)	32 (18.0)	23 (10.6)	45 (18.1)	58 (19.1)	
Systolic blood pressure	149.9 ± 28.8	153.3 ± 33.6	152.5 ± 30.1	148.3 ± 27.6	149.2 ± 28.8	148.8 ± 27.3	0.078
Diastolic blood pressure	85 ± 16.6	87.4 ± 21.1	86.3 ± 15.9	86.3 ± 16.6	84.1 ± 16.4	82.8 ± 15.3	0.018
Last normal to ED	144.3 ± 180.4	117.6 ± 159.2	131.7 ± 146.6	139.4 ± 178.3	148.9 ± 174.5	162.8 ± 213.8	0.015

Table 1. *Cont.*

	Total	Calendar Year						*p*-Value for Trends
		2012 (*n* = 103)	2013 (*n* = 231)	2014 (*n* = 284)	2015 (*n* = 302)	2017 (*n* = 306)		
ED to CT (*n* = 1212)	18.5 ± 21.7	21.5 ± 16.1	18.4 ± 42.3	16.5 ± 12.5	17.8 ± 11.6	20.1 ± 14.1		0.450
ED to t-PA infusion (*n* = 908)	47.1 ± 23.1	56.5 ± 24.9	47.8 ± 22	47.1 ± 21.8	48.7 ± 25.5	41.1 ± 20.6		<0.001
ED to groin puncture (*n* = 593)	124.1 ± 57.7	137.2 ± 63.7	133.7 ± 66.5	131.6 ± 50.8	123.1 ± 60.3	112.8 ± 53.1		0.009
ED to final recanalization (*n* = 497)	192.3 ± 76.8	240.1 ± 99.1	206.6 ± 89.1	208.8 ± 69.2	181.8 ± 78.4	172.9 ± 62.6		<0.001
Last normal to final recanalization (*n* = 497)	389.9 ± 244.2	401.3 ± 184.8	402.1 ± 206.9	395.0 ± 249.0	395.7 ± 257.0	367.8 ± 256.6		0.127
NIHSS score at stroke onset	12 (7–17)	13 (7–18)	13 (7–17)	13 (7–18)	12 (6–17)	12 (5–16)		0.004
Treatment modality								<0.001
IV t-PA alone	633 (51.6)	58 (56.3)	144 (62.3)	154 (54.2)	172 (57.0)	105 (34.3)		
EVT alone	318 (25.9)	25 (24.3)	49 (21.2)	71 (25.0)	73 (24.2)	100 (32.7)		
EVT + IV t-PA	275 (22.4)	20 (19.4)	38 (16.5)	59 (20.8)	57 (18.9)	101 (33.0)		
Use of stentriever *	499 (48.1)	31 (68.9)	60 (69.0)	107 (82.3)	115 (88.5)	186 (92.5)		<0.001

Values are presented as *n* (%), unless otherwise indicated. ICA, internal carotid artery; MCA, middle cerebral artery; VBA, vertebrobasilar artery; ED, emergency department; NIHSS, National Institutes of Health Stroke Scale; IV, intravenous; EVT, endovascular; t-PA, tissue plasminogen activator. * Among 499 patients who received EVT with/without IV t-PA.

3.2. Secular Trends of Functional and Radiologic Outcomes

There was an increase in the number of patients who received the reperfusion therapy and the number of patients was 103 in 2012, 231 in 2013, 284 in 2014, 302 in 2015, and 306 in 2017. When we compared the baseline characteristics annually, initial diastolic blood pressure, NIHSS score at admission, and frequency of atrial fibrillation or atrial flutter decreased, while frequency of dyslipidemia or preadmission disability (mRS score of >2 before stroke) increased (Table 1). However, there were no differences in demographics or other vascular risk factors between calendar years. In time parameters, the intervals from stroke onset to arrival to emergency department (ED) increased, while those from door to initiation of IV t-PA (in 908 patients who received IV t-PA) or groin puncture (in 593 patients who received EVT) decreased over the years (all $p < 0.05$, Table 1). Especially, in 497 patients who had achieved final recanalization using EVT, the intervals from door to final recanalization [decreased from 240.1 ± 99.1 min in 2012 to 172.9 ± 62.6 min in 2017 ($p < 0.001$). During the study period, total number of stroke neurologist of study hospitals slightly increased (34 in 2012, 37 in 2013, 38 in 2014, 40 in 2015, 41 in 2017), while the number of neurointerventionalists or neurosurgeons involving EVT was similar (35 in 2012, 37 in 2013, 36 in 2014, 35 in 2015, 37 in 2017).

During the study period, patients achieved favorable functional outcome (mRS score of 0–2) in 48.6% and excellent functional outcome (mRS score of 0–1) in 31.3% at discharge. Among 1203 patients with available mRS data at 90 days, 501 (41.8%) patients achieved favorable functional outcome and 703 (58.6%) patients did excellent functional outcome at 90 days. The improvement in functional outcome at discharge after reperfusion therapy was noted as calendar year increased (Figure 2). The proportion of patients who were discharged home significantly increased (from 45.6% in 2012 to 58.5% in 2017) ($p < 0.001$). Likewise, functional outcome at 90 days was also different between calendar years ($p < 0.05$). There was an increase in favorable functional outcome (mRS score of 0–2) or excellent outcome (mRS score of 0–1) at discharge or after 90 days (all $p < 0.05$) (Table 2). In addition, the mortality rate at discharge or after 90 days significantly decreased with an increase in calendar year (all $p < 0.05$). These secular trends were consistently observed regardless of treatment modalities (Figure 2).

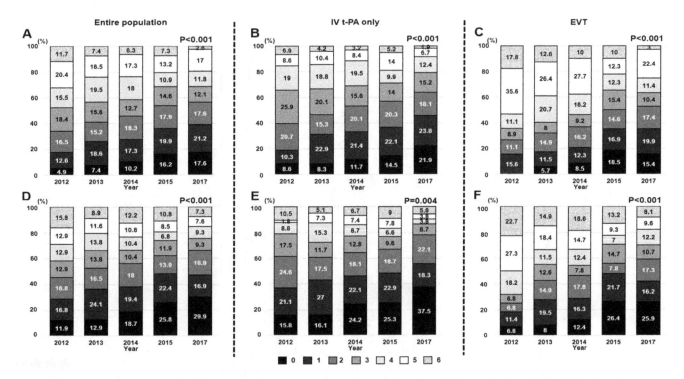

Figure 2. Secular trends in functional outcome at discharge (**A–C**) and after 90 days (**D–F**). Distribution of mRS scores of the entire population (A and D), those who received IV t-PA alone (**B,E**), and those who received EVT with/without IV t-PA (**C,F**).

Table 2. Clinical and radiologic outcome.

| | Total | Calendar Year | | | | | p-Value for Trends |
		2012	2013	2014	2015	2017	
mRS score of 0–1 at discharge	384 (31.3)	18 (17.5)	60 (26.0)	78 (27.5)	109 (36.1)	119 (38.9)	<0.001
mRS score of 0–2 at discharge	596 (48.6)	35 (34.0)	95 (41.1)	130 (45.8)	163 (54.0)	173 (56.5)	<0.001
Discharge route							0.001
Transfer to rehabilitation	168 (13.7)	18 (17.5)	25 (10.8)	42 (14.8)	27 (8.9)	56 (18.3)	
Home	662 (54.0)	47 (45.6)	114 (49.4)	140 (49.3)	182 (60.3)	179 (58.5)	
Transfer to other hospitals or departments	318 (25.9)	26 (25.2)	76 (32.9)	82 (28.9)	71 (23.5)	63 (20.6)	
Death	78 (6.4)	12 (11.7)	16 (6.9)	20 (7.0)	22 (7.3)	8 (2.6)	
mRS score of 0–1 at 90 days	501 (41.8)	29 (28.7)	83 (37.1)	106 (38.1)	142 (48.1)	141 (46.8)	<0.001
mRS score of 0–2 at 90 days	703 (58.6)	46 (45.5)	120 (53.6)	156 (56.1)	183 (62.0)	198 (65.8)	<0.001
Successful recanalization immediately after EVT	478 (80.6)	37 (82.2)	66 (75.9)	99 (76.2)	101 (77.7)	175 (87.1)	0.02
Successful recanalization within 24 h	628 (78.1)	47 (78.3)	95 (71.4)	135 (75.8)	143 (75.7)	208 (85.2)	0.004
Symptomatic intracranial hemorrhage	46 (3.8)	4 (3.9)	13 (5.6)	12 (4.2)	13 (4.3)	4 (1.3)	0.018

Values are presented as n (%), unless otherwise indicated. mRS, modified Rankin score; EVT, endovascular treatment.

Successful recanalization rate could be evaluated in 804 patients who had undergone follow-up angiographic studies within 24 h after IV t-PA therapy or EVT. The successful recanalization rate increased over time from 78.3% in 2012 to 85.2% in 2017 ($p = 0.004$) (Table 2). On the contrary, the development of symptomatic intracerebral hemorrhage has declined over time ($p = 0.018$).

3.3. Determinants of Functional Outcomes

We investigated the determinants associated with functional outcomes. The univariable analysis demonstrated that favorable outcome (mRS score of 0–2) at discharge was associated with age, male sex, diabetes, current smoking, atrial fibrillation or atrial flutter, previous stroke, preadmission disability, initial stroke severity, and intervals from stroke onset to ED or from ED to reperfusion therapy, along with the calendar year (all $p < 0.05$). Among 804 patients who had large vessel occlusion and underwent angiographic studies before and after reperfusion therapy, favorable outcome was associated with occlusion site or achievement of successful recanalization. After adjusting these significant variables ($p < 0.05$) in the univariable analysis, the independent and significant predictors for favorable functional outcome at discharge were age, diabetes, preadmission disability, initial stroke severity, intervals from door to reperfusion therapy, achievement of successful recanalization, and calendar year (Supplementary Table S1). When we investigated the independent factor for functional outcome at 90 days. the same variables were independently associated with favorable outcome at 90 days (Table 3).

Further, we performed the univariable and multivariable ordinal regression analysis to obtain a significant factor for a shift in mRS at discharge and 90 days. The independent determinants of mRS at discharge and 90 days included age, diabetes, previous stroke, preadmission disability, initial stroke severity, intervals from door to reperfusion therapy, and achievement of successful recanalization, along with the calendar year (Supplementary Table S1 and Table 3).

Table 3. Independent determinants for functional outcome at 90 days.

	Ordinal Logistic Regression (Increase in mRS)				Binary Logistic Regression (mRS ≤ 2 vs. mRS > 2)			
	OR (95% CI)	p-Value*	OR (95% CI)	p-Value†	OR (95% CI)	p-Value*	OR (95% CI)	p-Value†
Calendar year								
2012	1		1		1		1	
2013	0.882 (0.579–1.343)	0.559	0.686 (0.391–1.203)	0.188	1.209 (0.701–2.088)	0.495	1.776 (0.813–3.882)	0.15
2014	0.796 (0.529–1.198)	0.274	0.579 (0.339–0.991)	0.046	1.464 (0.857–2.501)	0.163	2.650 (1.241–5.661)	0.012
2015	0.626 (0.417–0.942)	0.025	0.525 (0.306–0.900)	0.019	1.706 (1.000–2.909)	0.05	2.014 (0.950–4.273)	0.068
2017	0.507 (0.337–0.762)	0.001	0.467 (0.276–0.791)	0.005	2.131 (1.246–3.645)	0.006	2.395 (1.142–5.023)	0.021
Age	1.03 (1.019–1.04)	<0.001	1.027 (1.014–1.039)	<0.001	0.966 (0.953–0.980)	<0.001	0.968 (0.951–0.985)	<0.001
Male sex	0.936 (0.746–1.173)	0.565	0.85 (0.642–1.125)	0.255	1.083 (0.802–1.461)	0.604	1.262 (0.857–1.859)	0.239
Diabetes	2.421 (1.955–2.997)	<0.001	2.791 (2.139–3.643)	<0.001	0.382 (0.290–0.503)	<0.001	0.329 (0.230–0.469)	<0.001
Current smoking	1.037 (0.785–1.369)	0.799	0.912 (0.634–1.313)	0.621	0.976 (0.673–1.417)	0.9	1.112 (0.672–1.842)	0.679
Atrial fibrillation or atrial flutter	0.721 (0.579–0.897)	0.003	0.8 (0.613–1.046)	0.103	1.468 (1.100–1.959)	0.009	1.216 (0.843–1.753)	0.296
Congestive heart failure	1.294 (0.823–2.035)	0.265	1.333 (0.801–2.219)	0.269				
Previous stroke	1.359 (1.05–1.759)	0.02	1.418 (1.05–1.914)	0.023	0.742 (0.530–1.039)	0.082	0.793 (0.526–1.195)	0.267
Preadmission disability	3.888 (2.268–6.673)	<0.001	2.855 (1.565–5.202)	0.001	0.094 (0.035–0.251)	<0.001	0.178 (0.062–0.510)	0.001
Last normal to ED	1.001 (1.000–1.001)	0.08	1.001 (1.000–1.001)	0.095	0.999 (0.999–1.000)	0.104	0.999 (0.999–1.000)	0.126
ED to treatment	1.003 (1.001–1.005)	0.002	1.003 (1.001–1.005)	0.002	0.996 (0.994–0.999)	0.002	0.995 (0.992–0.998)	0.001
NIHSS at stroke onset	1.119 (1.099–1.139)	<0.001	1.126 (1.100–1.152)	<0.001	0.878 (0.857–0.900)	<0.001	0.860 (0.832–0.890)	<0.001
Location site								
ICA			1				1	
MCA			0.871 (0.647–1.174)	0.365			0.834 (0.554–1.257)	0.386
VBA			1.215 (0.787–1.878)	0.379			0.723 (0.391–1.338)	0.302
Others			1.212 (0.608–2.414)	0.584			0.544 (0.211–1.403)	0.208
Successful recanalization within 24 h			0.221 (0.159–0.307)	<0.001			6.477 (4.056–10.345)	<0.001

ED, emergency department; NIHSS, National Institutes of Health Stroke Scale; ICA, internal carotid artery; MCA, middle cerebral artery; VBA, vertebrobasilar artery. * Adjusted for significant variables in the univariable analysis among the entire study population (n = 1199). † Adjusted for significant variables in the univariable analysis among patients who had arterial occlusion at initial angiographic studies and could determine whether a successful recanalization was achieved at follow-up angiographic studies (n = 783).

4. Discussion

We investigated whether clinical or radiologic outcomes after reperfusion therapy changed over time using nationwide, multicenter data covering real clinical practice between 2012 and 2017 in Korea. We demonstrated that there was an increase in the number of patients who received reperfusion therapy, especially EVT, and the clinical outcomes of patients who received reperfusion therapy significantly improved over the past five years. The favorable trend in functional outcomes may be partly ascribed to the increases in successful recanalization rate and decreases in the door-to-treatment intervals and hemorrhagic complications. Of note, the calendar year was a significant factor for functional outcome even after adjusting for significant determinants.

The rate of favorable outcome in this study was comparable to or even better than those of the previous randomized controlled trials. For example, in previous trials investigating the usefulness of IV t-PA, the proportions of patients with mRS score of 0–1 at 90 days were 39% in the National Institute of Neurological Disorders and Stroke study [13], 52.4% in ECASS III [12], and 39% in Safe Implementation of Thrombolysis in Stroke-Monitoring Study [17]. A previous study using the data of Get with the Guidelines-Stroke hospitals showed that in-hospital mortality and discharge-to-home rates were 8.25% and 42.7%, respectively, among patients received IV t-PA therapy [18].

In this analysis, 45.3% of patients had a mRS score of 0–1 at 90 days, and 62.4% of patients could be discharged to home among patients with IV t-PA alone.

The meta-analysis of pooled patient data from five randomized trials after 2015 showed that 46% of patients achieved mRS score of 0–2 at 90 days [4]. In our patients who received EVT with/without IV t-PA, 50.7% of patients had an mRS score of 0–2 at 90 days. In addition, successful recanalization rate in our study population was 83%–87%, which was similar to those in recent EVT trials [19]. Although comparison of clinical outcomes between studies might be difficult because of different patient characteristics, feasibilities of procedures, types of devices, or treatment modalities between studies, our data suggested the benefits of current reperfusion therapy can be reproduced in the real clinical practice.

Our study also demonstrated that some characteristics of patients who received the reperfusion therapy have changed. Although age, vascular risk factors other than dyslipidemia, and occlusion site did not change over time, stroke severity slightly decreased. This may be ascribed to the increase in reperfusion therapy for minor stroke and decrease in the prevalence of atrial fibrillation- or atrial flutter-related stroke [20,21]. Furthermore, time from stroke onset to ED was longer than those in previous studies because patient eligibility for EVT might be based more on imaging parameters recently, instead of the time window paradigm [22]. Increase in the intervals from stroke onset to arrival to ED over years might be partly because more patients with delayed presentation to ED might have been treated with the reperfusion therapy over the years, thanks to advances in selection of patients by multimodal neuroimaging.

In this study, we reaffirm the importance of earlier treatment and achieving successful recanalization to improve patient outcome. Reducing the time from stroke onset to treatment is beneficial to not only reduce the ischemic core but also to remove thrombus [23–25]. Earlier treatment would also reduce the risk of symptomatic intracranial hemorrhage. [26,27] In Korea, there have been continuing efforts on reducing the time delay for patients with stroke using the stroke code system based on the computerized physician order entry system [9,27]. Actually, our data showed that mean time from door to initiation of treatment was continuously decreasing (up to 41.1 min for IV t-PA or 113 min for groin puncture).

Moreover, completely reopening the occluded artery is known as one of the essential components in reperfusion therapy [5]. Currently, the stentriever is the most commonly preferred device in approximately 90% of hospitals in Korea [8]. Stentriever use had some advantages such as easy handling, faster and complete reperfusion, temporal opening, and lesser bleeding complications [28,29]. There were increasing trends in successful recanalization (up to 87% in 2017) and rapid recanalization (mean intervals from door to final recanalization from 240.1 min in 2014 to 173 min in 2017) and decreasing trends in symptomatic intracranial hemorrhage, which might be related with growing use of stentriever over time in Korea.

The calendar year was one of significant factors for favorable outcome even after adjusting for significant variables including age, initial stroke severity, comorbidities, and time from door to needle or achievement of successful recanalization. This implied that the advances in certain factors over time could also play a role for these trends. First, optimal medical treatment before and after reperfusion therapy would prevent complications or early neurologic deterioration and favorably affect the outcome. In this context, the role of the stroke team is important even in the era of EVT for acute stroke. Over the past decades, there has been an improvement in stroke care in Korea: Increase in stroke unit-based centers, multidisciplinary stroke team, guideline-based clinical practice, certification of stroke center, use of antithrombotics or statin in preventing stroke, development of networks among regional comprehensive and primary stroke centers, and provision of nationwide quality care for stroke [10,30–32]. Additionally, there was a possibility of advancement in the selection of eligible candidates who would benefit from reperfusion therapy. Many stroke centers in Korea use imaging parameters, such as collateral status, diffusion/perfusion mismatch, clot characteristics, or ASPECTS score, for identifying patients who are more suitable for reperfusion therapy [8,33].

There are some limitations to this study. First, the decision regarding the method of reperfusion therapy was based on discretion of the stroke neurologist or neurointerventionalist at each study center. The selection of EVT device, number of EVT passes, and use of balloon-guided catheter was not standardized. However, most stroke centers are collaborative in terms of sharing experience and protocols. Second, there were some unmeasured variables, such as socioeconomic status, educational level, and medication adherence before/after stroke, that could affect the functional outcome after stroke.

5. Conclusions

Our analysis demonstrated the increase in favorable outcomes among patients who received reperfusion therapy in Korea. There were a changing patterns, such as an improvement in time parameters, increase in successful recanalization rate, and decrease in bleeding complication rate, leading to the improvement in stroke metrics. However, there is still room for additional efforts, such as rapid notification or communication, for reduction in time delay before arrival to the hospital. Our data also suggest the need for support of personnel or infrastructure to continue the optimum treatment.

Author Contributions: Conceptualization: Y.D.K., H.S.N.; methodology: Y.D.K., J.H.H., H.S.L., H.S.N.; formal analysis: Y.D.K., H.S.L.; investigation: Y.D.K., J.H.H., J.Y., H.P., B.M.K., O.Y.B., H.C.K., E.H., D.J.K., J.H., M.K., J.K.C., K.-Y.L., H.S.L., D.H.S., H.-Y.C., S.-I.S., J.-H.H., J.-H.B., G.S.K., W.-K.S., J.-W.C., S.H.K., T.-J.S., S.W.H., J.H.P., J.K., Y.H.J., H.-J.C., S.H.A., S.I.L., K.-D.S., H.S.N.; data curation: Y.D.K., J.H.H., J.Y., H.P., B.M.K., O.Y.B., H.C.K., E.H., D.J.K., J.H., M.K., J.K.C., K.-Y.L., H.S.L., D.H.S., H.-Y.C., S.-I.S., J.-H.H., J.-H.B., G.S.K., W.-K.S., J.-W.C., S.H.K., T.-J.S., S.W.H., J.H.P., J.K., Y.H.J., H.-J.C., S.H.A., S.I.L., K.-D.S., H.S.N.; writing—original draft preparation: Y.D.K., H.S.N.; writing—review and editing: Y.D.K., J.H.H., J.Y., H.P., B.M.K., O.Y.B., H.C.K., E.H., D.J.K., J.H., M.K., J.K.C., K.-Y.L., H.S.L., D.H.S., H.-Y.C., S.-I.S., J.-H.H., J.-H.B., G.S.K., W.-K.S., J.-W.C., S.H.K., T.-J.S., S.W.H., J.H.P., J.K., Y.H.J., H.-J.C., S.H.A., S.I.L., K.-D.S., H.S.N.; supervision: H.J.J., H.S.N.; funding acquisition: H.S.N. All authors have read and agreed to the published version of the manuscript.

References

1.   Wang, H.; Naghavi, M.; Allen, C.; Barber, R.M.; Bhutta, Z.A. Global, regional, and national life expectancy, all-cause mortality, and cause-specific mortality for 249 causes of death, 1980–2015: A systematic analysis for the global burden of disease study 2015. *Lancet (Lond. Engl.)* **2016**, *388*, 1459–1544. [CrossRef]

2.   Kassebaum, N.J.; Arora, M.; Barber, R.M.; Bhutta, Z.A.; Brown, J.; Carter, A.; Casey, D.C.; Charlson, F.J.; Coates, M.M.; Coggeshall, M.; et al. Global, regional, and national disability-adjusted life-years (dalys) for 315 diseases and injuries and healthy life expectancy (hale), 1990–2015: A systematic analysis for the global burden of disease study 2015. *Lancet* **2016**, *388*, 1603–1658. [CrossRef]

3.   Donnan, G.A.; Fisher, M.; Macleod, M.; Davis, S.M. Stroke. *Lancet (Lond. Engl.)* **2008**, *371*, 1612–1623. [CrossRef]

4.   Goyal, M.; Menon, B.K.; van Zwam, W.H.; Dippel, D.W.; Mitchell, P.J.; Demchuk, A.M.; Davalos, A.; Majoie, C.B.; van der Lugt, A.; de Miquel, M.A.; et al. Endovascular thrombectomy after large-vessel ischaemic stroke: A meta-analysis of individual patient data from five randomised trials. *Lancet (Lond. Engl.)* **2016**, *387*, 1723–1731. [CrossRef]

5.   Rha, J.H.; Saver, J.L. The impact of recanalization on ischemic stroke outcome: A meta-analysis. *Stroke* **2007**, *38*, 967–973. [CrossRef] [PubMed]

6.   Fargen, K.M.; Meyers, P.M.; Khatri, P.; Mocco, J. Improvements in recanalization with modern stroke therapy: A review of prospective ischemic stroke trials during the last two decades. *J. Neurointerv. Surg.* **2013**, *5*, 506–511. [CrossRef]

7.   Jansen, I.G.H.; Mulder, M.; Goldhoorn, R.B.; investigators, M.C.R. Endovascular treatment for acute ischaemic stroke in routine clinical practice: Prospective, observational cohort study (mr clean registry). *BMJ* **2018**, *360*, k949. [CrossRef]

8.   Seo, K.-D.; Suh, S.H. Endovascular treatment in acute ischemic stroke: A nationwide survey in korea. *Neurointervention* **2018**, *13*, 84–89. [CrossRef]

9.   Heo, J.H.; Kim, Y.D.; Nam, H.S.; Hong, K.S.; Ahn, S.H.; Cho, H.J.; Choi, H.Y.; Han, S.W.; Cha, M.J.; Hong, J.M.; et al. A computerized in-hospital alert system for thrombolysis in acute stroke. *Stroke* **2010**, *41*, 1978–1983. [CrossRef]

10. Kim, J.Y.; Kang, K.; Kang, J.; Koo, J.; Kim, D.H.; Kim, B.J.; Kim, W.J.; Kim, E.G.; Kim, J.G.; Kim, J.M.; et al. Executive summary of stroke statistics in korea 2018: A report from the epidemiology research council of the korean stroke society. *J. Stroke* **2019**, *21*, 42–59. [CrossRef]

11. Goldstein, L.B.; Samsa, G.P.; Matchar, D.B.; Horner, R.D. Charlson index comorbidity adjustment for ischemic stroke outcome studies. *Stroke* **2004**, *35*, 1941–1945. [CrossRef]

12. Hacke, W.; Kaste, M.; Bluhmki, E.; Brozman, M.; Dávalos, A.; Guidetti, D.; Larrue, V.; Lees, K.R.; Medeghri, Z.; Machnig, T.; et al. Thrombolysis with alteplase 3 to 4.5 h after acute ischemic stroke. *N. Engl. J. Med.* **2008**, *359*, 1317–1329. [CrossRef] [PubMed]

13. Tissue Plasminogen Activator for Acute Ischemic Stroke. The national institute of neurological disorders and stroke rt-pa stroke study group. *N. Engl. J. Med.* **1995**, *333*, 1581–1587.

14. Jauch, E.C.; Saver, J.L.; Adams, H.P.; Bruno, A.; Connors, J.J.; Demaerschalk, B.M.; Khatri, P.; McMullan, P.W.; Qureshi, A.I.; Rosenfield, K.; et al. Guidelines for the early management of patients with acute ischemic stroke: A guideline for healthcare professionals from the american heart association/american stroke association. *Stroke* **2013**, *44*, 870–947. [CrossRef] [PubMed]

15. Kernan, W.N.; Ovbiagele, B.; Black, H.R.; Bravata, D.M.; Chimowitz, M.I.; Ezekowitz, M.D.; Fang, M.C.; Fisher, M.; Furie, K.L.; Heck, D.V.; et al. Guidelines for the prevention of stroke in patients with stroke and transient ischemic attack: A guideline for healthcare professionals from the american heart association/american stroke association. *Stroke* **2014**, *45*, 2160–2236. [CrossRef] [PubMed]

16. Higashida, R.T.; Furlan, A.J. Trial design and reporting standards for intra-arterial cerebral thrombolysis for acute ischemic stroke. *Stroke* **2003**, *34*, e109–e137. [CrossRef] [PubMed]

17. Wahlgren, N.; Ahmed, N.; Davalos, A.; Ford, G.A.; Grond, M.; Hacke, W.; Hennerici, M.G.; Kaste, M.; Kuelkens, S.; Larrue, V.; et al. Thrombolysis with alteplase for acute ischaemic stroke in the safe implementation of thrombolysis in stroke-monitoring study (sits-most): An observational study. *Lancet* **2007**, *369*, 275–282. [CrossRef]

18. Fonarow, G.C.; Zhao, X.; Smith, E.E.; Saver, J.L.; Reeves, M.J.; Bhatt, D.L.; Xian, Y.; Hernandez, A.F.; Peterson, E.D.; Schwamm, L.H. Door-to-needle times for tissue plasminogen activator administration and clinical outcomes in acute ischemic stroke before and after a quality improvement initiative. *JAMA* **2014**, *311*, 1632–1640. [CrossRef]

19. Hong, K.S.; Ko, S.B.; Lee, J.S.; Yu, K.H.; Rha, J.H. Endovascular recanalization therapy in acute ischemic stroke: Updated meta-analysis of randomized controlled trials. *J. Stroke* **2015**, *17*, 268–281. [CrossRef]

20. Baek, J.H.; Kim, B.M. Angiographical identification of intracranial, atherosclerosis-related, large vessel occlusion in endovascular treatment. *Front. Neurol.* **2019**, *10*, 298. [CrossRef]

21. Yoo, J.; Sohn, S.I.; Kim, J.; Ahn, S.H.; Lee, K.; Baek, J.H.; Kim, K.; Hong, J.H.; Koo, J.; Kim, Y.D.; et al. Delayed intravenous thrombolysis in patients with minor stroke. *Cerebrovasc. Dis.* **2018**, *46*, 52–58. [CrossRef] [PubMed]

22. Kim, J.T.; Cho, B.H.; Choi, K.H.; Park, M.S.; Kim, B.J.; Park, J.M.; Kang, K.; Lee, S.J.; Kim, J.G.; Cha, J.K.; et al. Magnetic resonance imaging versus computed tomography angiography based selection for endovascular therapy in patients with acute ischemic stroke. *Stroke* **2019**, *50*, 365–372. [CrossRef] [PubMed]

23. Meretoja, A.; Keshtkaran, M.; Saver, J.L.; Tatlisumak, T.; Parsons, M.W.; Kaste, M.; Davis, S.M.; Donnan, G.A.; Churilov, L. Stroke thrombolysis: Save a minute, save a day. *Stroke* **2014**, *45*, 1053–1058. [CrossRef] [PubMed]

24. Kim, Y.D.; Nam, H.S.; Kim, S.H.; Kim, E.Y.; Song, D.; Kwon, I.; Yang, S.H.; Lee, K.; Yoo, J.; Lee, H.S.; et al. Time-dependent thrombus resolution after tissue-type plasminogen activator in patients with stroke and mice. *Stroke* **2015**, *46*, 1877–1882. [CrossRef]

25. Bourcier, R.; Goyal, M.; Liebeskind, D.S.; Muir, K.W.; Desal, H.; Siddiqui, A.H.; Dippel, D.W.J.; Majoie, C.B.; van Zwam, W.H.; Jovin, T.G.; et al. Association of time from stroke onset to groin puncture with quality of reperfusion after mechanical thrombectomy: A meta-analysis of individual patient data from 7 randomized clinical trials. *JAMA Neurol.* **2019**, *76*, 405–411. [CrossRef] [PubMed]

26. Fonarow, G.C.; Smith, E.E.; Saver, J.L.; Reeves, M.J.; Bhatt, D.L.; Grau-Sepulveda, M.V.; Olson, D.M.; Hernandez, A.F.; Peterson, E.D.; Schwamm, L.H. Timeliness of tissue-type plasminogen activator therapy in acute ischemic stroke: Patient characteristics, hospital factors, and outcomes associated with door-to-needle times within 60 min. *Circulation* **2011**, *123*, 750–758. [CrossRef] [PubMed]

27. Jeon, S.B.; Ryoo, S.M.; Lee, D.H.; Kwon, S.U.; Jang, S.; Lee, E.J.; Lee, S.H.; Han, J.H.; Yoon, M.J.; Jeong, S.; et al. Multidisciplinary approach to decrease in-hospital delay for stroke thrombolysis. *J. Stroke* **2017**, *19*, 196–204. [CrossRef]

28. Song, D.; Heo, J.H.; Kim, D.I.; Kim, D.J.; Kim, B.M.; Lee, K.; Yoo, J.; Lee, H.S.; Nam, H.S.; Kim, Y.D. Impact of temporary opening using a stent retriever on clinical outcome in acute ischemic stroke. *PLoS ONE* **2015**, *10*, e0124551. [CrossRef]

29. Touma, L.; Filion, K.B.; Sterling, L.H.; Atallah, R.; Windle, S.B.; Eisenberg, M.J. Stent retrievers for the treatment of acute ischemic stroke: A systematic review and meta-analysis of randomized clinical trials. *JAMA Neurol.* **2016**, *73*, 275–281. [CrossRef]

30. Choi, H.Y.; Cha, M.J.; Nam, H.S.; Kim, Y.D.; Hong, K.S.; Heo, J.H.; Korean Stroke Unit Study, C. Stroke units and stroke care services in korea. *Int. J. Stroke* **2012**, *7*, 336–340. [CrossRef]

31. Kim, Y.D.; Jung, Y.H.; Saposnik, G. Traditional risk factors for stroke in east asia. *J. Stroke* **2016**, *18*, 273–285. [CrossRef] [PubMed]

32. Kim, J.; Hwang, Y.H.; Kim, J.T.; Choi, N.C.; Kang, S.Y.; Cha, J.K.; Ha, Y.S.; Shin, D.I.; Kim, S.; Lim, B.H. Establishment of government-initiated comprehensive stroke centers for acute ischemic stroke management in south korea. *Stroke* **2014**, *45*, 2391–2396. [CrossRef] [PubMed]

33. Yoo, J.; Baek, J.H.; Park, H.; Song, D.; Kim, K.; Hwang, I.G.; Kim, Y.D.; Kim, S.H.; Lee, H.S.; Ahn, S.H.; et al. Thrombus volume as a predictor of nonrecanalization after intravenous thrombolysis in acute stroke. *Stroke* **2018**, *49*, 2108–2115. [CrossRef] [PubMed]

10

Utility of Leptomeningeal Collaterals in Predicting Intracranial Atherosclerosis-Related Large Vessel Occlusion in Endovascular Treatment

Jang-Hyun Baek [1,2]**, Byung Moon Kim** [3,*]**, Jin Woo Kim** [4]**, Dong Joon Kim** [3]**, Ji Hoe Heo** [2]**, Hyo Suk Nam** [2] **and Young Dae Kim** [2]

[1] Department of Neurology, Kangbuk Samsung Hospital, Sungkyunkwan University School of Medicine, Seoul 03181, Korea; janghyun.baek@gmail.com

[2] Department of Neurology, Severance Stroke Center, Severance Hospital, Yonsei University College of Medicine, Seoul 03722, Korea; jhheo@yuhs.ac (J.H.H.); hsnam@yuhs.ac (H.S.N.); neuro05@yuhs.ac (Y.D.K.)

[3] Interventional Neuroradiology, Severance Stroke Center, Severance Hospital, Department of Radiology, Yonsei University College of Medicine, Seoul 03722, Korea; djkimmd@yuhs.ac

[4] Department of Radiology, Gangnam Severance Hospital, Yonsei University College of Medicine, Seoul 06273, Korea; sunny-cocktail@hanmail.net

* Correspondence: bmoon21@hanmail.net

Abstract: Earlier or preprocedural identification of occlusion pathomechanism is crucial for effective endovascular treatment. As leptomeningeal collaterals tend to develop well in chronic ischemic conditions such as intracranial atherosclerosis (ICAS), we investigated whether leptomeningeal collaterals can be a preprocedural marker of ICAS-related large vessel occlusion (ICAS-LVO) in endovascular treatment. A total of 226 patients who underwent endovascular treatment were retrospectively reviewed. We compared the pattern of leptomeningeal collaterals between patients with ICAS-LVO and without. Leptomeningeal collaterals were assessed by preprocedural computed tomography angiography (CTA) and basically categorized by three different collateral assessment methods. Better leptomeningeal collaterals were significantly associated with ICAS-LVO, although they were not independent for ICAS-LVO. When leptomeningeal collaterals were dichotomized to incomplete (<100%) and complete (100%), the latter was significantly more frequent in patients with ICAS-LVO (52.5% versus 20.4%) and remained an independent factor for ICAS-LVO (odds ratio, 3.32; 95% confidence interval, 1.52–7.26; p = 0.003). The area under the curve (AUC) value of complete leptomeningeal collateral supply was 0.660 for discrimination of ICAS-LVO. Incomplete leptomeningeal collateral supply was not likely ICAS-LVO, based on the high negative predictive value (88.6%). Considering its negative predictive value and the independent association between complete leptomeningeal collateral supply and ICAS-LVO, leptomeningeal collaterals could be helpful in the preprocedural determination of occlusion pathomechanism.

Keywords: atherosclerosis; computed tomography angiography; stroke; thrombectomy

1. Introduction

Mechanical thrombectomy has been primarily considered in most cases of endovascular treatment of acute intracranial large vessel occlusion [1]. However, mechanical thrombectomy might not be an optimal modality for a specific occlusion pathomechanism—that is, an in situ thrombo-occlusion of underlying intracranial atherosclerosis (intracranial atherosclerosis-related large vessel occlusion (ICAS-LVO)) [2,3]. ICAS-LVO is not a rare condition. In the Asian population, up to 30% of patients might have ICAS-LVO for their occlusion pathomechanism in endovascular treatment of anterior circulation [4]. More importantly, conventional mechanical thrombectomy modalities, such as stent retriever and thrombaspiration, are ineffective in ICAS-LVO. Mechanical thrombectomy was effective only in less than 20% of ICAS-LVO cases. Due to frequent reocclusion events, specific rescue endovascular modalities (i.e., intra-arterial glycoprotein IIb/IIIa inhibitor, balloon angioplasty, and intracranial stenting) were inevitable in most cases to achieve significant recanalization in ICAS-LVO [5–9].

On this point, earlier strategical consideration is crucial to shorten the time to recanalization [4]. For earlier strategical consideration, it could be more helpful if the occlusion pathomechanism is determined before endovascular treatment. However, the completion of such a preprocedural determination is challenging as the information available before endovascular treatment can be limited. In clinical practice, we are able to rely on only a few preprocedural clinical and imaging findings [7,10]. However, further reliable methods are sparse.

Leptomeningeal collaterals are one of the preprocedural factors which are potentially able to predict occlusion pathomechanism. Nevertheless, their association has not been clearly evaluated yet. Several experimental and clinical findings led us to focus on leptomeningeal collaterals. In these experimental findings, the vascular bed was more developed in chronic or long-term ischemic conditions [11–13]. Similarly, in patients with an intracranial stenosis due to ICAS, leptomeningeal collaterals were prominently developed to compensate for the diminished cerebral blood flow under chronic ischemia [11,12]. In one report, full and rapid leptomeningeal collateral filling was commented on as a finding, which suggests ICAS-LVO [7]. However, no specific evidence supported this comment. Instead, it was reported that initial infarct volume was smaller among patients with an ICAS-LVO. This merely indirectly suggested that leptomeningeal collaterals were better in ICAS-LVO [7,14].

If leptomeningeal collaterals are discriminatorily developed in patients with ICAS, we believe that they may be an indirect finding for ICAS-LVO. Thus, we hypothesized that (1) leptomeningeal collaterals would be different according to the occlusion pathomechanism—that is, robust or better leptomeningeal collaterals are associated with ICAS-LVO, and (2) based on this association, we could predict ICAS-LVO before endovascular treatment. Accordingly, this study aimed to evaluate (1) the association between leptomeningeal collaterals and ICAS-LVO, and (2) the predictability of preprocedural leptomeningeal collaterals for ICAS-LVO.

2. Methods

We retrospectively reviewed consecutive acute stroke patients between January 2010 and December 2018 who underwent endovascular treatment of intracranial vessel occlusion. Patients were selected from a prospective registry of a tertiary stroke center (Severance Stroke Center, Severance Hospital, Seoul, Korea). The registry consists of consecutive patients who underwent endovascular treatment, which was considered by the following criteria: (1) a computed tomography angiography (CTA)-determined, endovascularly accessible intracranial LVO associated with neurological symptoms; (2) within 8 h from stroke onset, though, in the later study period, patients falling within the window of 8 h to 12 h from stroke onset were also considered if they had an Alberta Stroke Program Early CT Score of seven points or more on initial non-contrast CT; and (3) a baseline National Institutes of Health Stroke Scale (NIHSS) score of four points or more. For patients eligible for intravenous tissue-type plasminogen activator treatment, the full dose of tissue-type plasminogen activator (0.9 mg/kg) was administered.

For this study, patients who had an M1 occlusion and CTA performed before endovascular treatment were selected from the registry. Conversely, those who presented with an internal carotid artery occlusion were excluded, as collateral flows through anterior or posterior communicating arteries can contribute to lesion-side cerebral flow. Additionally, patients with an occlusion of the distal artery or posterior circulation were also excluded because leptomeningeal collaterals could not be determined reliably in this population. We did not include patients with multiple intracranial artery occlusions because they could also affect leptomeningeal collaterals on middle cerebral artery territory.

The institutional review board approved this study and waived the requirement for obtaining informed consent prior to study inclusion based on the retrospective design.

2.1. Assessment of Leptomeningeal Collaterals (Collateral Assessment Methods)

Leptomeningeal collaterals were determined by CTA performed immediately before endovascular treatment. CTA collateral grade was assessed on 20-mm thickness maximum intensity projection images of single-phase CTA. In patients who underwent multiphase CTA imaging, we only used the first-phase images to evaluate leptomeningeal collaterals.

From among the various existing CTA-based collateral assessment methods, three different methods were adopted [15–17]. First, leptomeningeal collaterals were primarily assessed by a four-scale method previously reported as follows: (1) absent collateral supply to the occluded middle cerebral artery (MCA) territory of 0%, (2) collateral supply of greater than 0% but less than or equal to 50%, (3) collateral supply of greater than 50% but less than 100%, and (4) complete collateral supply of 100% (collateral assessment method 1; Tan's method; Figure 1) [15]. Second, the four grades were regrouped into a three-scale grade system as follows: (1) absent collateral supply to the occluded MCA territory of 0%, (2) collateral supply of greater than 0% but less than 100%, and (3) complete collateral supply of 100% (collateral assessment method 2; shortened from Mass' method) [16]. Third, the four grades were simply dichotomized into (1) collateral supply of 50% or less of the occluded MCA territory and (2) collateral supply of more than 50% (collateral assessment method 3; modified Tan's method) [17]. The four-scale grade of leptomeningeal collaterals was determined by two independent interventional neuroradiologists who were blinded to the clinical and procedural information. The kappa value for the interrater agreement was 0.85 (95% confidence interval, 0.79–0.91), which was similar to its original report [15]. Discrepant cases were resolved by consensus.

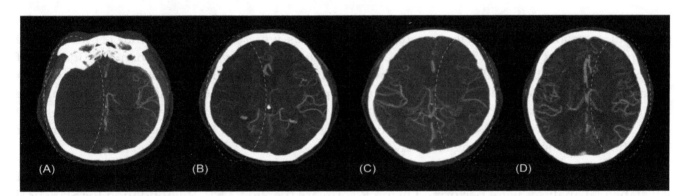

Figure 1. Assessment of leptomeningeal collaterals according to collateral assessment method 1 (Tan et al.'s method). Four computed tomography angiography maximum intensity projection axial images from different patients showing leptomeningeal collaterals. (**A**) Absent collateral supply to the occluded middle cerebral artery territory (circle), compared to the contralateral normal side. (**B**) Collateral supply of greater than 0% but less than or equal to 50%. (**C**) Collateral supply of greater than 50% but less than 100%. (**D**) Complete collateral supply of 100%.

2.2. Identification of ICAS-LVO

ICAS-LVO was determined angiographically. If the occlusion site was completely recanalized without any residual stenosis and reocclusion tendency, the occlusion pathomechanism was not considered as ICAS. In contrast, when significant fixed focal stenosis was noted on angiography, the case was considered as positive for ICAS-LVO [7]. For intractable cases whose occlusion was never recanalized, so that the focal stenosis could not be evaluated, occlusion at the arterial trunk was determined as indicative of ICAS-LVO [6]. ICAS-LVO was assessed independently by two other interventional neuroradiologists who were blinded to the CTA findings and clinical information. The kappa value for the interrater agreement was 0.92 (95% confidence interval, 0.86–0.98). Discrepant cases were also resolved by consensus.

2.3. Statistical Analysis

Based on the identification of ICAS-LVO, patients were assigned to the ICAS group or the non-ICAS group. First, we evaluated the association between leptomeningeal collaterals as determined by the three collateral assessment methods and ICAS-LVO. In this process, (1) basic demographics (age and sex), risk factors for atherosclerosis (hypertension diabetes, dyslipidemia, smoking, and coronary artery disease), typical clinical factors associated with occlusion pathomechanism (atrial fibrillation and initial NIHSS score), and leptomeningeal collaterals by each collateral assessment method were compared between the ICAS and non-ICAS groups. The Mann–Whitney U test, chi-squared test, and Fisher's exact test were used for comparison. Also, we summarized the study population by descriptive statistics. Continuous variables were expressed by a mean value with standard deviation or a median value with interquartile range, as appropriate. Categorical variables were expressed by a frequency with its percentage. Then, (2) to see whether better leptomeningeal collaterals were associated with ICAS-LVO, we performed binary logistic regression analyses for each collateral assessment method. To determine whether better leptomeningeal collaterals can be an independent variable for ICAS-LVO, variables with a p-value < 0.10 in the univariable analysis were entered into the multivariable model. Finally, (3) to evaluate the predictive power of leptomeningeal collaterals for ICAS-LVO, we calculated the sensitivity, specificity, positive predictive value (PPV), negative predictive value (NPV), and accuracy of each collateral assessment method. Receiver operating characteristic curve analyses were also performed to calculate the area under the curve (AUC) values and cutoff points, which were determined based on Youden's index.

Second, based on the results of logistic regression analyses and calculated cutoff points of each collateral assessment method, leptomeningeal collaterals were dichotomized into (1) incomplete collateral supply of less than 100% or (2) complete collateral supply of 100%. Then, the findings of complete and incomplete collateral supplies were compared between the ICAS and non-ICAS groups. To see whether complete leptomeningeal collateral supply was associated with ICAS-LVO, univariable and multivariable binary logistic regression analyses were performed in the same manner as the three collateral assessment methods. We also calculated sensitivity, PPV, NPV, accuracy, and AUC value for the dichotomization in predicting ICAS-LVO.

A p-value < 0.05 was considered statistically significant for the 95% confidence interval. All statistical analyses were performed using R software (version 3.5.0; R Foundation for Statistical Computing, Vienna, Austria).

3. Results

Among the 604 patients that underwent endovascular treatment for an intracranial vessel occlusion, 226 patients (mean age 69.0 ± 12.1 years; 54.4% male) were included (Figure 2). Patients with arterial dissection ($n = 5$), distal artery occlusion ($n = 132$), internal carotid artery occlusion ($n = 154$), and vertebrobasilar artery occlusion ($n = 79$) were excluded. In eight patients, leptomeningeal collaterals could not be determined by CTA because the arterial target was changed between CTA and endovascular treatment ($n = 2$; internal carotid artery occlusion on initial CTA was changed to M1 occlusion on cerebral angiography) or CTA was not performed before endovascular treatment ($n = 6$). Leptomeningeal collaterals were 0% in the occluded MCA territory in 15 patients (6.6%), greater than 0% but less than or equal to 50% in 57 (25.2%), greater than 50% but less than 100% in 95 (42.1%), and 100% in 59 (26.1%).

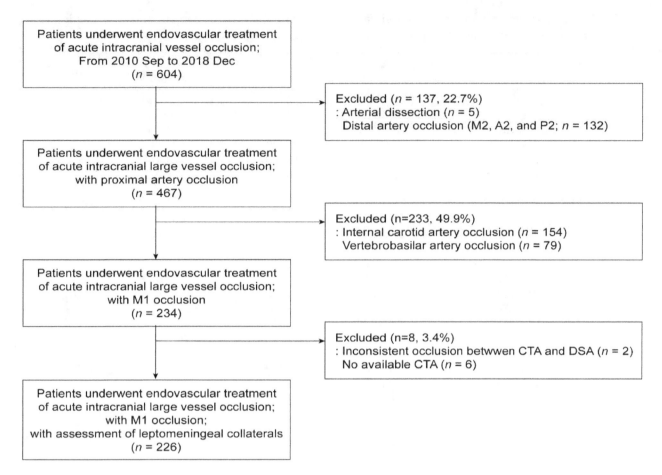

Figure 2. Patients selection flow chart. DSA, digital subtraction angiography.

3.1. Association Between Leptomeningeal Collaterals and ICAS-LVO

A total of 40 patients (17.7%) showed an ICAS-LVO as the occlusion pathomechanism. Based on the use of collateral assessment methods 1 and 2, patients with leptomeningeal collaterals of 0%, greater than 0% but less than or equal to 50%, and greater than 50% but less than 100% of occluded MCA territory were less common in the ICAS group, whereas cases of complete (100%) leptomeningeal collaterals were significantly more frequently found in the ICAS group (52.5% versus 20.4%; $p < 0.001$; Table 1). For collateral assessment method 3, more patients in the ICAS group had leptomeningeal collaterals of greater than 50% than the non-ICAS group (85.0% versus 64.5%; $p = 0.012$).

Table 1. Comparison of demographics, risk factors for stroke and atherosclerosis, and leptomeningeal collaterals between intracranial atherosclerosis (ICAS) and non-ICAS groups.

	All (n = 226)	ICAS (n = 40)	Non-ICAS (n = 186)	p-Value
Age, years	69.0 (±12.1)	66.2 (±16.4)	69.6 (±10.9)	0.222
Male sex	123 (54.4)	20 (50.0)	103 (55.4)	0.536
Hypertension	166 (73.5)	32 (80.0)	134 (72.0)	0.301
Diabetes	66 (29.2)	13 (32.5)	53 (28.5)	0.613
Dyslipidemia	48 (21.2)	12 (30.0)	36 (19.4)	0.135
Current smoking	42 (18.6)	16 (40.0)	26 (14.0)	<0.001
Coronary artery disease	52 (23.0)	11 (27.5)	41 (22.0)	0.457
Atrial fibrillation	119 (52.7)	11 (27.5)	108 (58.1)	<0.001
Initial NIHSS score	15.0 (11.0; 19.0)	12.0 (7.0; 17.0)	15.0 (12.0; 19.0)	0.001
Leptomeningeal collaterals Three assessment methods Method 1 (Tan)				
0%	15 (6.6)	1 (2.5)	14 (7.5)	<0.001
>0% but ≤50%	57 (25.2)	5 (12.5)	52 (28.0)	
>50% but <100%	95 (42.1)	13 (32.5)	82 (44.1)	
100%	59 (26.1)	21 (52.5)	38 (20.4)	
Method 2 (shortened Maas)				
0%	15 (6.6)	1 (2.5)	14 (7.5)	<0.001
>0% but <100%	152 (67.3)	18 (45.0)	134 (72.1)	
100%	59 (26.1)	21 (52.5)	38 (20.4)	
Method 3 (modified Tan)				
≤50%	72 (31.9)	6 (15.0)	66 (35.5)	0.012
>50%	154 (68.1)	34 (85.0)	120 (64.5)	
Dichotomization by cutoff				
Incomplete (<100%)	167 (73.9)	19 (47.5)	148 (79.6)	<0.001
Complete (100%)	59 (26.1)	21 (52.5)	38 (20.4)	

Age is represented by a mean value (±standard deviation); initial National Institutes of Health Stroke Scale (NIHSS) score by a median value (first and third quartile); all other variables by the number of patients (frequency, %).

On the logistic regression analyses for collateral assessment methods 1, 2, and 3, odds ratios for ICAS-LVO gradually increased as leptomeningeal collaterals improved (Figure 3). However, none were statistically significant in univariable and multivariable analyses (Table S1 and Figure 3). For multivariable analyses, each collateral assessment method was adjusted by current smoking, atrial fibrillation, and initial NIHSS score.

(A)

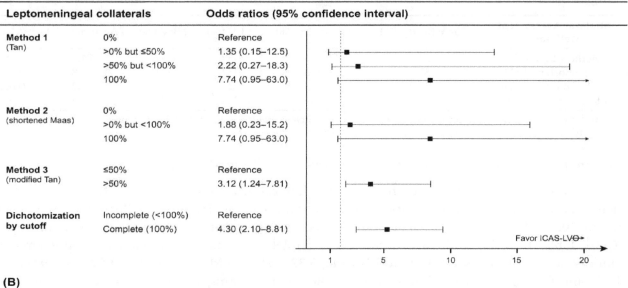

(B)

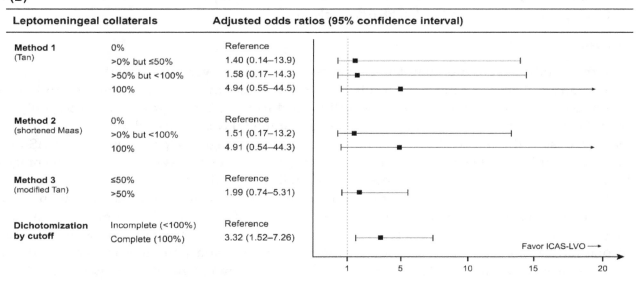

Figure 3. Univariable and multivariable logistic regression analyses of leptomeningeal collaterals for intracranial atherosclerosis-related large vessel occlusion (ICAS-LVO). Odds ratios with 95% confidence intervals from (**A**) univariable and (**B**) multivariable logistic regression analyses are plotted. In multivariable analyses, each leptomeningeal collateral assessment method was adjusted by current smoking, atrial fibrillation, and initial NIHSS score.

3.2. Predictive Power of Leptomeningeal Collaterals for ICAS-LVO

For collateral assessment methods 1 and 2, the calculated sensitivity, specificity, PPV, and NPV of leptomeningeal collaterals to predict ICAS-LVO were 52.5%, 79.6%, 35.6%, and 88.6%, respectively (Table 2). Collateral assessment method 3 showed higher sensitivity and lower specificity for ICAS-LVO than collateral assessment methods 1 and 2. AUC values of leptomeningeal collaterals were below 0.7 for all collateral assessment methods (each $p < 0.001$).

Table 2. Diagnostic performance of leptomeningeal collaterals for intracranial atherosclerosis-related large vessel occlusion.

Collateral Assessment Methods	Sensitivity (%)	Specificity (%)	PPV (%)	NPV (%)	Accuracy (%)	AUC
Method 1 (Tan) [1]	52.5	79.6	35.6	88.6	74.8	0.686
Method 2 (shortened Maas) [1]	52.5	79.6	35.6	88.6	74.8	0.668
Method 3 (modified Tan) [2]	85.0	35.5	22.1	91.7	44.2	0.602
Dichotomization by cutoff [1]	52.5	79.6	35.6	88.6	74.8	0.660

[1] For leptomeningeal collaterals of 100%; [2] for leptomeningeal collaterals of > 50%; PPV, positive predictive value; NPV, negative predictive value; AUC, area under curve.

3.3. Significance of Complete Leptomeningeal Collaterals in Predicting ICAS-LVO

Based on the results from the analyses of collateral assessment methods 1, 2, and 3, study participants' leptomeningeal collaterals were dichotomized to incomplete (less than 100%) and complete (100%). Patients in the ICAS group showed more complete leptomeningeal collateral supply ($p < 0.001$; Table 1). During multivariable analysis, complete leptomeningeal collateral supply remained an independent factor for ICAS-LVO (odds ratio, 3.32; 95% confidence interval, 1.52–7.26; $p = 0.003$; Table S1 and Figure 3). An AUC value for complete leptomeningeal collaterals was 0.660 (95% CI, 0.595–0.722; $p < 0.001$), with an NPV of 88.6% (Table 2).

4. Discussion

In this study, we found that leptomeningeal collaterals were associated with occlusion pathomechanism. Better leptomeningeal collaterals were significantly associated with ICAS-LVO in common collateral assessment methods. Nevertheless, during logistic regression analyses, only the use of a dichotomization method (incomplete versus complete) was independently associated with ICAS-LVO. Despite the independence, it achieved only a modest degree of predictability of ICAS-LVO. To the best of our knowledge, this study is the first study to evaluate the association of leptomeningeal collaterals with ICAS-LVO and its preprocedural possibility to predict ICAS-LVO.

This study was originally contrived from the necessity to enhance the preprocedural determination of occlusion pathomechanism in endovascular treatment of LVO. Because the optimal endovascular strategy—which includes selection of the most effective endovascular modality and when to switch from one modality to another—depends on the type of occlusion pathomechanism, the earlier determination of occlusion pathomechanism can be crucial in attaining significant recanalization [18,19]. However, unfortunately, there have been only a few practical factors identified that we can rely on to identify occlusion pathomechanism before an endovascular procedure. Common cardioembolic sources such as atrial fibrillation or valvular heart diseases are typically considered as evidence of an embolic occlusion of an intracranial artery [7]. Specific imaging findings—for example, a hyperdense artery sign on CT or a blooming artifact on magnetic resonance imaging—have also been regarded as markers of embolic occlusion [14,20]. Uniquely, the occlusion type observed on preprocedural CTA was significantly associated with occlusion pathomechanism. The occlusion type was superior to the atrial fibrillation and hyperdense artery sign in predicting the occlusion pathomechanism [10]. Patient demographics or a few risk factors for atherosclerosis can be referred to in order to assume the occlusion pathomechanism; however, they are quite indirect means [7]. Particular infarct patterns could also be helpful in determining the occlusion pathomechanism. However, the infarct pattern is less evident and may be limited in the preprocedural condition [14].

As we expected, leptomeningeal collaterals were significantly associated with occlusion pathomechanism in this study. In particular, complete leptomeningeal collaterals were consistently associated with ICAS-LVO with a modest level of predictability. In comparison with other preprocedural findings used to predict ICAS-LVO, the discriminative power of complete leptomeningeal collaterals seemed not so inferior. In this study population, the AUC value of complete leptomeningeal collaterals for ICAS-LVO was not lower than that of atrial fibrillation (0.653; 95% confidence interval, 0.587–0.715).

Furthermore, the AUC value of CTA-determined occlusion type for stent retriever success, one of the preprocedural findings presumed to be highly associated with ICAS-LVO, was less than 0.7 [5].

To the best of our knowledge, only one other study has commented on the association between leptomeningeal collaterals and ICAS-LVO in endovascular treatment [7]. In the literature, full and rapid leptomeningeal collaterals were significantly more frequent in patients with ICAS-LVO, which was consistent with our study. However, the result was unofficial from a small number of patients, so it was merely a piece of unpublished data in a review article. Additionally, leptomeningeal collaterals were not considered as a predictor of ICAS-LVO in the literature. Leptomeningeal collaterals were assessed by initial cerebral angiogram during endovascular treatment, not preprocedurally.

Complete leptomeningeal collaterals showed low sensitivity and PPV with a relatively higher NPV in discriminating ICAS-LVO. For practical use, the statistical parameters can be interpreted as follows: (1) in patients with ICAS-LVO, the probability of showing complete leptomeningeal collaterals was about 50% (low sensitivity); (2) even among cases showing complete leptomeningeal collaterals, ICAS-LVO was only present in about 40% of them (low PPV); and (3) if a patient showed incomplete leptomeningeal collaterals, occlusion pathomechanism was not likely to be ICAS-LVO up to 90% (high NPV).

The study results might be substantially affected by the chosen collateral assessment method. However, there has been no consensual grading system established to evaluate leptomeningeal collaterals on CTA. To avoid arbitrary grading, we tried to choose collateral assessment methods that have all been widely used in previous studies [21,22]. Based on the consistent findings from those collateral assessment methods, we regrouped the leptomeningeal collaterals by its cutoff value into incomplete or complete. Cerebral angiography can be a good modality with which to assess leptomeningeal collaterals. However, in most endovascular procedures, initial leptomeningeal collateral flow is not assessed on cerebral angiography because the arterial target is directly approached without taking the angiography of other cerebral vessels. We think that CTA might be the most rational modality to use to assess leptomeningeal collaterals in daily clinical practice. Multiphase CTA could be another collateral assessment method. However, multiphase CTA cannot be deployed in all centers; indeed, multiphase CTA was not performed in the early period of this study.

This study had a few limitations. First, it was performed retrospectively in a single tertiary stroke center. However, all patients were prospectively registered with a detailed description of their endovascular procedure. Furthermore, this study focused on objective findings, including imaging markers and angiographic findings rather than on clinical outcomes, thereby minimizing this limitation. Nevertheless, based on the retrospective nature of this study, there might be a possibility that the patients with better leptomeningeal collaterals were preferentially chosen for endovascular treatment. Although the predetermined protocol in our center did not regulate the leptomeningeal collateral status for endovascular treatment eligibility, the physician's clinical decision might be partly affected by the leptomeningeal collateral status.

Second, this study included patients only with M1 occlusion. Thus, the generalization of our study results to all anterior circulation strokes might be inappropriate. However, as described earlier, such use of this strict inclusion criterion was to ensure the improved evaluation of uncontaminated leptomeningeal collaterals. Study findings should be understood as providing verification of a general hypothesis that better leptomeningeal collaterals are associated with ICAS-LVO. In addition, generalization of the study results could also be limited because this study was performed in an Asian country where ICAS is more prevalent. As statistical power might be affected by the number of patients with ICAS-LVO, no one could precisely figure out the association of leptomeningeal collaterals with ICAS-LVO in other countries where ICAS is much less prevalent.

Third, this study also included patients with a tandem occlusion (M1 occlusion with cervical ICA occlusion/stenosis). Chronic ischemia, even due to severe cervical ICA stenosis, might be associated with robust leptomeningeal collaterals. Thus, theoretically, for the tandem occlusion, leptomeningeal collaterals could be abundant or complete, although its M1 occlusion is embolic from a cervical ICA lesion. In fact, about 5% patients of this study had an atherosclerotic cervical ICA occlusion. Fortunately, even after excluding the patients with tandem occlusions, the significance of the study results was not changed.

5. Conclusions

Leptomeningeal collaterals determined by preprocedural CTA were significantly associated with occlusion pathomechanism. Specifically, complete leptomeningeal collateral supply was independently associated with ICAS-LVO. Despite the association, however, leptomeningeal collaterals were simply predictive of ICAS-LVO in a modest degree. In clinical practice, one could assume that incomplete leptomeningeal collateral supply is not likely ICAS-LVO based on high NPV. In this way, leptomeningeal collaterals could be helpful in the preprocedural determination of occlusion pathomechanism.

Author Contributions: Conceptualization, J.-H.B. and B.M.K.; data curation, J.-H.B., B.M.K., J.W.K., D.J.K., J.H.H., H.S.N., and Y.D.K.; formal analysis, J.-H.B. and J.W.K.; funding acquisition, B.M.K.; methodology, J.-H.B. and B.M.K.; writing—original draft, J.-H.B.; writing—review and editing, J.-H.B. and B.M.K. All authors have read and agreed to the published version of the manuscript.

References

1.   Powers, W.J.; Rabinstein, A.A.; Ackerson, T.; Adeoye, O.M.; Bambakidis, N.C.; Becker, K.; Biller, J.; Brown, M.; Demaerschalk, B.M.; Hoh, B. Guidelines for the early management of patients with acute Ischemic stroke: 2019 Update to the 2018 guidelines for the early management of acute ischemic stroke: A auideline for healthcare professionals from the American Heart Association/American Stroke Association. *Stroke* **2019**, *50*, e344–e418. [PubMed]

2.   Kang, D.-H.; Yoon, W.; Baek, B.H.; Kim, S.K.; Lee, Y.Y.; Kim, J.-T.; Park, M.-S.; Kim, Y.-W.; Hwang, Y.-H.; Kim, Y.-S. Front-line thrombectomy for acute large-vessel occlusion with underlying severe intracranial stenosis: Stent retriever versus contact aspiration. *J. Neurosurg.* **2020**, *132*, 1202–1208. [CrossRef] [PubMed]

3.   Lee, J.S.; Lee, S.-J.; Hong, J.M.; Choi, J.W.; Yoo, J.; Hong, J.-H.; Kim, C.-H.; Kim, Y.-W.; Kang, D.-H.; Hwang, Y.-H.; et al. Solitaire thrombectomy for acute stroke due to intracranial atherosclerosis-related occlusion: ROSE ASSIST study. *Front. Neurol.* **2018**, *9*, e9. [CrossRef]

4.   Tsang, A.C.O.; Orru, E.; Klostranec, J.M.; Yang, I.-H.; Lau, K.K.; Tsang, F.C.P.; Lui, W.M.; Pereira, V.M.; Krings, T. Thrombectomy outcomes of intracranial atherosclerosis-related occlusions. *Stroke* **2019**, *50*, 1460–1466. [CrossRef] [PubMed]

5.   Baek, J.-H.; Kim, B.; Heo, J.H.; Nam, H.S.; Song, D.; Bang, O.Y.; Kim, D.J. Importance of truncal-type occlusion in stentriever-based thrombectomy for acute stroke. *Neurology* **2016**, *87*, 1542–1550. [CrossRef]

6.   Baek, J.-H.; Kim, B.; Heo, J.H.; Kim, D.J.; Nam, H.S.; Kim, Y.D. Outcomes of endovascular treatment for acute intracranial atherosclerosis–related large vessel occlusion. *Stroke* **2018**, *49*, 2699–2705. [CrossRef]

7.   Lee, J.S.; Hong, J.M.; Kim, J.S. Diagnostic and therapeutic strategies for acute intracranial atherosclerosis-related occlusions. *J. Stroke* **2017**, *19*, 143–151. [CrossRef]

8.   Park, H.; Baek, J.-H.; Kim, B. Endovascular treatment of acute stroke due to intracranial atherosclerotic stenosis-related large vessel occlusion. *Front. Neurol.* **2019**, *10*, e308. [CrossRef]

9.   Kang, D.-H.; Yoon, W. Current opinion on endovascular therapy for emergent large vessel occlusion due to underlying intracranial atherosclerotic stenosis. *Korean J. Radiol.* **2019**, *20*, 739–748. [CrossRef]

10. Baek, J.-H.; Kim, B.; Yoo, J.; Nam, H.S.; Kim, Y.D.; Kim, D.J.; Heo, J.H.; Bang, O.Y. Predictive value of computed tomography angiography-determined occlusion type in stent retriever thrombectomy. *Stroke* **2017**, *48*, 2746–2752. [CrossRef]

11. Brozici, M.; Van Der Zwan, A.; Hillen, B. Anatomy and functionality of leptomeningeal anastomoses: A review. *Stroke* **2003**, *34*, 2750–2762. [CrossRef] [PubMed]

12. Shuaib, A.; Butcher, K.; A Mohammad, A.; Saqqur, M.; Liebeskind, D.S. Collateral blood vessels in acute ischaemic stroke: A potential therapeutic target. *Lancet Neurol.* **2011**, *10*, 909–921. [CrossRef]

13. Liebeskind, D.S. Collateral circulation. *Stroke* **2003**, *34*, 2279–2284. [CrossRef] [PubMed]
14. Suh, H.I.; Hong, J.M.; Lee, K.S.; Han, M.; Choi, J.W.; Kim, J.S.; Demchuk, A.M.; Lee, J.S. Imaging predictors for atherosclerosis-related intracranial large artery occlusions in acute anterior circulation stroke. *J. Stroke* **2016**, *18*, 352–354. [CrossRef]
15. Tan, I.; Demchuk, A.; Hopyan, J.; Zhang, L.; Gladstone, D.J.; Wong, K.-K.; Martin, M.; Symons, S.; Fox, A.; Aviv, R. CT angiography clot burden score and collateral score: Correlation with clinical and radiologic outcomes in acute middle cerebral artery infarct. *AJNR Am. J. Neuroradiol.* **2009**, *30*, 525–531. [CrossRef]
16. Maas, M.B.; Lev, M.H.; Ay, H.; Singhal, A.B.; Greer, D.M.; Smith, W.S.; Harris, G.J.; Halpern, E.; Kemmling, A.; Koroshetz, W.J.; et al. Collateral vessels on CT angiography predict outcome in acute ischemic stroke. *Stroke* **2009**, *40*, 3001–3005. [CrossRef]
17. Kim, B.; Baek, J.-H.; Heo, J.H.; Nam, H.S.; Kim, Y.D.; Yoo, J.; Kim, D.J.; Jeon, P.; Baik, S.K.; Suh, S.; et al. Collateral status affects the onset-to-reperfusion time window for good outcome. *J. Neurol. Neurosurg. Psychiatry* **2018**, *89*, 903–909. [CrossRef]
18. Tian, C.; Cao, X.; Wang, J. Recanalisation therapy in patients with acute ischaemic stroke caused by large artery occlusion: Choice of therapeutic strategy according to underlying aetiological mechanism? *Stroke Vasc. Neurol.* **2017**, *2*, 244–250. [CrossRef]
19. Kim, B.M. Causes and solutions of endovascular treatment failure. *J. Stroke* **2017**, *19*, 131–142. [CrossRef]
20. Kim, S.K.; Baek, B.H.; Lee, Y.; Yoon, W. Clinical implications of CT hyperdense artery sign in patients with acute middle cerebral artery occlusion in the era of modern mechanical thrombectomy. *J. Neurol.* **2017**, *264*, 2450–2456. [CrossRef]
21. McVerry, F.; Liebeskind, D.; Muir, K.W. Systematic review of methods for assessing leptomeningeal collateral flow. *AJNR Am. J. Neuroradiol.* **2012**, *33*, 576–582. [CrossRef] [PubMed]
22. Kim, B.; Chung, J.; Park, H.-K.; Kim, J.Y.; Yang, M.-H.; Han, M.-K.; Jeong, C.; Hwang, G.; Kwon, O.-K.; Bae, H.-J. CT angiography of collateral vessels and outcomes in endovascular-treated acute ischemic stroke patients. *J. Clin. Neurol.* **2017**, *13*, 121–128. [CrossRef] [PubMed]

11

One-Stop Management of 230 Consecutive Acute Stroke Patients: Report of Procedural Times and Clinical Outcome

Marios-Nikos Psychogios [1,2,*], Ilko L. Maier [3], Ioannis Tsogkas [1], Amélie Carolina Hesse [1], Alex Brehm [1,2], Daniel Behme [1], Marlena Schnieder [3], Katharina Schregel [1], Ismini Papageorgiou [4], David S. Liebeskind [5], Mayank Goyal [6], Mathias Bähr [3], Michael Knauth [1] and Jan Liman [3]

[1] Department of Neuroradiology, University Medical Center Goettingen, 37075 Goettingen, Germany; ioannis.tsogkas@usb.ch (I.T.); amelie.hesse@med.uni-goettingen.de (A.C.H.); alex.brehm@usb.ch (A.B.); daniel.behme@med.uni-goettingen.de (D.B.); katharina.schregel@med.uni-goettingen.de (K.S.); michael.knauth@med.uni-goettingen.de (M.K.)

[2] Department of Neuroradiology, Clinic for Radiology & Nuclear Medicine, University Hospital Basel, 4031 Basel, Switzerland

[3] Department of Neurology, University Medical Center Goettingen, 37075 Goettingen, Germany; ilko.maier@med.uni-goettingen.de (I.L.M.); marlena.schnieder@med.uni-goettingen.de (M.S.); mbaehr@gwdg.de (M.B.); jliman@gwdg.de (J.L.)

[4] Department of Neuroradiology, Südharz Klinikum, 99734 Nordhausen, Germany; ismini.e.papageorgiou@gmail.com

[5] Neurovascular Imaging Research Core and Stroke Center, Department of Neurology, University of California Los Angeles, Los Angeles, CA 90095, USA; davidliebeskind@yahoo.com

[6] Calgary Stroke Program, Department of Clinical Neurosciences, University of Calgary, Calgary, AB 2500, Canada; mgoyal@ucalgary.ca

[*] Correspondence: marios.psychogios@usb.ch

Abstract: Background and purpose: Rapid thrombectomy for acute ischemic stroke caused by large vessel occlusion leads to improved outcome. Optimizing intrahospital management might diminish treatment delays. To examine if one-stop management reduces intrahospital treatment delays and improves functional outcome of acute stroke patients with large vessel occlusion. Methods: We performed a single center, observational study from June 2016 to November 2018. Imaging was acquired with the latest generation angiography suite at a comprehensive stroke center. Two-hundred-thirty consecutive adults with suspected acute stroke presenting within 6 h after symptom onset with a moderate to severe National Institutes of Health Stroke Scale ($\geq$10 in 2016; $\geq$7 since January 2017) were directly transported to the angiography suite by bypassing multidetector CT. Noncontrast flat-detector CT and biphasic flat-detector CT angiography were acquired with an angiography system. In case of a large vessel occlusion patients remained in the angiography suite, received intravenous rtPA therapy and underwent thrombectomy. As primary endpoints, door-to-reperfusion times and functional outcome at 90 days were recorded and compared in a case-control analysis with matched prior patients receiving standard management. Results: A total of 230 patients (123 women, median age of 78 years (Interquartile Range (IQR) 69–84)) were included. Median symptom-to-door time was 130 min (IQR 70–195). Large vessel occlusion was diagnosed in 166/230 (72%) patients; 64/230 (28%) had conditions not suitable for thrombectomy. Median door-to-reperfusion time for M1 occlusions was 64 min (IQR 56–87). Compared to 43 case-matched patients triaged with multidetector CT, median door-to-reperfusion time was reduced from 102 (IQR 85–117) to 68 min (IQR 53–89; $p < 0.001$). Rate of good functional outcome was significantly better in the one-stop management group ($p = 0.029$). Safety parameters (mortality, sICH, any hemorrhage) did not differ significantly between groups. Conclusions: One-stop management for stroke triage reduces intrahospital time delays in our specific hospital setting.

Keywords: stroke; hemorrhage; thrombectomy; cone-beam computed tomography; cerebral angiography

---

1. Introduction

Swift and complete reperfusion of the occluded vessel territory is the key of every revascularization therapy in stroke patients with large vessel occlusion (LVO) [1,2]. Thrombectomy became the new standard of LVO-therapy after publication of multiple trials showing higher reperfusion rates and improved functional outcomes in patients receiving the combination of thrombectomy and medical therapy as opposed to medical therapy alone [3–7]. However, door-to-groin times have been consistently longer than one hour, even in trials focusing on rapid treatment of stroke patients [2,6]. The primary limitation leading to time-delays in the treatment of LVO-patients is the lack of a fast, reliable and affordable prehospital screening tool in stroke treatment akin to e.g., the electrocardiogram in patients with an acute coronary syndrome. While STEMI-patients with a positive electrocardiogram are directly transported to the angiography-suite, stroke patients are usually first triaged with a noninvasive imaging method in one room, or even hospital, and then transported to a different room, or even different hospital, for thrombectomy.

In order to minimize intrahospital times at the treating hospital, we recently proposed a method of noninvasive triage with a flat-detector computed tomography (FDCT) capable angiography-suite, IV lysis and thrombectomy in the same room (one-stop management) with the potential of significant reduction of door-to-groin and door-to-reperfusion times [8]. We demonstrated in prior work, that a rather simple, fast and commercially available non-enhanced FDCT protocol can be used to detect intracranial hemorrhage (ICH) with a very high sensitivity, which is comparable to multi-detector CT (MDCT) [9]. Furthermore, biphasic FDCT angiography enabled us to reliable detect LVOs and grade collaterals [10]. These advancements made the aforementioned paradigm feasible for the triage of mothership, who are eligible for IV lysis, as well as transfer patients.

In this study, we report the first 230 consecutive stroke patients diagnosed and treated with a one-stop management and analyze the 90 days functional outcomes, compared to patients managed with an optimized stroke workflow previously published [11].

2. Materials and Methods

2.1. Patient Selection

This observational study includes all 230 consecutive adult patients treated with one-stop management in our hospital from June 2016 to November 2018. All patients presented with clinical signs of an ischemic stroke within 6 h after symptom onset and a National Institutes of Health Stroke Scale (NIHSS) ($\geq$10 in 2016; $\geq$7 since January 2017) were included in our study. Unknown symptom onset, prolonged time from symptom onset, a low NIHSS (<10 in 2016; <7 since January 2017) or occupation of the FDCT-capable angiography-suite during admission were exclusion criteria. Data were prospectively collected and documented in an Institutional Review Board-approved database. A neurological assessment was performed (i) at hospital admission, (ii) hospital discharge and (iii) 90 days after stroke by a certified stroke neurologist. The imaging data were documented by the treating physician and re-evaluated by a core-team, consisting of an experienced neurointerventionalist (>10 years of experience) and a neuroradiology resident. A patient's consent for treatment was obtained according to the institutional guidelines. The local ethics committee waived the need for a formal application or a separate consent concerning the inclusion in our observational database.

2.2. Image Acquisition and Processing

Images were acquired using an Artis Q angiography system (Siemens Healthcare GmbH, Forchheim, Germany) as described before [8,12]. First, an FDCT was acquired to exclude intracranial hemorrhage. A commercially available 20 s rotational acquisition was used (20 s DCT Head, 109 kV, 1.8 µGy/frame, 200° angle, 0.4°/frame angulation step; effective dose ~2.5 mSv; Siemens Healthineers AG, Erlangen, Germany) and raw data were instantly and automatically reconstructed in 5 mm multiplanar reconstructions on a commercially available workstation (syngo × Workplace; Siemens Healthineers AG, Erlangen, Germany). Next, a commercially available biphasic FDCT-angiography (biFDCTA) was acquired for detection of arterial occlusion and evaluation of intracranial collaterals (2 × 10 s DSA, 70kV, 1.2 µGy/frame, 200° angle, 0.8°/frame angulation step; effective dose ~ 2.5 mSv; Siemens Healthineers AG, Erlangen, Germany) after intravenous injection of 60 mL contrast media (Imeron 400; Bracco Imaging Inc, Konstanz, Germany) at a flow rate of 5 mL/s followed by 60 mL saline chaser at 5 mL/s. Both FDCTA datasets were instantly and automatically reconstructed on the aforementioned workstation and 24 mm transversal maximal intensity projections of the first and second phase were simultaneously viewable on the workstation. Timing for the start of the first (arterial) phase acquisition was determined using a bolus-tracking acquisition. The second (venous) phase was acquired automatically with a delay of 5 s from the end of the first rotation. The acquisition, reconstruction and evaluation of all datasets do not require more than 2 min.

2.3. Management After Imaging

Patients with no hemorrhage and with an LVO were treated, if eligible, with intravenous recombinant tissue plasminogen activator (IV rtPA) and with thrombectomy. As per institutional guidelines, a low Alberta Stroke Program Early CT Scale (ASPECTS) or low collateral score was not an exclusion criterion for thrombectomy in the first 6 h after symptom onset. Patients with no hemorrhage and with a small vessel occlusion (SVO) were treated with IV rtPA only, if eligible. Patients with no hemorrhage and with no arterial occlusion were started on IV rtPA, if eligible, and received an additional stroke MRI to decide on further treatment. Patients with an intracranial hemorrhage and no occlusion were treated as per institutional standards. Lastly, patients with an intracranial hemorrhage (ICH) and LVO were treated with thrombectomy after an individualized case discussion between the neurologist, interventional neuroradiologist and patient or his/her next of kin.

2.4. Statistical Analysis

Characteristics and time-metrics of the one-stop database are reported by descriptive statistics. Time-intervals are documented with median, interquartile range (IQR) and 90th percentile, as recently proposed [13]. A case-matched analysis is performed between the one-stop database and the standard workflow (multidetector CT (MDCT)-triaged patients) database with the following criteria: patient's age, admission NIHSS, ASPECTS and symptom-to-door time. Only standard-workflow-patients that arrived in our hospital with an NIHSS ≥7 while the angiography-suite was not occupied were included in the case-matched analysis in order to simulate a similar scenario for matching purposes. The maximum allowed difference for case-matching was chosen arbitrarily and was 10 years for age, six points for NIHSS, 3 points for ASPECTS and 45 min for symptom-to-door time. Continuous variables were compared between one-stop management and optimized workflow patients either by t-test, in the case of normal distribution, or by the Wilcoxon test, in the case of non-normal or ordinal distribution. Categorical variables were compared between the 2 groups by the Fisher's exact test.

The probability of favorable outcome (modified Rankin scale (mRS) ≤ 2) between the two groups at 90 days was further assessed by logistic regression using selected variables. Statistical analyses were performed with the MedCalc Statistical Software version 18 (MedCalc Software bv, Ostend, Belgium; http://www.medcalc.org; 2018).

3. Results

Two-hundred-thirty one-stop managed patients were included in our study (123 women; median age of 78 years (IQR 69–84)). The overall admission NIHSS was 15 (IQR 12–19) and 166/230 (72%) patients were diagnosed with an LVO, 25/230 (11%) with an SVO, 24/230 (10%) with an ICH, 11/230 (5%) with a Todd's paresis and 4/230 (2%) with a recanalized LVO after transfer, respectively (Table 1). One-hundred-twenty-seven out of 230 (55%) cases were direct admissions, while 103/230 (45%) were transfer patients from a peripheral stroke center with a confirmed LVO. Of the 127 direct admission patients 74/127 (58%) were LVOs, 19/127 (15%) were SVOs, 23/127 (18%) were ICHs and 11/127 (9%) were Todd's paresis. Of the 103 transfer patients, 61/103 (59%) received IV rtPA at the peripheral stroke center ("drip and ship"), 1/103 (1%) was diagnosed with a new subdural hematoma on FDCT that was not present on the initial external MDCT and 4/103 (4%) showed complete revascularization on baseline FDCTA at our center. The median time required between the external MDCT and the FDCT was 124 min (110–155; 90th percentile 218).

The overall door-to-FDCT time was 15 min (IQR 10–20; 90th percentile 26) and door-to-IVrtPA was 22 min (IQR 20–30; 90th percentile 41). The median door-to-groin time for LVO patients was 29 min (IQR 22–39; 90th percentile 50) with a median door-to-reperfusion time of 72 min (IQR 58–91; 90th percentile 117; Table 2). Patients with an M1 occlusion had a median door-to-reperfusion time of 64 min (IQR 56–87; 90th percentile 102). Any hemorrhage was depicted in 25/166 (15%), a parenchymal hematoma type-2 in 2/166 (1%) and a symptomatic intracranial hemorrhage (sICH) in 6/166 (4%) of the LVOs on follow-up imaging. Overall mortality was 22%. A favorable outcome was documented in 65/166 (39%) of the LVO patients at discharge. Nineteen LVO patients were lost to follow-up; favorable outcome and mortality for mothership patients with a pre-stroke mRS less than three were 57% and 31% while overall favorable outcome and mortality of mothership LVO patients were 51% and 32% respectively at 90 days after stroke onset.

The case-control analysis revealed 43 LVO matches for each group (one-stop vs. traditional management). Matching variables were not significantly different between one-stop and traditional workflow patients; other baseline and imaging characteristics (e.g., collaterals) were also balanced between the two groups (Table 3). We observed a significant reduction of door-to-groin and door-to-reperfusion times, both during working and off-duty hours, for direct admission and transfer patients. Safety variables, such as sICH, any hemorrhage on follow-up imaging or mortality were comparable between the two groups. Median discharge and 90 d mRS in the one-stop group was three (IQR 1–5) and two (IQR 1–5), respectively. The rate of good functional outcome at 90 days was significantly higher in the one-stop management group with 58% (25/43) as compared to 33% (14/43) in the normal workflow group ($p = 0.029$). In the logistic regression model comparing predictors of favorable clinical outcome in the matched population, the one-stop management (odds ratio (OR) 3.75; 95% confidence interval (CI) 1.13–12.44; $p = 0.031$) and successful reperfusion (OR 2.58; 95% CI 1.19–5.55; $p = 0.015$) were significant contributors to the prediction of a favorable outcome (Figure 1).

Table 1. Clinical, angiographic, and procedural details of the 100 one-stop-management patients.

	All, n = 230	LVO, n = 166	SVO, n = 25	ICH, n = 24	Todd's, n = 11	RLVO, n = 4
Age, median (IQR)	78 (69–84)	77 (68–84)	79 (71–87)	78 (75–83)	79 (73–82)	81 (77–86)
Admission NIHSS	15 (12–19)	16 (13–19)	13 (11–15)	15 (10–17)	12 (11–15)	13 (11–13)
Female	123 (54%)	90 (54%)	12 (48%)	12 (50%)	5 (46%)	4 (100%)
IV-rtPA	144 (63%)	112 (68%)	23 (92%)	1	4 (36%)	4 (100%)
Hemorrhage on initial FDCT	25 (11%)	1 (1%)	0 (0%)	24 (100%)	0 (0%)	0 (0%)
Occlusion site						
ICA-T		41 (25%)				
M1		88 (53%)				
M2		15 (9%)				
Other		22 (13%)				
Tandem occlusion		34 (21%)				
Times, min (IQR; 90th Percentile)						
Symptom to door	130 (70–195; 253)	154 (67–205; 264)	82 (66–134; 205)	105 (69–129; 204)	131 (95–146; 186)	229 (181–259)
Door to FDCT	15 (10–20; 26)	14 (9–19; 25)	16 (12–24; 32)	17 (14–22; 30)	21 (13–23; 31)	16 (14–16)
Door to IV-rtPA	22 (20–30; 41)	22 (20–29; 38)	26 (20–45; 53)			
Door to treatment start[α]				21 (18–33; 34)	27 (19–32; 37)	
Door to groin		29 (22–39; 50)				
Groin to reperfusion		40 (28–60; 80)				
FDCT to reperfusion		59 (45–82; 101)				
Door to reperfusion		72 (58–91; 117)				
Door to reperfusion M1		64 (56–87; 102)				
extCT to FDCT	124 (110–155; 218)					

Table 1. *Cont.*

	All, n = 230	LVO, n = 166	SVO, n = 25	ICH, n = 24	Todd's, n = 11	RLVO, n = 4
Direct admission	127 (55%)	74 (45%)	19 (76%)	23 (96%)	11 (100%)	0 (0%)
Working hours β	95 (41%)	68 (41%)	13 (52%)	11 (46%)	2 (18%)	1 (25%)
Reperfusion, mTICI2b-3		142 (86%)				
Any hemorrhage on FU	49 (21%)	25 (15%)	0 (0%)	24 (100%)	0 (0%)	
PH-2 hematoma on FU		2 (1%)				
sICH		6 (4%)				
Discharge NIHSS	5 (2–10)	5 (2–12)	7 (4–10)	5 (1–9)	4 (1–6)	6 (4–7)
Discharge mRS	4 (1–5)	4 (1–5)	4 (2–5)	2 (2–6)	3 (1–4)	3 (3–4)
Mortality	45/230 (20%)	36 (22%)	2 (8%)	5 (30%)	2 (18%)	0 (0%)
90 d mRS		4 (1–6)				
90 d favorable outcome	54/147 (37%)					

LVO, large vessel occlusion; SVO, small vessel occlusion; ICH, intracranial hemorrhage; RLVO, recanalized LVO during transfer; IQR, interquartile range; NIHSS, National Institutes of Health Stroke Scale; IV-rtPA, intravenous recombinant tissue plasminogen activator; FDCT, flat-detector CT; extCT, external CT; mTICI, modified thrombolysis in cerebral infarction score; FU, follow-up; mRS, modified Rankin scale; α, intravenous injection of antihypertensive drugs in case of ICB or sedative drugs in case of seizures; β, weekdays 08:00 to 17:00.

Table 2. Procedural details of one-stop-management patients with large vessel occlusion.

Direct Admission $n = 74$	Min (IQR; 90th Percentile)
Door to FDCT	15 (12–20; 24)
Door to IV–rtPA	22 (20–29; 38)
Door to groin	34 (28–45; 51)
Groin to reperfusion	41 (26–55; 73)
FDCT to reperfusion	61 (47–81; 93)
Door to reperfusion	76 (61–92; 116)
Door to reperfusion of M1	68 (58–89; 101)
Occluded vessel	ICA-T 13 (18%), M1 42 (58%), M2 9 (12%)
Tandem occlusions	15 (20%)
Transfer patients $n = 92$	
extCT to FDCT	124 (110–155; 218)
Door to FDCT	10 (8–17; 25)
Door to groin	25 (19–33; 41)
Groin to reperfusion	38 (29–65; 87)
FDCT to reperfusion	56 (44–86; 110)
Door to reperfusion	68 (53–90; 126)
Door to reperfusion of M1	59 (52–84; 118)
Occluded vessel	ICA-T 28 (30%), M1 46 (50%), M2 6 (7%)
Tandem occlusions	19 (20%)
Working hours $n = 68$	
Door to FDCT	12 (7–16; 21)
Door to IV–rtPA	22 (20–26; 34)
Door to groin	25 (19–33; 41)
Groin to reperfusion	38 (25–53; 85)
FDCT to reperfusion	61 (42–69; 101)
Door to reperfusion	66 (52–85; 105)
Off-hours $n = 98$	
Door to FDCT	15 (10–21; 27)
Door to IV–rtPA	23 (19–29; 38)
Door to groin	33 (25–42; 60)
Groin to reperfusion	38 (25–53; 86)
FDCT to reperfusion	52 (42–69; 101)
Door to reperfusion	66 (52–85; 105)

Table 3. Case-control study of FDCT vs. MDCT patients, n =86.

	MDCT, $n = 43$	FDCT, $n = 43$	p-Value
*Age median (IQR) *	*77 (69–81)*	*77 (69–82)*	*0.962*
*Admission NIHSS *	*17 (14–20)*	*16 (13–20)*	*0.796*
*CT ASPECTS *	*8 (7–9)*	*9 (7–10)*	*0.138*
*Onset to door, min (IQR; 90th) *	*129 (76–200; 244)*	*160 (74–202; 221)*	*0.511*
Female	26 (61%)	26 (61%)	1.000
IV-rtPA	36 (84%)	30 (70%)	0.201
Hypertension	35 (81%)	33 (77%)	0.791
Hyperlipidemia	14 (33%)	20 (47%)	0.266
PAD	2 (5%)	5 (12%)	0.433
DM	11 (26%)	17 (40%)	0.249
Collateral grading	7 (5–8)	7 (4–8)	0.699
Direct admissions	30 (70%)	18 (42%)	**0.016**
Working hours	22 (51%)	19 (44%)	0.666
Door to CT, min (IQR; 90th)	15 (11–20; 24)	9 (6–14; 16)	**<0.001**
Door to IV-rtPA	27 (22–34; 35)	19 (12–22; 34)	**0.016**
Door to groin	60 (48–68; 79)	25 (19–30; 38)	**<0.001**
Working hours	60 (42–65; 85)	21 (17–25; 41)	**<0.001**
Off-hours	62 (53–69; 75)	25 (21–32; 38)	**<0.001**
Direct admissions	61 (54–67; 83)	26 (25–38; 44)	**<0.001**
Transfer patients	40 (30–69; 75)	21 (19–26; 35)	**<0.001**
Groin to reperfusion	42 (27–62; 94)	43 (33–60; 78)	0.866
CT to reperfusion	84 (71–99; 144)	59 (44–75; 96)	**<0.001**
Door to reperfusion	102 (85–117; 166)	68 (53–89; 104)	**<0.001**
Working hours	102 (79–145; 191)	62 (52–81; 104)	**0.006**
Off-hours	103 (93–116; 126)	74 (55–90; 109)	**<0.001**
Direct admissions	103 (85–121; 184)	72 (58–87; 103)	**0.001**
Transfer patients	102 (68–109; 120)	64 (51–88; 108)	**0.05**
ICA-T	7 (16%)	13 (30%)	0.179
M1	26 (61%)	25 (58%)	0.888
M2	9 (21%)	3 (7%)	0.117
Tandem occlusion	6 (14%)	7 (16%)	1
Successful reperfusion (mTICI2b-3)	31 (72%)	38 (88%)	0.102
sICH	3 (7%)	2 (5%)	1
Any hemorrhage	11 (26%)	7 (16%)	0.427
PH–2 hemorrhage	1 (2%)	1 (2%)	1
Discharge mRS	4 (2–5)	3 (1–5)	0.374
90d mRS	4 (1–5)	2 (1–5)	0.153
90d mRS of 0–2	14 (33%)	25 (58%)	**0.029**
Mortality	9 (21%)	10 (23%)	1

* Matching variables.

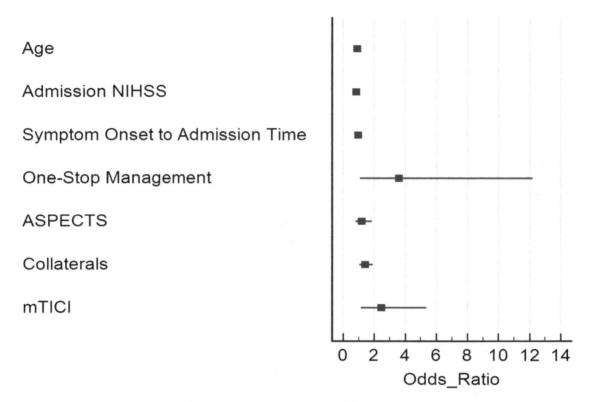

Figure 1. Logistic regression model comparing predictors of favorable clinical outcome in the matched population (one-stop management vs. normal management with MDCT).

4. Discussion

Our observational study establishes on a large scale the results from prior brief reports with median door-to-groin times under 30 min and median door-to-reperfusion times under 90 min for patients triaged with a one-stop management [8]. The proposed fast and commercially available protocol is safe for both direct admission and transfer patients. Intravenous rtPA was administered in 63% of our patients, with rates of any hemorrhage, symptomatic ICH and mortality comparable to larger trials. Regarding outcome results it should be noted that our observational study had no restrictions regarding pre-stroke mRS or initial ASPECTS. Compared to the thrombectomy trial from 2015 with focus on rapid endovascular treatment we observed markedly lower door-to-groin times with a 90th percentile of 50 min in our study vs. 147 min in the ESCAPE trial [6]. Door-to-reperfusion times were also markedly lower in our study with a 90th percentile of 117 min compared to 190 min in the ESCAPE trial [6]. Even in comparison to recent trials published in 2018 and performed in large-volume centers with daily training and standardized workflows, our median intrahospital times were more than 30 min lower with 29 min door-to-groin time (106 min in the 3D-Separator trial) and 59 min imaging-to-reperfusion time (97 min in the DEFUSE 3 trial) in our study [14,15].

In the period from 2014 to 2015 we were able to significantly reduce intrahospital times from a median door-to-groin time of 121 to 64 min by standardizing interdisciplinary operating procedures, conducting frequent team meetings, and providing mutual feedback [11]. However, despite the increased workload and training in the consecutive years we were not able to further reduce the intrahospital times through the MDCT-route [16]. The current case-matched analysis shows, indeed, that a one-stop management allows for and additional reduction of intrahospital times (Table 3). The decreased handling times together with the increased rates of successful reperfusion in the one-stop arm patient pool led to a significant increase in rates of favorable functional outcome at 90 days.

While the increased reperfusion rates are probably a result of increased use of sophisticated thrombectomy techniques [17], the earlier groin puncture times may also play a role in increased rates of complete reperfusion in one-stop patients. A recent study of the HERMES dataset has shown a decreased probability of successful reperfusion with prolonged intrahospital times in LVO patients [18]. Another interesting aspect of the one-stop management in stroke is the interaction of IV rtPA and remaining thrombi after incomplete thrombectomy. In the meta-analysis of the five positive thrombectomy trials in 2015, the median door-to-needle time was 35 min and the median door-to-reperfusion time 148 min [2]. As the thrombolytic effect of IV lysis is rapidly lost after termination of the 60 min infusion there is usually no effect of IV rtPA on distal emboli after incomplete mechanical reperfusion. In our setting, both the IV rtPA infusion and thrombectomy are initiated within a narrow time frame which frequently leads to substantial reperfusion prior to completion of the IV rtPA infusion. This fact could lead to resolution of emboli in new territories or distal emboli with a positive effect on functional outcome.

In order to establish a one-stop management of stroke patients with the proposed protocol there is obviously a need for angio-time capacity within the stroke center. Angiography suite capacity should not be a problem in off-hours. We did not encounter a relevant problem in our effort to establish a one-stop management as more than half of the interventions performed in our center are mechanical thrombectomies. For other centers with limited angiography availability, possible solutions include the installation of a dedicated stroke angiography or a pre-notification system. Even with a dedicated stroke angiography-suite there is always the possibility of another stroke patient arriving while performing mechanical thrombectomy on the 'stroke machine'. Regarding workload and safety, it should be noted that we decided to involve the senior physician in the exclusion of an ICH on FDCT images at all times, after a case of profound ICH which was missed by the resident on duty during off-hours (Figure 2). Discrepancies between residents and seniors in the interpretation of overnight head CTs and the detection of hemorrhages have been studied before for MDCT. The reported frequency of 1/230 cases in our study is comparable to the 141/22,590 cases in a study by Vagal et al. [19]. The workload of the stroke angiography can also be influenced by the NIHSS threshold chosen for the one-stop management. As of January 2017, we lowered our one-stop threshold to an admission NIHSS of ≥7 as a recent publication suggested that the best predictor for LVO is the NIHSS score with the aforementioned cut-off [20]. Other possibilities for a one-stop management include the combination of MDCT and C-arm in one room (so called MIYABI system) or the use of a mobile C-arm within the CT room [21]. Both systems have the disadvantages of a monoplanar angio system. The first solution has an additional drawback due to the increased costs for two machines, while with the second option the usually heavily utilized CT scanner is being blocked during thrombectomy. Our door-to-groin times were slightly higher (29 min) compared to the time metrics reported by Ribo et al. (17 min) and Jovin et al. (22 min). However, their door-to-reperfusion times (73 and 66 min respectively) were similar to ours (72 min) [22,23]. Furthermore, as we used non-invasive FDCT angiography for the delineation of LVOs, no unnecessary groin punctures were performed compared to a reported rate of 7% by Ribo et al. [24].

The main limitation of our study is the observational single-center design. All time metrics are prospectively documented in a stroke database, but the documentation is not performed in a blinded fashion. As this study was performed in a comprehensive stroke center, the number of LVO may be increased compared to regional stroke centers, which leads to an increased number of ischemic strokes compared to other centers. However, based on the observations including a significant reduction of door-to-groin times and secure triage of patients with hemorrhagic strokes, we have started a prospective, randomized trial in order to prove the effectiveness and safety of the proposed one-stop protocol.

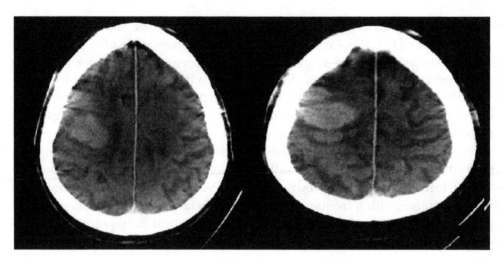

Figure 2. FDCT scan of intracranial hemorrhage which was missed by resident during off-hours.

5. Conclusions

One-stop management of stroke patients with a modern, FDCT-supporting angiography suite is feasible and allows for significantly shorter intrahospital times.

Author Contributions: Conception and Design of the work (M.-N.P., M.K., J.L., M.B.), Acquisition of the data (I.L.M., I.T., A.C.H., A.B., D.B., M.S., K.S.), Analysis and interpretation of the data (M.-N.P., I.P., D.S.L., M.G.), Drafting the work (M.-N.P.), Revising it critically for important intellectual property (All Authors), Final approval of the version to be published (All Authors), Accountable for all aspects of the work (M.-N.P., J.L.).

References

1.   Goyal, M.; Menon, B.K.; van Zwam, W.H.; Dippel, D.W.J.; Mitchell, P.J.; Demchuk, A.M.; Dávalos, A.; Majoie, C.B.L.M.; van der Lugt, A.; de Miquel, M.A.; et al. Endovascular thrombectomy after large-vessel ischaemic stroke: A meta-analysis of individual patient data from five randomised trials. *Lancet* **2016**, *387*, 1723–1731. [CrossRef]

2.   Saver, J.L.; Goyal, M.; van der Lugt, A.; Menon, B.K.; Majoie, C.B.; Dippel, D.W.; Campbell, B.C.; Nogueira, R.G.; Demchuk, A.M.; Tomasello, A.; et al. Time to Treatment With Endovascular Thrombectomy and Outcomes From Ischemic Stroke: A Meta-analysis. *JAMA* **2016**, *316*, 1279–1288. [CrossRef] [PubMed]

3.   Berkhemer, O.A.; Fransen, P.S.; Beumer, D.; van den Berg, L.A.; Lingsma, H.F.; Yoo, A.J.; Schonewille, W.J.; Vos, J.A.; Nederkoorn, P.J.; Wermer, M.J.; et al. A randomized trial of intraarterial treatment for acute ischemic stroke. *N. Engl. J. Med.* **2015**, *372*, 11–20. [CrossRef]

4.   Campbell, B.C.V.; Mitchell, P.J.; Kleinig, T.J.; Dewey, H.M.; Churilov, L.; Yassi, N.; Yan, B.; Dowling, R.J.; Parsons, M.W.; Oxley, T.J.; et al. Endovascular Therapy for Ischemic Stroke with Perfusion-Imaging Selection. *N. Engl. J. Med.* **2015**, *372*, 1009–1018. [CrossRef] [PubMed]

5.   Saver, J.L.; Goyal, M.; Bonafe, A.; Diener, H.C.; Levy, E.I.; Pereira, V.M.; Albers, G.W.; Cognard, C.; Cohen, D.J.; Hacke, W.; et al. Stent-retriever thrombectomy after intravenous t-PA vs. t-PA alone in stroke. *N. Engl. J. Med.* **2015**, *372*, 2285–2295. [CrossRef] [PubMed]

6.   Goyal, M.; Demchuk, A.M.; Menon, B.K.; Eesa, M.; Rempel, J.L.; Thornton, J.; Roy, D.; Jovin, T.G.; Willinsky, R.A.; Sapkota, B.L.; et al. Randomized Assessment of Rapid Endovascular Treatment of Ischemic Stroke. *N. Engl. J. Med.* **2015**, *372*, 1019–1030. [CrossRef]

7.   Jovin, T.G.; Chamorro, A.; Cobo, E.; de Miquel, M.A.; Molina, C.A.; Rovira, A.; San Roman, L.; Serena, J.; Abilleira, S.; Ribo, M.; et al. Thrombectomy within 8 hours after symptom onset in ischemic stroke. *N. Engl. J. Med.* **2015**, *372*, 2296–2306. [CrossRef]

8. Psychogios, M.N.; Behme, D.; Schregel, K.; Tsogkas, I.; Maier, I.L.; Leyhe, J.R.; Zapf, A.; Tran, J.; Bahr, M.; Liman, J.; et al. One-Stop Management of Acute Stroke Patients: Minimizing Door-to-Reperfusion Times. *Stroke* **2017**, *48*, 3152–3155. [CrossRef]

9. Leyhe, J.R.; Tsogkas, I.; Hesse, A.C.; Behme, D.; Schregel, K.; Papageorgiou, I.; Liman, J.; Knauth, M.; Psychogios, M.-N. Latest generation of flat detector CT as a peri-interventional diagnostic tool: A comparative study with multidetector CT. *J. Neurointerv. Surg.* **2017**, *9*, 1253–1257. [CrossRef]

10. Maier, I.L.; Scalzo, F.; Leyhe, J.R.; Schregel, K.; Behme, D.; Tsogkas, I.; Psychogios, M.-N.; Liebeskind, D.S. Validation of collateral scoring on flat-detector multiphase CT angiography in patients with acute ischemic stroke. *PLoS ONE* **2018**, *13*, e0202592. [CrossRef]

11. Schregel, K.; Behme, D.; Tsogkas, I.; Knauth, M.; Maier, I.; Karch, A.; Mikolajczyk, R.; Hinz, J.; Liman, J.; Psychogios, M.N. Effects of Workflow Optimization in Endovascularly Treated Stroke Patients—A Pre-Post Effectiveness Study. *PLoS ONE* **2016**, *11*, e0169192. [CrossRef] [PubMed]

12. Psychogios, M.N.; Bahr, M.; Liman, J.; Knauth, M. One Stop Management in Acute Stroke: First Mothership Patient Transported Directly to the Angiography Suite. *Clin. Neuroradiol.* **2017**, *27*, 389–391. [CrossRef] [PubMed]

13. Holodinsky, J.K.; Kamal, N.; Wilson, A.T.; Hill, M.D.; Goyal, M. Workflow in Acute Stroke: What Is the 90th Percentile? *Stroke* **2017**, *48*, 808–812. [CrossRef] [PubMed]

14. Albers, G.W.; Marks, M.P.; Kemp, S.; Christensen, S.; Tsai, J.P.; Ortega-Gutierrez, S.; McTaggart, R.A.; Torbey, M.T.; Kim-Tenser, M.; Leslie-Mazwi, T.; et al. Thrombectomy for Stroke at 6 to 16 Hours with Selection by Perfusion Imaging. *N. Engl. J. Med.* **2018**, *379*, 708–718. [CrossRef] [PubMed]

15. Nogueira, R.G.; Frei, D.; Kirmani, J.F.; Zaidat, O.; Lopes, D.; Turk, A.S., 3rd; Heck, D.; Mason, B.; Haussen, D.C.; Levy, E.I.; et al. Safety and Efficacy of a 3-Dimensional Stent Retriever With Aspiration-Based Thrombectomy vs Aspiration-Based Thrombectomy Alone in Acute Ischemic Stroke Intervention: A Randomized Clinical Trial. *JAMA Neurol.* **2018**, *75*, 304–311. [CrossRef] [PubMed]

16. Schregel, K.; Behme, D.; Tsogkas, I.; Knauth, M.; Maier, I.; Karch, A.; Mikolajczyk, R.; Bähr, M.; Schäper, J.; Hinz, J.; et al. Optimized Management of Endovascular Treatment for Acute Ischemic Stroke. *J. Vis. Exp.* **2018**, *131*, e56397. [CrossRef]

17. Maus, V.; Behme, D.; Kabbasch, C.; Borggrefe, J.; Tsogkas, I.; Nikoubashman, O.; Wiesmann, M.; Knauth, M.; Mpotsaris, A.; Psychogios, M.N. Maximizing First-Pass Complete Reperfusion with SAVE. *Clin. Neuroradiol.* **2017**, *28*, 327–338. [CrossRef]

18. Bourcier, R.; Goyal, M.; Liebeskind, D.S.; Muir, K.W.; Desal, H.; Siddiqui, A.H.; Dippel, D.W.J.; Majoie, C.B.; van Zwam, W.H.; Jovin, T.G.; et al. Association of Time From Stroke Onset to Groin Puncture With Quality of Reperfusion After Mechanical Thrombectomy: A Meta-analysis of Individual Patient Data From 7 Randomized Clinical Trials. *JAMA Neurol* **2019**, *76*, 405–411. [CrossRef]

19. Strub, W.M.; Leach, J.L.; Tomsick, T.; Vagal, A. Overnight preliminary head CT interpretations provided by residents: Locations of misidentified intracranial hemorrhage. *AJNR Am. J. Neuroradiol.* **2007**, *28*, 1679–1682. [CrossRef]

20. Heldner, M.R.; Hsieh, K.; Broeg-Morvay, A.; Mordasini, P.; Buhlmann, M.; Jung, S.; Arnold, M.; Mattle, H.P.; Gralla, J.; Fischer, U. Clinical prediction of large vessel occlusion in anterior circulation stroke: Mission impossible? *J. Neurol.* **2016**, *263*, 1633–1640. [CrossRef]

21. Pfaff, J.; Schonenberger, S.; Herweh, C.; Pham, M.; Nagel, S.; Ringleb, P.A.; Heiland, S.; Bendszus, M.; Mohlenbruch, M.A. Influence of a combined CT/C-arm system on periprocedural workflow and procedure times in mechanical thrombectomy. *Eur. Radiol.* **2017**, *27*, 3966–3972. [CrossRef] [PubMed]

22. Ribo, M.; Boned, S.; Rubiera, M.; Tomasello, A.; Coscojuela, P.; Hernández, D.; Pagola, J.; Juega, J.; Rodriguez, N.; Muchada, M.; et al. Direct transfer to angiosuite to reduce door-to-puncture time in thrombectomy for acute stroke. *J. Neurointerv. Surg.* **2018**, *10*, 221–224. [CrossRef] [PubMed]

23. Jadhav, A.P.; Kenmuir, C.L.; Aghaebrahim, A.; Limaye, K.; Wechsler, L.R.; Hammer, M.D.; Starr, M.T.; Molyneaux, B.J.; Rocha, M.; Guyette, F.X.; et al. Interfacility Transfer Directly to the Neuroangiography Suite in Acute Ischemic Stroke Patients Undergoing Thrombectomy. *Stroke* **2017**, *48*, 1884–1889. [CrossRef] [PubMed]
24. Mendez, B.; Requena, M.; Aires, A.; Martins, N.; Boned, S.; Rubiera, M.; Tomasello, A.; Coscojuela, P.; Muchada, M.; Rodríguez-Luna, D.; et al. Direct Transfer to Angio-Suite to Reduce Workflow Times and Increase Favorable Clinical Outcome. *Stroke* **2018**, *49*, 2723–2727. [CrossRef] [PubMed]

12

Interhemispheric Functional Connectivity in the Primary Motor Cortex Assessed by Resting-State Functional Magnetic Resonance Imaging Aids Long-Term Recovery Prediction among Subacute Stroke Patients with Severe Hand Weakness

Yu-Sun Min [1,2,3,†], Jang Woo Park [4,†], Eunhee Park [1,2], Ae-Ryoung Kim [1,2], Hyunsil Cha [4], Dae-Won Gwak [2], Seung-Hwan Jung [2], Yongmin Chang [4,5,6,*] and Tae-Du Jung [1,2,*]

[1] Department of Rehabilitation Medicine, School of Medicine, Kyungpook National University, Daegu 41944, Korea; ssuni119@naver.com (Y.-S.M.); ehmdpark@naver.com (E.P.); ryoung20@hanmail.net (A.-R.K.)
[2] Department of Rehabilitation Medicine, Kyungpook National University Hospital, Daegu 41944, Korea; eodnjs108@naver.com (D.-W.G.); pyromyth@naver.com (S.-H.J.)
[3] Department of Biomedical Engineering, Seoul National University College of Medicine, Seoul 03080, Korea
[4] Department of Medical & Biological Engineering, Kyungpook National University, Daegu 41944, Korea; giantstar.jw@gmail.com (J.W.P.); hscha1002@daum.net (H.C.)
[5] Department of Radiology, Kyungpook National University Hospital, Daegu 41944, Korea
[6] Department of Molecular Medicine, School of Medicine, Kyungpook National University, Daegu 41944, Korea
* Correspondence: ychang@knu.ac.kr (Y.C.); teeed0522@hanmail.net (T.-D.J.)
† Contributed equally to this work.

Abstract: This study aimed to evaluate the usefulness of interhemispheric functional connectivity (FC) as a predictor of motor recovery in severe hand impairment and to determine the cutoff FC level as a clinically useful parameter. Patients with stroke ($n = 22$; age, 59.9 ± 13.7 years) who presented with unilateral severe upper-limb paresis and were confirmed to elicit no motor-evoked potential responses were selected. FC was measured using resting-state functional magnetic resonance imaging (rsfMRI) scans at 1 month from stroke onset. The good recovery group showed a higher FC value than the poor recovery group ($p = 0.034$). In contrast, there was no statistical difference in FC value between the good recovery and healthy control groups ($p = 0.182$). Additionally, the healthy control group showed a higher FC value than that shown by the poor recovery group ($p = 0.0002$). Good and poor recovery were determined based on Brunnstrom stage of upper-limb function at 6 months as the standard, and receiver operating characteristic curve indicated that a cutoff score of 0.013 had the greatest prognostic ability. In conclusion, interhemispheric FC measurement using rsfMRI scans may provide useful clinical information for predicting hand motor recovery during stroke rehabilitation.

Keywords: functional magnetic resonance imaging; neuronal plasticity; recovery of function; stroke; motor cortex

1. Introduction

Stroke is the leading cause of adult disability worldwide, accounting for a majority of patients with upper-limb impairment. The degrees of spontaneous improvement vary according to the severity of upper-limb paresis. In patients with mild-to-moderate upper-limb paresis, spontaneous recovery, as reflected by improvements in clinical parameters including Fugl-Meyer assessment of the upper extremity (FMA-UE) scores, is mainly restricted to the first 4 weeks post-stroke [1].There is evidence in the literature that in stroke patients with mild-to-moderate impairment, the degree of initial deficits predicts outcome. In contrast to mildly impaired patients, it is relatively difficult to predict the spontaneous recovery pattern of upper-limb motor function in severely impaired patients. Clinical data alone cannot accurately predict arm recovery, particularly in patients with initial severe upper-limb impairment [2–4]. High inter-individual variability associated with recovery makes it difficult to predict arm recovery. However, very few severely impaired patients show late-onset motor recovery of the upper-limb [5]. Therefore, a prognostic biomarker reflecting functional long-term motor recovery is urgently required to decide the manner in which rehabilitation treatment strategies, including goal setting and effective treatment duration, for upper-limb recovery in severe hemiplegic stroke patients can be modified.

Recently, we reported that initial power spectral density (PSD) analysis of resting-state functional magnetic resonance imaging (rsfMRI) data can provide a sensitive prognostic predictor for patients with subacute stroke combined with severe hand disability [6]. PSD is measured as resting-state intrinsic neuronal activity in the frequency domain. In contrast to PSD, functional connectivity (FC) analysis is another approach to measure the resting-state intrinsic neuronal activity in the time domain using rsfMRI. Changes in FC value in the interhemispheric motor cortex (M1) after stroke are reportedly reflective of long-term recovery, and patients with good functional outcomes have greater FC values than patients with poor outcomes [7–9]. However, a recent study reported that differences in FC value in the interhemispheric M1 did not change over time with recovery [10]. Therefore, whether motor recovery after stroke can be predicted by the change in interhemispheric FC still remains controversial.

This study aimed to evaluate whether interhemispheric FC is useful for predicting upper-limb motor recovery among patients with severe hand impairment for whom it was difficult to predict the recovery pattern based on an initial clinical parameter. Therefore, addition of FC as a prognostic parameter for patients with severe hand deficits may eventually be useful for setting individualized therapeutic goals and strategies as well as for selecting patients for future trials.

2. Materials and Methods

2.1. Subjects

Twenty-two patients (59.9 ± 13.7 years; 9 males and 13 females) and 12 healthy subjects (60.2 ± 6.8 years; 8 males, 4 females) were included in this study. They were all right-handed. The inclusion criteria for patients were as follows: (1) unilateral ischemic stroke in the middle cerebral artery (MCA) territory confirmed by MRI, (2) first stroke, (3) age over 20, (4) hemiplegic motor deficit less than Gr 1 by manual muscle test present at the time of admission (Table 1). Patients with unstable medical conditions and those lost to follow-up were excluded.

All patients underwent resting functional magnetic resonance imaging about 1 month (27.8 ± 8.4) from stroke onset. We used Brunnstrom stage (hand score) as a parameter to assess clinical outcome at 1 month and 6 months after stroke onset. We included the patients with Brunnstrom stage 1 (flaccidity or absence of an active finger movement) but without any motor-evoked potential (MEP) responses of the affected hand at 1 month after stroke. Patients with severely impaired cognitive function [Mini-Mental State Examination (MMSE) < 24], severe visual or perceptual impairment, previous musculoskeletal abnormality, or damaged upper-limbs were excluded. All patients received individual physiotherapy training as well as cognitive training every day. The physiotherapy treatments comprised 30-min sessions two times per day for five days a week and included walking and balance training as well as individual exercise. Informed consent was provided to all patients according to OO University Institutional Review Board (2012-05-023).

Table 1. Demographics and baseline characteristics of enrolled patients.

Subject	Group	Sex	Age	Lesion Territory	Total Lesion Volume (cc)	Lesion Volume (CST-Overlapped) (cc)	BS-Hand (Pre)	BS-Hand (Post)	Hand Dominance	BDI	MMSE	NIHSS
1	Good	F	57	MCA	4.8	0.247	1	4	Rt	10	28	8
2	Good	F	67	MCA	58.3	0.359	1	4	Rt	12	25	3
3	Good	F	70	MCA	13.1	0.439	1	4	Rt	22	27	9
4	Good	F	32	MCA	75	0.683	1	4	Rt	12	30	9
5	Good	F	80	MCA	4.7	0.226	1	4	Rt	10	27	5
6	Good	M	67	MCA	11.2	0.177	1	5	Rt	16	28	7
7	Good	F	75	MCA	7.1	0.241	1	4	Rt	24	26	9
8	Good	F	75	MCA	2.1	0.305	1	4	Rt	16	23	4
9	Good	M	40	MCA	9.0	0.216	1	4	Rt	23	27	9
10	Good	M	57	MCA	7.5	0.189	1	4	Rt	8	18	6
11	Good	M	44	MCA	130.4	0.544	1	5	Rt	5	14	7
12	Poor	F	66	MCA	84.5	0.522	1	1	Rt	33	5	16
13	Poor	M	42	MCA	273.8	0.246	1	1	Rt	20	24	7
14	Poor	M	59	MCA	268.7	0.680	1	2	Rt	4	24	9
15	Poor	F	75	MCA	78.3	0.291	1	1	Rt	29	-	13
16	Poor	F	75	MCA	25.0	0.257	1	1	Rt	13	25	13
17	Poor	M	68	MCA	23.6	0.247	1	1	Rt	5	21	15
18	Poor	M	40	MCA	334.2	0.442	1	1	Rt	-	-	21
19	Poor	F	69	MCA	121.4	0.683	1	1	Rt	15	24	14
20	Poor	F	44	MCA	164.4	0.571	1	1	Rt	-	-	12
21	Poor	M	53	MCA	5.1	0.302	1	2	Rt	2	30	6
22	Poor	F	64	MCA	5.3	0.245	1	3	Rt	28	30	11

CST; CorticoSpinal Tract, BS, Brunnstrom stage; BDI, Beck Depression Inventory; MMSE, Mini Mental State Examination; NIHSS, National Institutes of Health Stroke Scale MCA, Middle Cerebral Artery.

2.2. Motor Task Functional Magnetic Resonance Imaging

Region of interest (ROI) of M1 for each participant was defined using motor task functional magnetic resonance imaging (fMRI). Motor task fMRI alternatively comprised three active periods and three rest periods, and each period was 30-s long. A light touch on the leg or hand was used to give a start signal at the start point of each period. Participants performed the motor task twice with the right and left hands and repeated flexion–extension during scanning. If any of the participants could not move their hand, they received assistance to perform passive movement.

To perform motor task fMRI data acquisition, T2-weighted echo-planar imaging sequences were used with the following parameters: TE (echo time) = 40 ms, TR (repetition time) = 3000 ms, Flip Angle (FA) = 90°, FOV (field-of-view) = 21 cm, acquisition matrix = 64 × 64, 4-mm thickness with no gap, and total scan time = 4 min and 12 s, with four dummy scans.

2.3. Resting-State fMRI

All fMRI data were obtained on a Signa Exite 3.0-T scanner (GE Healthcare, Milwaukee, WI, USA). All applicants were instructed to lie down comfortably and close their eyes during MRI scanning, but not fall asleep. The rsfMRI data were obtained using T2-weighted echo-planar imaging sequences using the following parameters: TE = 40 ms, TR = 2000 ms, FA = 90°, FOV = 22 cm, acquisition matrix = 64 × 64, 4-mm thickness with no gap, and total scan time= 8 min and 12 s, with six dummy scans.

Three-dimensional-fast spoiled gradient echo sequence [repetition time (TR) = 7.8 ms; echo time (TE) = 3 ms; inversion time = 450 ms; flip angle = 20; matrix = 256 × 256; field-of-view (FOV) = 24 mm; 1.3 mm thickness] was used for the acquisition of T1-weighted high-resolution anatomical images.

2.4. fMRI Data Analysis

Image preprocessing and statistical analyses of fMRI data were conducted using the statistical parametric mapping software SPM12 (http://www.fil.ion.ucl.ac.uk/spm/), implemented in MATLAB (Mathworks, Inc., Sherborn, MA, USA). By slice-timing, realignment, co-registration, and normalization, functional images were preprocessed into the Montreal Neurological Institute (MNI) template based on a standard stereotaxic coordinate system and spatial smoothing with 8-mm full-width at half-maximum (FWHM) Gaussian kernel. FMRI data are superimposed onto MNI space. The seed MNI coordinates for the patients were summarized in Table S1 (Supplementary Materials).

2.5. Rest State Functional Connectivity

The seed-based method was used to determine resting-state functional connectivity (rsFC). In brief, FC CONN15 toolbox (http://web.mit.edu/swg/software.htm) was used to show a strong temporal correlation between bilateral M1 and supplementary motor area (SMA). The contralesion and ipsilesion (namely M1 and SMA; spheres of 5-mm radius) were identified using MarsBar ROI tool (http://marsbar.sourceforge.net/) on MNI coordinates. Four ROI positions (spheres of 5 mm radius), namely contralesional M1, ipsilesional M1, contralesional SMA, and ipsilesional SMA, were selected based on individual motor task results. Noise, cerebrospinal fluid, white matter, and motion parameters were used to correct time fluctuations in blood-oxygen-level-dependent (BOLD) signals as nuisance covariates, and a band-pass filter (range, 0.008 Hz–0.09 Hz) was used. FC scores between pairs of ROIs on each subject were calculated using the FC SPM12 toolbox.

2.6. Lesion Volume Analysis

The lesion volume associated with hand motor function in the stroke area was calculated based on the overlapping area of the lesion mask between the T1-weighted images and the template of the corticospinal tract (CST). T1-weighted images were taken by preprocessing, which involves co-registration and normalization to a T1-weighted template using the SPM12 software package. A stroke physiatrist, who was blinded to the study, manually drew the lesions by using MRIcro (http:

//www.mccauslandcenter.sc.edu/crnl/mricro). The CST template was constructed using a previously reported method of probabilistic tractography [11,12]. Probabilistic tractography was conducted for 26 healthy controls to reconstruct CST. The seed, target, waypoint, and exclusion mask were drawn as follows. Individual seed masks for each hemisphere were placed in the hand knob area of M1 (MNI coordinates (37, −25, 62); (−37, −25, 62)), and each participant used an established semi-automated pipeline. The target masks were basis pontis. The waypoint masks included the posterior limb of the internal capsules and cerebral peduncles. For CST, a mask covering trajectories at the tegmentum pontis was added to the mid-sagittal and basal ganglia exclusion masks as an additional exclusion mask. A total of 50,000 streamlines were sent from M1 to the spinal target masks in the ventral medulla oblongata. Three different thresholds at 0.5%, 1%, and 2% were established for CST output distributions. The average of each tract was calculated for each of the three thresholds by summing all individual threshold- and subject-specific trajectories.

2.7. Statistical Analysis

To assess differences in FC scores between the three groups for each pair of ROIs, an ANOVA F-test was performed; subsequently, post-hoc two-sample t-tests were conducted for carrying out further comparisons. All statistical analyses were performed using the Statistical Package for the Social Sciences (SPSS, Chicago, IL, USA). A p value of <0.05 was considered to be statistically significant.

Receiver-operating characteristic (ROC) curve analysis was performed to determine the cutoff value for the prognostic model of upper-limb stroke recovery by using the difference in FC score between ipsilesional and contralesional M1 at 1 month.

True-positive rate (sensitivity) and false-positive rate (1-specificity) were computed and plotted as ROC curves. In an ROC space, a diagonal line corresponds to random discrimination. The area under the ROC curve (AUC) is commonly used to quantify classifier discriminability, with a value of 0.5 corresponding to random classification and a value of 1 corresponding to perfect classification.

3. Results

At 6 months after stroke onset, 11 patients (60.3 ± 15.9 years; seven males, four females) with Brunnstrom stage 4 (lateral prehension with release by thumb movement or semi-voluntary finger extension of a small range of motion) or 5 (palmar prehension or cylindrical/spherical grasp with limited function or voluntary mass finger extension of variable range) were categorized into the good recovery group and 11 patients (59.5 ± 12.9 years; six males, five females) with Brunnstrom stage 1, 2, and 3 were categorized into the poor recovery group. There were no age and sex-based differences between the good recovery and the poor recovery groups and the healthy control group ($p = 0.986$ and $p = 0.827$, respectively). Additionally, there was no statistical difference ($p = 0.158$) in lesion overlap volume between the good recovery group (0.33 ± 0.15 cc) and the poor recovery group (0.40 ± 0.17 cc). However, there was statistical difference ($p = 0.019$) in total lesion volume between the good recovery group (29.37 ± 41.31 cc) and the poor recovery group (125 ± 118.73 cc) (Figure 1). The demographic and clinical characteristics of 22 patients with stroke are summarized in Table 1.

Among the three groups, ANOVA F-test results reveal a statistically significant difference in FC between ipsilesional M1–contralesional M1 ($p = 0.00039$) (Figure 2). Post-hoc two-sample t-tests were performed for comparing the three groups further. The good recovery group showed a higher FC than that of the poor recovery group ($p = 0.034$). Contrastingly, the good recovery group showed no statistical difference in FC when compared with the healthy control group ($p = 0.182$), but the latter had a higher FC than that of the poor recovery group ($p = 0.0002$).

Moreover, according to the ANOVA F-test, the FC between ipsilesional SMA and contralesional SMA was significantly different among the three groups ($p = 0.003$) (Figure 1). In the post-hoc two-sample t-test, the FC between ipsilesional SMA and contralesional SMA was higher in the healthy control group compared with that in the good recovery group and the poor recovery group ($p = 0.019$

and $p = 0.004$, respectively), but there was no difference in the FC value between the good recovery group and the poor recovery group ($p = 0.804$).

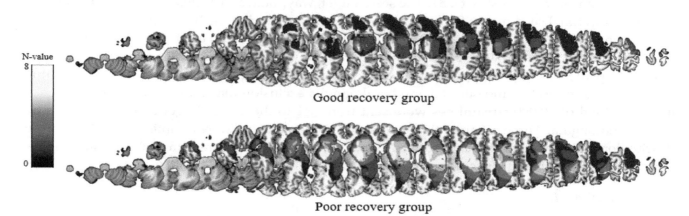

Figure 1. Total lesion overlay maps for the good recovery group and the poor recovery group.

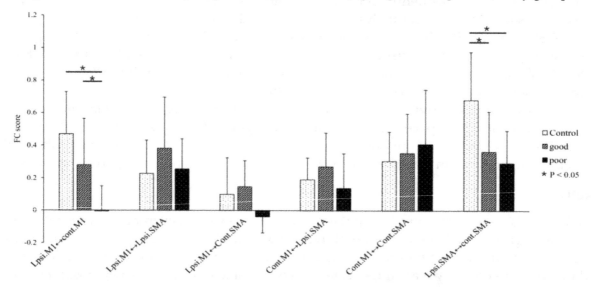

Figure 2. ANOVA F-tests showed significant differences in functional connectivity (FC) between ipsilesional M1-contralesional M1 among the three groups ($p = 0.00039$). Post-hoc two-sample t-tests were performed for further comparing between the groups. The good recovery group showed a higher FC than that shown by the poor recovery group ($p = 0.034$). In contrast, no significant difference in FC was seen between the good recovery and the healthy control groups ($p = 0.182$). Additionally, the healthy control group showed a higher FC than that of the poor recovery group ($p = 0.0002$).

Contrastingly, the ANOVA F-test result reveals no significant difference in FC among ipsilesional M1-SMA ($p = 0.318$), ipsilesional M1-contralesional SMA ($p = 0.056$), contralesional M1-ipsilesional SMA ($p = 0.297$), and contralesional M1-contralesional SMA ($p = 0.656$).

When the total lesion volume was included as a covariate in statistical analysis, ANOVA F-test results reveal a statistically significant difference in FC between ipsilesional M1–contralesional M1 among the three groups ($p = 0.018$) and in FC between ipsilesional M1–contralesional SMA among the three groups ($p = 0.015$). In the post-hoc two-sample t-test, however, there was no difference in the FC value between the good recovery group and poor recovery group ($p = 0.232$).

FC between ipsilesional and contralesional M1 positively correlated with hand function prognosis, as evaluated by Brunnstrom motor stages (BMS) (r = 0.581 and $p = 0.005$, respectively) (Figure 3). However, FC between ipsilesional and contralesional SMA did not correlate with hand function prognosis, as evaluated by BMS (r = −0.006, $p = 0.979$).

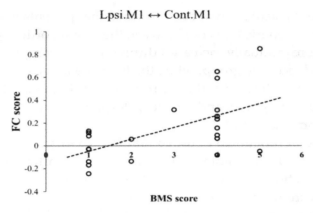

Figure 3. FC between ipsilesional and contralesional M1 is positively correlated with prognosis of hand function, as evaluated by Brunnstrom motor stages (BMS) (r = 0.581, p = 0.005).

Good and poor recovery outcomes based on the Brunnstrom stage of upper-limb function at 6 months were determined as the standard, and the ROC curve indicated that a cutoff score of 0.013 had the greatest prognostic ability (maximum sensitivity and specificity) (Figure 4). The sensitivity of this model for predicting good recovery was 81.8% and the specificity was 63.6%. AUC value was 0.793, which is a fair level.

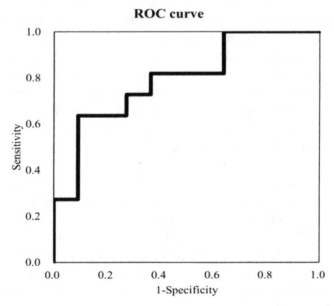

Figure 4. Good and poor recovery were determined based on Brunnstrom stage of upper-limb function at 6 months as the standard, and ROC (Receiver-operating characteristic) curve indicated that a cutoff score of 0.013 had the greatest prognostic ability (maximum sensitivity and specificity).

4. Discussion

Here, we demonstrated the predictive value of FC for long-term motor outcomes in subacute stroke patients with stroke, predominantly in the MCA territory. The FC between ipsilateral and contralateral M1 was lower in the poor recovery group compared with that in the good recovery and healthy control groups, and it was also well correlated with hand function prognosis, evaluated by BMS. Our study demonstrated that the interhemispheric FC score calculated at 1 month after stroke has a good predictive value for recovery over a 6-month period in patients with severe hand impairment. However, the total lesion volume showed a tendency to swallow a large amount of explanatory variance of the outcome parameter. We also suggested an FC cutoff score for discriminating the good recovery group from the poor recovery group with high sensitivity and specificity.

Previous rsfMRI studies on acute stroke demonstrated that patients with mild-to-moderate motor deficits showed low interhemispheric FC score between the motor cortices [8,9,13]. These studies also revealed that the low FC score gradually increased during the recovery process and finally restored to near-normal levels in a good recovery group, while the FC score in the poor recovery group continued to decrease. Our findings are in line with these previous studies, i.e., interhemispheric FC score is useful for assessing the stroke prognosis and recovery despite varying scanning times (e.g., 3 days vs. 4 weeks) and evaluation domains [7,14,15].

These results suggest that functional neuroadaptation (reorganization) may be occurring in the most severely injured brains. One possible explanation for this finding is the physiological balance in reciprocal inhibitory projections between both of the hemispheres [16]. This explanation suggests that an abnormal inhibitory influence of the undamaged contralesional motor cortex on the damaged ipsilesional motor cortex disturbs the balance between the hemispheres, which is important for voluntarily generating paretic hand movement in poor recovery patients [16–19]. Here, the patients in the good recovery group had a higher rsFC between the motor cortex, which enhanced motor ability in the paretic hand. Our findings are consistent with those of previous studies, which demonstrated that rsFC within either the ipsilesional primary sensorimotor cortex or contralesional primary sensorimotor cortex reduced at an early stage after stroke, after which, in those patients who showed an improvement in motor impairment, the rsFC gradually increased to near-normal levels during recovery.

However, Nijboer et al. reported that ipsilesional rsFC between motor areas was lower than the contralesional rsFC, but this difference did not change over time [10]; they demonstrated that no relations were observed between individual changes in rsFC and upper-limb motor recovery. In that study, patient population presented with mild upper-limb impairments as opposed to the patients in our study who had severe motor impairment at 4 weeks after stroke. The patients only showed a limited amount of improvement (i.e., ceiling effect) after the first 4 weeks. The changes in brain activation patterns (i.e., cerebral reorganization) might have a different impact on a mild patient population compared with that on a population comprising severely impaired patients [20]. Here, patients were completely motor deficit with no hand movement and MEP response.

Using rsfMRI, we elucidated the cutoff value of FC to be 0.013, and sensitivity and specificity rates for good recovery prediction were 81.8% and 63.6%, respectively. There have been many studies on modeling the prediction of function recovery after stroke. The representative models are the PREP algorithm and the proportional recovery model [2,21]. However, when the two models were validated, the predicted prognosis rate (sensitivity and specificity) remained around 73–88%. The reason is that fitting to that predictive model did not work well in patients with severe corticospinal tract damage early in the injury, clinically complete unilateral paralysis, and patients with no MEP response. That is, in the case of mild to moderate severity, the prediction through clinical data and infarction size fit well, but in severe cases, it was difficult to predict through the model, and these were called 'non-fitter'. In this study, we included relatively homogenous patients with MCA infarction, clinically no hand movement at all, and neurophysiologically no MEP response. Therefore, measuring interhemispheric functional connectivity in these patient populations can help predict prognosis. The prediction power associated with the use of only one parameter, namely interhemispheric rsFC, was comparable to the power associated with the multi-parameter model, without causing any compromise in sensitivity and specificity rates.

The present study had some limitations. First of all, our study is limited by small numbers in the patient population. Due to this limitation, stroke patients included only those with cortical and subcortical stroke, and we could not definitely determine the differential impact of lesion location and stroke severity on rsFC. Hence, from our results, we could not fully elucidate the mechanisms responsible for the reduction in rsFC after stroke as well as its influence on patient behavior. However, a more important clinical implication would be the establishment of the prognostic power of rsFC at an early stage. Therefore, larger sample size and longitudinal follow-up are warranted to confirm these relationships in future studies.

5. Conclusions

Interhemispheric FC estimated via rsfMRI provides useful clinical information and has a predictive value for hand motor recovery during stroke rehabilitation.

Author Contributions: Conceptualization, J.W.P.; Data curation, D.-W.G. and S.-H.J.; Formal analysis, E.P.; Funding acquisition, Y.C.; Investigation, A.-R.K.; Methodology, J.W.P.; Resources, H.C. and Y.C.; Software, J.W.P.; Supervision, T.-D.J.; Validation, E.P.; Visualization, J.W.P.; Writing—original draft, Y.-S.M.; Writing—review & editing, Y.C. All authors have read and agreed to the published version of the manuscript.

References

1. Kwakkel, G.; Kollen, B.J.; van der Grond, J.; Prevo, A.J.H. Probability of regaining dexterity in the flaccid upper limb: Impact of severity of paresis and time since onset in acute stroke. *Stroke* **2003**, *34*, 2181–2186. [CrossRef]

2. Byblow, W.D.; Stinear, C.M.; Barber, P.A.; Petoe, M.A.; Ackerley, S.J. Proportional recovery after stroke depends on corticomotor integrity. *Ann. Neurol.* **2015**, *78*, 848–859. [CrossRef]

3. Feng, W.; Wang, J.; Chhatbar, P.Y.; Doughty, C.; Landsittel, D.; Lioutas, V.A.; Kautz, S.A.; Schlaug, G. Corticospinal tract lesion load: An imaging biomarker for stroke motor outcomes. *Ann. Neurol.* **2015**, *78*, 860–870. [CrossRef] [PubMed]

4. Buch, E.R.; Rizk, S.; Nicolo, P.; Cohen, L.G.; Schnider, A.; Guggisberg, A.G. Predicting motor improvement after stroke with clinical assessment and diffusion tensor imaging. *Neurology* **2016**, *86*, 1924–1925. [CrossRef] [PubMed]

5. Jung, T.D.; Kim, J.Y.; Seo, J.H.; Jin, S.U.; Lee, H.J.; Lee, S.H.; Lee, Y.S.; Chang, Y. Combined information from resting-state functional connectivity and passive movements with functional magnetic resonance imaging differentiates fast late-onset motor recovery from progressive recovery in hemiplegic stroke patients: A pilot study. *J. Rehabil. Med.* **2013**, *45*, 546–552. [CrossRef] [PubMed]

6. Min, Y.S.; Park, J.W.; Jang, K.E.; Lee, H.J.; Lee, J.; Lee, Y.S.; Jung, T.D.; Chang, Y. Power Spectral Density Analysis of Long-Term Motor Recovery in Patients With Subacute Stroke. *Neurorehabil. Neural Repair* **2019**, *33*, 38–46. [CrossRef] [PubMed]

7. Puig, J.; Blasco, G.; Alberich-Bayarri, A.; Schlaug, G.; Deco, G.; Biarnes, C.; Navas-Martí, M.; Rivero, M.; Gich, J.; Figueras, J.; et al. Resting-State Functional Connectivity Magnetic Resonance Imaging and Outcome After Acute Stroke. *Stroke* **2018**, *49*, 2353–2360. [CrossRef] [PubMed]

8. Carter, A.R.; Shulman, G.L.; Corbetta, M. Why use a connectivity-based approach to study stroke and recovery of function? *Neuroimage* **2012**, *62*, 2271–2280. [CrossRef] [PubMed]

9. Golestani, A.M.; Tymchuk, S.; Demchuk, A.; Goodyear, B.G. VISION-2 Study Group Longitudinal evaluation of resting-state FMRI after acute stroke with hemiparesis. *Neurorehabil. Neural Repair* **2013**, *27*, 153–163. [CrossRef]

10. Nijboer, T.C.W.; Buma, F.E.; Winters, C.; Vansteensel, M.J.; Kwakkel, G.; Ramsey, N.F.; Raemaekers, M. No changes in functional connectivity during motor recovery beyond 5 weeks after stroke; A longitudinal resting-state fMRI study. *PLoS ONE* **2017**, *12*, e0178017. [CrossRef]

11. Schulz, R.; Koch, P.; Zimerman, M.; Wessel, M.; Bönstrup, M.; Thomalla, G.; Cheng, B.; Gerloff, C.; Hummel, F.C. Parietofrontal motor pathways and their association with motor function after stroke. *Brain* **2015**, *138*, 1949–1960. [CrossRef] [PubMed]

12. Schulz, R.; Park, C.H.; Boudrias, M.H.; Gerloff, C.; Hummel, F.C.; Ward, N.S. Assessing the integrity of corticospinal pathways from primary and secondary cortical motor areas after stroke. *Stroke* **2012**, *43*, 2248–2251. [CrossRef] [PubMed]

13. Carter, A.R.; Astafiev, S.V.; Lang, C.E.; Connor, L.T.; Rengachary, J.; Strube, M.J.; Pope, D.L.W.; Shulman, G.L.; Corbetta, M. Resting interhemispheric functional magn0065tic resonance imaging connectivity predicts performance after stroke. *Ann. Neurol.* **2010**, *67*, 365–375. [CrossRef] [PubMed]

14. Park, C.; Chang, W.H.; Ohn, S.H.; Kim, S.T.; Bang, O.Y.; Pascual-Leone, A.; Kim, Y.-H. Longitudinal changes of resting-state functional connectivity during motor recovery after stroke. *Stroke* **2011**, *42*, 1357–1362. [CrossRef]

15. Yin, D.; Song, F.; Xu, D.; Peterson, B.S.; Sun, L.; Men, W.; Yan, X.; Fan, M. Patterns in cortical connectivity for determining outcomes in hand function after subcortical stroke. *PLoS ONE* **2012**, *7*, e52727. [CrossRef]

16. Ward, N.S.; Brown, M.M.; Thompson, A.J.; Frackowiak, R.S.J. Neural correlates of outcome after stroke: A cross-sectional fMRI study. *Brain* **2003**, *126*, 1430–1448. [CrossRef]

17. Cramer, S.C.; Riley, J.D. Neuroplasticity and brain repair after stroke. *Curr. Opin. Neurol.* **2008**, *21*, 76–82. [CrossRef]

18. Buma, F.E.; Lindeman, E.; Ramsey, N.F.; Kwakkel, G. Functional neuroimaging studies of early upper limb recovery after stroke: A systematic review of the literature. *Neurorehabil. Neural Repair* **2010**, *24*, 589–608. [CrossRef]

19. Fan, Y.; Wu, C.; Liu, H.; Lin, K.; Wai, Y.; Chen, Y. Neuroplastic changes in resting-state functional connectivity after stroke rehabilitation. *Front. Hum. Neurosci.* **2015**, *9*. [CrossRef]

20. Xu, H.; Qin, W.; Chen, H.; Jiang, L.; Li, K.; Yu, C. Contribution of the Resting-State Functional Connectivity of the Contralesional Primary Sensorimotor Cortex to Motor Recovery after Subcortical Stroke. *PLoS ONE* **2014**, *9*, e84729. [CrossRef]

21. Stinear, C.M.; Barber, P.A.; Petoe, M.; Anwar, S.; Byblow, W.D. The PREP algorithm predicts potential for upper limb recovery after stroke. *Brain* **2012**, *135*, 2527–2535. [CrossRef] [PubMed]

13

Twenty Years of Cerebral Ultrasound Perfusion Imaging—Is the Best yet to Come?

Jens Eyding [1,2,*], Christian Fung [3], Wolf-Dirk Niesen [4] and Christos Krogias [5]

[1] Department of Neurology, Klinikum Dortmund gGmbH, Beurhausstr 40, 44137 Dortmund, Germany
[2] Department of Neurology, University Hospital Knappschaftskrankenhaus, Ruhr University Bochum, 44892 Bochum, Germany
[3] Department of Neurosurgery, Universityhospital, University of Freiburg, 79106 Freiburg, Germany; christian.fung@uniklinik-freiburg.de
[4] Department of Neurology, Universityhospital, University of Freiburg, 79106 Freiburg, Germany; wolf-dirk.niesen@uniklinik-freiburg.de
[5] Department of Neurology, St. Josef-Hospital, Ruhr University Bochum, 44791 Bochum, Germany; christos.krogias@rub.de
* Correspondence: jens.eyding@rub.de

Abstract: Over the past 20 years, ultrasonic cerebral perfusion imaging (UPI) has been introduced and validated applying different data acquisition and processing approaches. Clinical data were collected mainly in acute stroke patients. Some efforts were undertaken in order to compare different technical settings and validate results to gold standard perfusion imaging. This review illustrates the evolution of the method, explicating different technical aspects and milestones achieved over time. Up to date, advancements of ultrasound technology as well as data processing approaches enable semi-quantitative, gold standard proven identification of critically hypo-perfused tissue in acute stroke patients. The rapid distribution of CT perfusion over the past 10 years has limited the clinical need for UPI. However, the unexcelled advantage of mobile application raises reasonable expectations for future applications. Since the identification of intracerebral hematoma and large vessel occlusion can also be revealed by ultrasound exams, UPI is a supplementary multi-modal imaging technique with the potential of pre-hospital application. Some further applications are outlined to highlight the future potential of this underrated bedside method of microcirculatory perfusion assessment.

Keywords: ultrasound; acute ischemic stroke; perfusion imaging; contrast agent; intracerebral hematoma; subarachnoid hemorrhage

1. Introduction: Cerebral Ultrasound Perfusion Imaging (UPI), First Clinical Applications

Ultrasound imaging is a key diagnostic tool in clinical medicine. Even if an expert examiner is needed to obtain and interpret the images, it is advantageous to other diagnostic entities for various reasons, two of them being the mobile bedside character of the examination and the absence of radiation exposure. Besides gray-scale B-mode imaging for tissue characterization, vessel imaging by Doppler-based duplex-sonography is the basis in most diagnostic work-up settings. After application of specific contrast enhancing substances, improved vessel imaging and contrast-enhanced tissue imaging (CEUS) can provide sophisticated information like vascular occlusion or tissue perfusion imaging in various indications. In neurosonology, ischemic stroke and its diagnostic work up is the leading indication for ultrasound imaging questioning the vessel status of extra- and intracranial arteries. With the invention of contrast-enhanced perfusion imaging, the question of transferability to cerebral imaging quickly emerged. In 1998, the first report on the ability of tracing contrast enhancer in the cerebral microcirculation of healthy volunteers by transient harmonic imaging was published [1], followed by a case report on two acute stroke patients displaying impaired contrast increase in later infarcted areas in 1999 [2]. The technical approach was adapted from echocardiography, where size of myocardial infarct had been visualized before [3]. Various case series could reproduce the initial results by demonstrating missing signal increase in affected ischemic brain areas [4–6]. In the cerebral application, the temporal bone hampers ultrasound transmission resulting in relatively poor imaging quality. Therefore, different variations of harmonic imaging techniques and data acquisition and processing approaches have been introduced since to improve imaging quality [7–10]. Hereby, a novel approach displaying both hemispheres in one examination for isochronal comparison of normal and ischemic brain areas (bilateral or mirror approach) was introduced in 2003 [11] (compare "Data Acquisition and Processing" below for comparison of unilateral and bilateral approach). Using a bolus kinetic approach, time-based parameters such as TPI (time-to-peak intensity) could distinguish between areas of normal, impaired, and nullified parenchymal perfusion [12,13]. Figure 1 illustrates the conventional transversal insonation plane using the transtemporal bone window. Figure 2 illustrates an early unilateral examination of an acute stroke patient displaying missing contrast enhancement in later infarction, and Figure 3 an up-to-date bilateral examination of a normal person and an acute stroke patient displaying different areas of impaired perfusion. A systematical review of the literature on the method has recently summarized an overview until early 2017 [14].

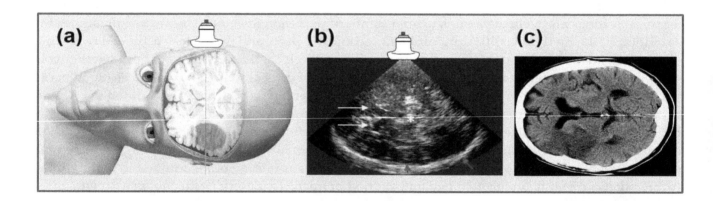

Figure 1. Schematic representation of insonation plane in transtemporal ultrasound imaging (**a**), adapted from [13] (with permission of copyright owner) with a corresponding "bilateral" B-mode image (**b**) with explanatory anatomical landmarks: white arrows = frontal horns of side ventricles; * = midline, third ventricle; red arrows = contralateral skull. Infarcted areas cannot be displayed in B-mode ultrasound. For orientation, comparison to conventional cerebral computed tomography scan, CCT, (**c**) with plane shifted by 90° accordingly, with an infarction in the hemisphere "contralateral" to the probe.

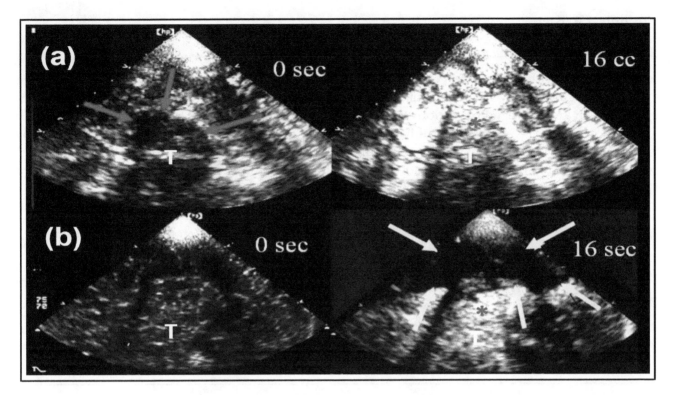

Figure 2. Ultrasound perfusion imaging in the course of time. Early "unilateral" gray-scale imaging in a healthy volunteer (**a**) and an acute stroke patient (**b**) corresponding to Figure 1: at baseline (0 s) and after contrast enhancer application at the time of maximal contrast enhancement (16 s). The thalamic region (red arrows) is marked with increase of brightness in both examples (*), whereas the regions of the lentiform nucleus and temporoparietal lobe are spared (yellow arrows), where later infarction was demonstrated in CCT follow-up. (T) indicates the third ventricle, adapted from [15] with permission from Elsevier.

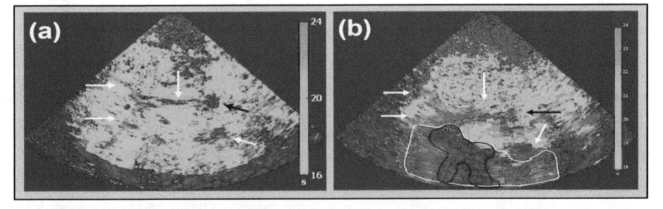

Figure 3. Up to date "bilateral" perfusion imaging corresponding to Figure 1: parametric image of time-to-peak intensity (TPI) in a healthy volunteer (**a**) with homogeneously distributed greenish parts of parenchymal structures (TPI 16 to 20 s) and the depiction of frontal and posterior horns of side ventricles as well as third ventricle (white arrows), and pineal gland (black arrow), adapted from [12]. Note the near field artifact. TPI parameter image of an acute stroke patient 2.5 h after symptom onset (**b**) of a severe stroke caused by occlusion of the M1 segment of the middle cerebral artery. Note the core of infarction (pink area, surrounded by black line) and hypo-perfused nature, and potentially salvageable area (orange area, surrounded by white line) due to collateral flow; adapted from [12] with the publisher's permission.

2. Technical Aspects

2.1. Microbubbles and Harmonic Imaging

The use of ultrasound contrast enhancers (US-CE) is a prerequisite in the application of ultrasound perfusion imaging (UPI). US-CEs consist of gaseous microbubbles (diameter ranging between 1 and 10 µm), which are stabilized by various types of shells, aiming to provide high microbubble stability with improved signal-to-noise ratio and a sufficient examination time [16]. These microbubbles show strong backscattering of beamed ultrasound pulses, not only with linear scattering, but mainly with non-linear scattering, which usually is not relevantly present in most tissues. The different composition of the US-CEs that have been used so far in UPI are displayed in Table 1.

Table 1. Ultrasound contrast enhancers having been used in brain perfusion studies (adapted from [16]).

Name	First Approved	Gas	Shell Material	Producer/Distributor
Levovist®	1993, withdrawn	Air	Galactose microparticles	Schering AG, Berlin, DE
Optison®	1998	Octafluoropropane, C_3F_8	Cross-linked serum albumin	GE healthcare, Buckinghamshire, UK
SonoVue®	2001	Sulphurhexafluoride, SF_6	Phospholipid	Bracco diagnostics, Milano, Italy

With increasing acoustic power, the microbubbles can be set into resonance vibrations, a process that results in the additional emission of harmonic frequencies—multiples of the fundamental frequency. This attribute enables various contrast harmonic imaging modes to detect the US-CE with high sensitivity and to differentiate it from the surrounding tissue. This goal is usually achieved by a band pass filter, which suppresses the fundamental frequencies.

Depending on the applied acoustic power, various interactions between the ultrasound beam and the US-CEs occur. By further increasing the ultrasound energy, the microbubbles can burst. This effect is referred to as "stimulated acoustic emission", since bursting microbubbles emit their own ultrasound, which in turn can be used for ultrasound imaging. The mechanical index (MI), originally defined to predict the onset of cavitation in fluids, gives an on-screen indication of the likelihood of microbubble destruction during examination. MI is defined as maximum value of the peak negative pressure divided by the square root of the acoustic center frequency. The threshold between a low MI and high MI is not clearly defined in cerebral imaging; however, an MI > 1.0 is needed for the destruction of the microbubbles to compensate for the ultrasound absorption of the skull [10]. Therefore, actual acoustic intensity in brain parenchyma is far less than in other organs as expected by mere MI values because of the strong absorption of the skull. Overall, data acquisition modes can be divided in "non-destructive" and "destructive" imaging modes:

2.1.1. "Non-Destructive Imaging Modes":

Conventional Harmonic Imaging

Conventional harmonic imaging is a single pulse modality based on the described stronger non-linear oscillation of US-CEs compared to the surrounding tissue. The non-linear oscillation results in harmonic frequencies (multiples of the fundamental frequency), enabling the differentiation between the signals of tissue and microbubbles by the use of band pass filters (Figure 4).

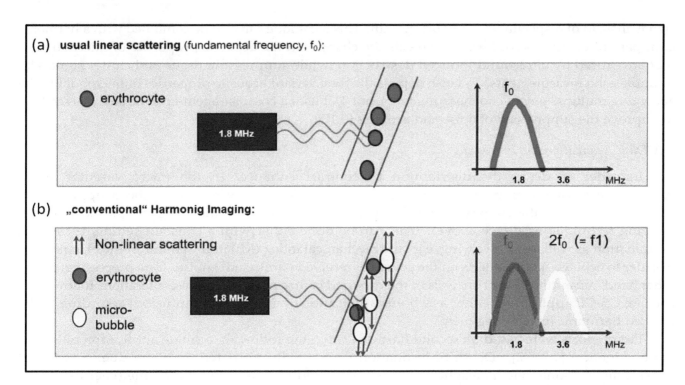

Figure 4. The basic principle of harmonic imaging. (**a**) When an ultrasound wave passes through tissue, the predominantly linear scattering of the erythrocytes results in a frequency, which is reflected back to the probe, which is equal to the transmitted frequency (here: fundamental frequency of 1.8 MHz). (**b**) "Harmonic imaging" due to non-linear scattering of the microbubbles: the resonance frequency of the microbubbles is typically a multiple of the transmitted (or fundamental) frequency. The harmonic frequencies are sent back to the probe, where they are used to create the image. Specifically, the second harmonic frequency (2f0) is used. The fundamental component is filtered out, so that that the received frequency of 3.6 MHz is two-fold higher than the transmitted frequency of 1.8 MHz.

Phase Inversion Harmonic Imaging

In phase (or pulse-) inversion harmonic imaging (PIHI), two echoes are acquired per line, resulting from a pair of mirror-inverted transmit pulses. An acoustic wave in a medium (i.e., the first transmit pulse) shows sinus-wave characteristics, so that a zone of overpressure is followed by a symmetric zone of negative pressure. In case of a linear scatterer, the summation of the two scattered and acquired echoes results in a reciprocative elimination, so that the fundamental is cancelled out. With the use of US-CEs, the non-linear oscillation changes according to the absolute pressure, so that the summation of the two echoes results in a mismatch, as the overpressure in the first echo will not be equal to the negative pressure in the second echo. This mismatch is the same for both half cycles, so that the result of the summation, in principle, is the second harmonic. Only this mismatch is visualized, so that PIHI performs the separation of the second harmonic from the fundamental [8].

Power Modulation Harmonic Imaging

Like in PIHI, power modulation harmonic imaging (PMHI) represents a further multi-pulse technique. Using multiple pulses with differences in amplitude, PMHI aims to detect the harmonic response by sending several pulses and subtracting the responses, as the linear response reduces with multi-pulsing and the harmonic response remains.

2.1.2. "Destructive Imaging modes":

Contrast Burst Imaging and Time Variance Imaging

Contrast burst imaging (CBI) and time variance imaging (TVI) are derived from Power Doppler in which pulses are broadband with high acoustic power. Power Doppler uses the Doppler shift in frequency induced by the movement of the scattering objects, displaying the amplitude of the Doppler signal, instead of displaying this frequency shift. This technique can also be combined with a harmonic bandpass filter. In this context, CBI detects the changes in the acoustic properties of microbubbles that are caused by ultrasound-induced destruction, while suppressing tissue and clutter signals by multiple echo measurements. TVI also depicts the time variant acoustic properties of microbubbles by analyzing multiple pulse echo measurements, but TVI uses a contrast-agent-specific analysis strategy to improve the suppression of noise and artifacts [9,17].

2.2. Data Acquisition and Processing

In order to detect the distribution of contrast enhancer in the micro vascular space, various approaches of data acquisition as well as data processing have been applied [14]. Data acquisition, in this context, means the kind of ultrasound application, i.e., the specific harmonic imaging technique used (see above). This can be done either with a constant setting during the examination as well as with varying, e.g., the mechanical index (MI) in the course of the examination in order to achieve specific effects on the course of received ("reflected") noise. Data processing, on the other hand, means the kind of analysis of the expected course of received noise alterations followed by specific US-CE application (either as a bolus application or as a constant infusion) according to the applied harmonic imaging regimen.

First reports were based on second harmonic imaging following a single application of US-CE (bolus kinetics) [1,2,4–7]. Depth of insonation was initially restricted to 10 cm due to technical constraints, i.e., only one hemisphere of the brain could be analyzed by the time (later called the "unilateral" approach). Received time intensity curves (TIC) were analyzed by dedicated algorithms, which derive specific parameters of wash-in and wash-out (such as time-to-peak intensity, TPI) by fitting the actual information (TIC) to the expected course defined by pre-described mathematical model functions [15] (compare Figure 5). Subsequent studies initially analyzed different harmonic imaging modes like phase inversion harmonic imaging (PIHI) [8] and also adapted "destructive" modes (applying higher MI) with the aim to increase signal-to-noise ratio (CBI and TVI) [10,17]. Due to the unilateral character of the examination, only qualitative information was extracted, i.e., perfusion could be classified as either normal or constricted. Another technical constraint of the unilateral approach is the fact that tissue close to the probe cannot be analyzed due to nearfield artifacts. Therefore, cortical areas of the brain cannot be evaluated.

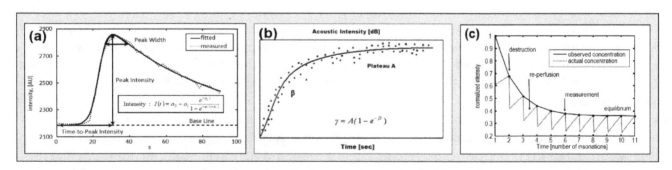

Figure 5. Theoretical course-of-time intensity curves in three different kinetic models as measured in models. Dotted lines represent measured concentration and straight lines represent course of fitted model function. (**a**) Bolus kinetic [8], (**b**) refill kinetic [18], and (**c**) depletion kinetic [15] with permission of the original publishers.

Further technical approaches intended to extract qualitative information (i.e., the degree of perfusion restriction) by applying different acquisition and processing approaches. The refill kinetics approach applied a combination of low MI and high MI imaging during a constant infusion of contrast enhancer [18]. The hypothesis was to destroy the US-CE by an ultra-quick series of high MI pulses and then to display the "refilling" of tissue perfusion by low MI imaging, which should be dependent on the state of perfusion. A given algorithm extracts specific parameters, which have been proven to represent semi-quantitative parameters in myocardial perfusion imaging. A different approach was to apply a longer series of relatively slow frequent and high MI pulses during a constant infusion of US-CE and thereby to evaluate the "depletion" of tissue perfusion, which should also be dependent on the state of perfusion (CODIM) [9]. Figure 5 displays considerations on the mathematical function describing three theoretical courses of time intensity curves of different kinetic models.

Another attempt to extract (semi-) quantitative data was introduced as the so-called bilateral approach [8]. Here, imaging depth was set to 15 cm, visualizing not only one but both hemispheres in one examination (compare Figures 2 and 3). This became possible due to improved ultrasound machines and the introduction of second generation US-CEs (Optison®, SonoVue®), improving signal-to-noise ratio. Two potential advantages were claimed. First, utilizing the so-called mirror approach, intra-individual comparison of perfusion parameters in both affected and unaffected hemispheres could facilitate semi-quantitative analyses. A prerequisite would be the depth-independence of at least one relevant parameter, which could especially be proven for the time dependent parameter, time-to-peak intensity (TPI) [11]. Second, once the affected hemisphere was on the far side of the probe, cortical areas of the affected hemisphere could also be evaluated for perfusion impairments. Since cortical areas are frequently involved in territorial infarction, this was seen as a relevant improvement.

Irrespective of data acquisition and processing modality, the evaluation of specific parameters can be performed two-fold, either by the analysis of pre-defined regions of interest (ROI) or by the presentation of parametric images, where data analysis is carried out by pixel-wise presentation according to one specific parameter (e.g., time-to-peak intensity) [8]. Both processing modalities are offered by industrial providers by now and have been tested against dedicated solutions recently [13]. Figure 6 displays both ROI-wise analysis and a parametric image in an acute stroke patient.

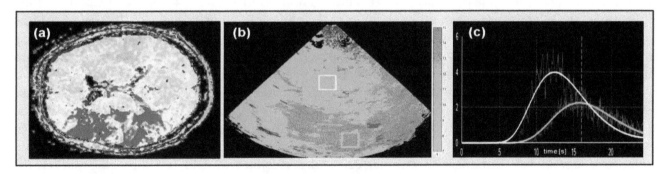

Figure 6. Perfusion MRI time-to-peak (TTP) map of an acute stroke patient with expanded penumbral perfusion delay in the territory of the middle cerebral artery (MCA) omitting basal ganglia (**a**). Ultrasonic cerebral perfusion imaging UPI parametric image with a corresponding depiction of time-to-peak intensity (TPI) delay in the MCA territory omitting basal ganglia (**b**). Exemplary depiction of ROI-wise course-of-time intensity curve in normal perfused brain tissue (yellow curve corresponding yellow box in (**c**) in basal ganglia of the unaffected hemisphere) and penumbral tissue (green curve and box) in an acute stroke patient with MCA occlusion and apparent collateral compensation.

3. Validation to Standard Imaging

Validating different UPI approaches to standard imaging has been crucial from the beginning. In the early studies, patients presenting with ischemic strokes were evaluated in a sub-acute time window up to 24–48 h after symptom onset [1,2,4–7]. Therefore, the actual target was the identification of already infarcted tissue, which was tested mainly against follow-up, non-contrast CCT. Since the focus of interest shifted toward the differentiation between ischemic and penumbral tissue, validation tools needed to become more sophisticated. However, CT (or MRI) perfusion imaging has not always been as well accessible as it is today. Hence, one approach was to define parenchymal tissue as normal, delayed-, or not-perfused in the acute UPI examination and correlate this classification to infarcted and non-infarcted tissue in follow-up CCT according to early clinical course [12]. The hypothesis was that both delayed- and not-perfused tissue of initial UPI should be infarcted in follow-up CCT once there had not been clinical improvement in the meantime. Once there had been distinctive clinical improvement, only not-perfused tissue of the initial UPI exam should be infarcted in the follow-up CCT.

As a matter of fact, especially CT perfusion imaging gained a lot of interest at that time and started its impressive road of success not just in clinical stroke medicine. Nowadays, CT perfusion imaging is widely accessible, probably being the most important factor why the significance of UPI has not further evolved. However, later UPI studies employed timely, correlated CT or MRI perfusion imaging and recently proved that the bilateral approach of high MI bolus imaging, in particular, could distinguish between unimpaired, delayed, and nullified perfusion [19]. Pre specified ROIs in both hemispheres were determined; TPI values of the unaffected hemisphere served as an intra-individual normal value. Values of the affected hemisphere yielded the perfusion status, either for specified ROIs or displayed as parameter image for the whole imaging plane. Once TPI was within ±4 s as compared with the intra-individual normal value, perfusion was unimpaired; a delay of more than 4 s indicated critically hypo-perfused tissue, and nullified rise of TIC indicated infarction. Hereby, the ability of the method to detect penumbral tissue in acute stroke was claimed.

4. Clinical Applications up to Date and Future Indications

Most of the UPI studies have been so far performed in acute stroke patients as described above. Besides contrast-enhanced imaging of cerebral vessels, UPI has already been mentioned in the EFSUMB guidelines and recommendations on the clinical practice of contrast-enhanced ultrasound (CEUS) in 2012 [20]. Studies have mainly been performed in territorial infarction due to main vessel occlusion. One study proved that infarctions as small as 2 cm in diameter can be reliably detected [21]. Case series have demonstrated detectable perfusion impairments in non-occlusive diseases as well [22,23]. In these applications, the bilateral approach utilizing a high MI setting following a bolus application of contrast enhancer seems to deliver the most robust information on the clinical questioning, focusing on vessel occlusion and penumbral imaging. Future challenges of UPI in acute stroke should focus on multicenter validation of up-to-date study results as well as the potential of mobile application. First attempts of mobile cerebral ultrasound imaging in acute stroke have focused on vessel imaging [24], but also basic perfusion imaging is challenged in one industrial project [25]. In addition to being a bedside method, UPI may also be used for serial studies in order to follow-up on brain perfusion. One indication may be early detection of successful recanalization. Serial assessment of UPI may also be used for the guidance of hemodynamic therapy to optimize cerebral perfusion with UPI as a surrogate marker. In a small study in stroke patients, improvement of cerebral perfusion detected by UPI was achieved due to systemic hemodynamic optimization [26].

However, different indications may require different technical settings. Whilst ischemic stroke remains the domain of UPI, it also has been used for identifying different acute or subacute cerebral lesions other than ischemic. There are a few studies on patients with intracranial hemorrhage (ICH) where UPI was used either to improve sonographic detectability of ICH or to describe perihemorrhagic penumbral perfusion (compare Figure 7). ICH can be detected as a hyperechogenic mass lesion within the brain parenchyma with a high sensitivity and specificity [27]. Detection and especially clear distinction of ICH from the adjacent tissue may be difficult in severe cerebral microangiopathy, in lobar hemorrhage, or in only small lesions. Comparable to CT-perfusion studies with a recess or severe hypo-perfusion of contrast media within the hemorrhagic lesion [28], UPI shows a recess of ultrasound contrast media especially within the ICH core and massive reduction of contrast media within the hemorrhagic lesion. Consecutively, ICH appears hypo-echogenic compared to the adjacent tissue, which is perfused normally as shown by the contrast agent with a clear delineation of the border of ICH from the surrounding tissue. Thus, detection of ICH volume may be improved significantly, especially in serial measurements [29]. Despite perihemorrhagic edema, the area of hypo-perfusion or non-perfusion in ICH is fairly restricted to the hemorrhagic lesion itself with no or a very narrow area of hypo-perfused tissue, e.g., perifocal penumbral perfusion. Conversely, parenchymal hemorrhagic transformation of ischemic stroke due to early spontaneous recanalization is difficult to distinguish from primary ICH on native scan but is characterized by a significantly larger perifocal penumbral zone of hypo-perfused tissue exceeding the hemorrhagic lesion by far [30]. Thus, UPI not only helps delineating the border of ICH for more valid volume measurement but also allows distinction of primary ICH from PHI.

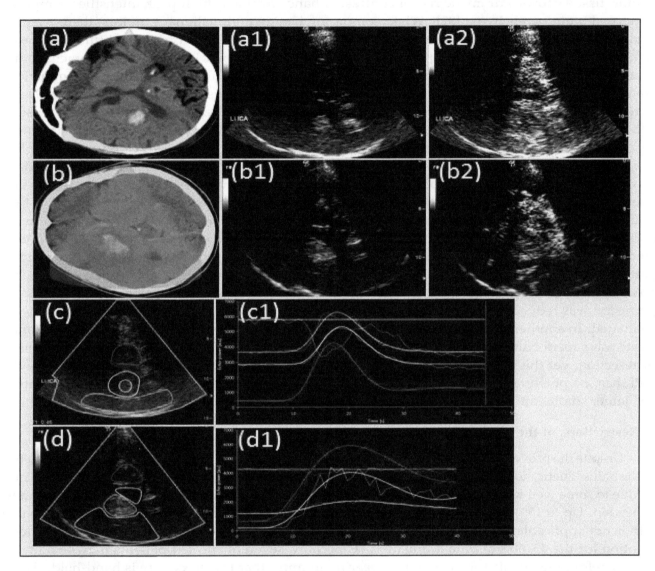

Figure 7. Perfusion imaging in intracerebral hemorrhage and hemorrhagic transformation of cerebral infarction. Cerebral CT of intracerebral hemorrhage (ICH) of the right basal ganglia, (**a**) native transcranial gray-scale sonography with hyperechogenic depiction of ICH (**a1**) and UPI with relative hypo-echogenicity of ICH compared to contrast perfusion of cerebral tissue (**a2**) due to non-perfusion constricted to the hemorrhagic lesion (**c,c1**). Cerebral CT of ICH due to hemorrhagic transformation (**b**), native transcranial gray-scale sonography with hyperechogenic depiction of hemorrhagic transformation (**b1**) and UPI with persistent hyperechogenicity of the hemorrhagic lesion due to omitted perfusion of the surrounding tissue due to acute stroke (**b2**) with slowed or missing tissue perfusion (**b2,d,d1**).

Even though bedside monitoring of cerebral perfusion in brain trauma and acute or chronic subdural hematoma is extremely interesting and theoretically may help in guiding therapy—for instance by defining a surgical need in chronic SDH by detection of cortical hypo-perfusion due to venous compromise—studies on UPI are lacking and data on brain perfusion in these patients generally are scarce. Another application of UPI currently under scientific evaluation is the setting of aneurysmal subarachnoid hemorrhage (NCT02907879). UPI is evaluated with respect to its potential to diagnose cerebral hypo-perfusion in the course of cerebral vasospasm.

Various authors have evaluated cerebral tumors and their ultrasound perfusion patterns [31–35]. UPI is not only able to increase the differentiation of normal brain tissue from brain tumors but it is also helpful to differentiate different tumor types according to their perfusion pattern [32]. Tumor tissue shows a dramatic rise of contrast enhancement and high peak intensities compared to normal brain parenchyma [32]. When comparing benign and malignant tumors, there were no significant differences in peak intensities of the time–intensity curves, yet malignant tumors showed shorter times-to-peak intensities [32]. In the eyes of the authors, UPI is a rapid, practical and cost-effective technique, especially in critically ill patients or if multiple consecutive examinations are necessary. During intraoperative application, ultrasound allows the surgeon to localize a lesion in real-time even before the opening of the dura. This facilitates the surgical access and is a useful add-on to neuronavigation [36,37]. In addition, UPI enables the surgeon to assess tumor enhancement, vascularity, and perfusion, and to control for completeness of resection [38–40]. UPI has been applied in a variety of different brain tumors, e.g., gliomas and metastases [40,41]. In a recent study, Prada et al. characterized intraoperative contrast-enhanced ultrasound images of various brain tumors [40]. They also found a high accuracy between US-based real-time neuronavigation and preoperative MRI findings. The authors concluded that contrast application is useful for the localization, definition of borders, and depiction of the vascularization and perfusion pattern of brain tumors [40]. In another study, UPI was specifically evaluated in brain space-occupying lesions and could identify specific patterns of brain perfusion [42]. It could be shown that meningeomas and glioblastomas, if no large areas of necrosis were present, showed an increased perfusion, while in tumors with necrosis the perfusion was reduced as compared to normal tissue, although in total only 15 brain tumors were evaluated. In another study, it was shown that the differentiation between tumor and normal brain tissue was superior after administration of US-CE [41]. US-CE also enabled the control of completeness of resection, yet this was dependent on technical aspects like the position of the resection cavity. UPI has the potential to become a helpful tool for the surgeon during intraoperative application, yet larger studies are needed.

5. Restrictions of the Method and Safety Considerations

Despite the proven evidence of reproducibility and robustness, especially of time-based parameters of the bolus kinetic, no widespread application of UPI modalities has yet been achieved. Partly, this may be due to some well-known limitations of the method. First, a sonolucent transtemporal bone window is needed. Up to 15%–20% of the elderly patients present with an insufficient bone window, so that UPI is not applicable. Second, patients need to be compliant, so that the transducer can be held in position for the 45–60 s of data acquisition. Especially, severely affected patients may be agitated and therefore unsuitable for the method, bearing in mind that the procedure is hand-held. Third, using the bolus kinetic approach only one two-dimensional imaging plane can be evaluated per bolus application. Therefore, quantification is restricted to an investigation plane that has to be chosen beforehand. However, future development of three-dimensional insonation systems may overcome these limitations. Fourth, quantification is yet only semi-quantitative, i.e., no absolute values can be determined. However, quantification (in acute stroke) as described above utilizes the mirror approach, which is also common in CT and MRI perfusion imaging. In addition, quantification has only been proven for one parameter (TPI). Other parameters have to be challenged in future studies. Regarding safety of UPI, there have been apprehensions of side effects of both US-CE and administration of ultrasound pulses on brain integrity. These have mainly been triggered by results of studies applying long-lasting, whole brain, low-frequency insonation in the setting of ultrasound-enhanced thrombolysis, resulting in massive hemorrhage and blood–brain barrier disruption [43,44]. However, applying standard settings of transcranial insonation, UPI is regarded safe with no evidence of blood–brain barrier affection [45,46].

6. Conclusions

Cerebral ultrasound perfusion imaging has the potential to serve as a supplementary tool to conventional diagnostics in various clinical questionings. As long as temporal bone window is present, a multi-modal approach of vascular imaging for the detection of vessel occlusion, microvascular perfusion impairment or intracerebral hemorrhage is covered by the method. In addition, conventional contrast-enhanced imaging omitting the quantification of perfusion may serve as an extension of diagnostic properties. The unique feature of mobility facilitates application at the bedside. This could enable pre-hospital diagnostics, but also easy-to-apply follow-up diagnostics in the intensive care unit or stroke unit as well as in the operating room. Future developments should focus on multi-center studies to validate the findings described in this manuscript and the development of automated algorithms for examiner independence.

Author Contributions: Conceptualization, J.E., C.F., W.-D.N., and C.K.; methodology, J.E., C.F., W.-D.N., and C.K.; writing—original draft preparation, J.E., C.F., W.-D.N., and C.K.; writing—review and editing, J.E., C.F., W.-D.N., and C.K. All authors have read and agree to the published version of the manuscript.

References

1. Postert, T.; Muhs, A.; Meves, S.; Federlein, J.; Przuntek, H.; Büttner, T. Transient response harmonic imaging: An ultrasound technique related to brain perfusion. *Stroke* **1998**, *29*, 1901–1907. [CrossRef] [PubMed]
2. Postert, T.; Federlein, J.; Weber, S.; Przuntek, H.; Büttner, T. Second harmonic imaging in acute middle cerebral artery infarction: Preliminary results. *Stroke* **1999**, *30*, 1702–1706. [CrossRef]
3. Firschke, C.; Lindner, J.R.; Wie, K.; Goodman, N.C.; Skyba, D.M.; Kaul, S. Myocardial perfusion imaging in the setting of coronary artery stenosis and acute myocardial infarction using venous injection of a second generation echocardiographic contrast agent. *Circulation* **1997**, *96*, 959–967. [PubMed]
4. Federlein, J.; Postert, T.; Meves, S.; Weber, S.; Przuntek, H.; Büttner, T. Ultrasonic evaluation of pathological brain perfusion in acute stroke using second harmonic imaging. *J. Neurol. Neurosurg. Psychiatry* **2000**, *69*, 616–622. [CrossRef]
5. Wiesmann, M.; Meyer, K.; Albers, T.; Seidel, G. Parametric imaging with contrast-enhanced ultrasound in acute ischemic stroke. *Stroke* **2004**, *35*, 508–513. [CrossRef] [PubMed]
6. Seidel, G.; Meyer-Wiethe, K.; Berdien, G.; Hollstein, D.; Toth, D.; Aach, T. Ultrasound perfusion imaging in acute middle cerebral artery infarction predicts outcome. *Stroke* **2004**, *35*, 1107–1111. [CrossRef]
7. Postert, T.; Hoppe, P.; Federlein, J.; Helbeck, S.; Ermert, H.; Przuntek, H.; Büttner, T.; Wilkening, W. Contrast agent specific imaging modes for the ultrasonic assessment of parenchymal cerebral echo contrast enhancement. *J. Cereb. Blood Flow. Metab.* **2000**, *20*, 1709–1716. [CrossRef]
8. Eyding, J.; Krogias, C.; Wilkening, W.; Meves, S.; Ermert, H.; Postert, T. Parameters of cerebral perfusion in phase inversion harmonic imaging (PIHI) ultrasound examinations. *Ultrasound. Med. Biol.* **2003**, *29*, 1379–1385. [CrossRef]
9. Eyding, J.; Wilkening, W.; Reckhardt, M.; Schmid, G.; Meves, S.; Ermert, H.; Przuntek, H.; Postert, T. Contrast Burst Depletion Imaging (CODIM): A new imaging procedure and analysis method for semi-quantitative ultrasonic perfusion imaging. *Stroke* **2003**, *34*, 77–83. [CrossRef]
10. Kern, R.; Perren, F.; Schoeneberger, K.; Gass, A.; Hennerici, M.; Meairs, S. Ultrasound microbubble destruction imaging in acute middle cerebral artey stroke. *Stroke* **2004**, *35*, 1665–1670. [CrossRef]
11. Krogias, C.; Postert, T.; Wilkening, W.; Meves, S.; Przuntek, H.; Eyding, J. Semiquantitative analysis of ultrasonic cerebral perfusion imaging. *Ultrasound Med. Biol.* **2005**, *31*, 1007–1012. [CrossRef] [PubMed]
12. Eyding, J.; Schöllhammer, M.; Eyding, D.; Wilkening, W.; Meves, S.; Schröder, A.; Przuntek, H.; Krogias, C.; Postert, T. Contrast-enhanced ultrasonic parametric perfusion imaging detects tissue at risk in acute stroke. *J. Cereb. Blood Flow. Metab.* **2006**, *26*, 576–582. [CrossRef] [PubMed]

13. Reitmeir, R.; Eyding, J.; Oertel, M.F.; Wiest, R.; Gralla, J.; Fischer, U.; Giquel, P.Y.; Weber, S.; Raabe, A.; Mattle, H.P.; et al. Is ultrasound perfusion imaging capable of detecting mismatch? A proof of- concept study in acute stroke patients. *J. Cereb. Blood Flow. Metab.* **2017**, *37*, 1517–1526. [CrossRef] [PubMed]

14. Vinke, E.J.; Kortenbout, J.; Eyding, J.; Slump, C.H.; van der Hoeven, J.G.; de Korte, C.L.; Hoedemaekers, C.W.E. Potential of contrast enhanced ultrasound as a bedside monitoring technique of cerebral perfusion: A systematic review. *Ultrasound Med. Biol.* **2017**, *43*, 2751–2757. [CrossRef]

15. Eyding, J.; Wilkening, W.; Postert, T. Brain perfusion and ultrasonic imaging techniques. *Eur. J. Ultrasound.* **2002**, *16*, 91–104. [CrossRef]

16. Paefgen, V.; Doleschel, D.; Kiessling, F. Evolution of contrast agents for ultrasound imaging and ultrasound-mediated drug delivery. *Front. Pharmacol.* **2015**, *6*, 197. [CrossRef]

17. Meves, S.H.; Wilkening, W.; Thies, T.; Eyding, J.; Holscher, T.; Finger, M.; Schmid, G.; Ermert, H.; Postert, T. Ruhr Center of Competence for Medical Engineering. Comparison between echo contrast agent specific imaging modes and perfusion-weighted magnetic resonance imaging for the assessment of brain perfusion. *Stroke* **2002**, *33*, 2433–2437. [CrossRef]

18. Kern, R.; Diels, A.; Pettenpohl, J.; Kablau, M.; Brade, J.; Hennerici, M.G.; Meairs, S. Real-time ultrasound brain perfusion imaging with analysis of microbubble replenishment in acute MCAstroke. *J. Cereb. Blood Flow. Metab.* **2011**, *31*, 1716–1724. [CrossRef]

19. Eyding, J.; Reitmair, R.; Oertel, M.; Fischer, U.; Wiest, R.; Gralla, J.; Raabe, A.; Zubak, I.; Z'Graggen, W.; Beck, J. Ultrasonic quantification of cerebral perfusion in acute arterial occlusive stroke-a comparative challenge of the refill- and the bolus-kinetics approach. *PLoS ONE* **2019**, *14*, e0220171. [CrossRef]

20. Piscaglia, F.; Nolsøe, C.; Dietrich, C.F.; Cosgrove, D.O.; Gilja, O.H.; Bachmann Nielsen, M.; Albrecht, T.; Barozzi, L.; Bertolotto, M.; Catalano, O.; et al. The EFSUMB Guidelines and Recommendations on the Clinical Practice of Contrast Enhanced Ultrasound (CEUS). Update 2011 on non-hepatic applications. *Ultraschall Med.* **2012**, *33*, 33–59. [CrossRef]

21. Nolte, C.H.; Gruss, J.; Steinbrink, J.; Jungehulsing, G.J.; Brunecker, P.; Hopt, A.M.; Schreiber, S.J. Ultrasound Perfusion Imaging of Small Stroke Involving the Thalamus. *Ultraschall Med.* **2008**, *29*, 1–5. [CrossRef] [PubMed]

22. Krogias, C.; Henneböhl, C.; Geier, B.; Hansen, C.; Hummel, T.; Meves, S.H.; Lukas, C.; Eyding, J. Transcranial ultrasound perfusion imaging and perfusion-MRI–a pilot study on the evaluation of cerebral perfusion in severe carotid artery stenosis. *Ultrasound Med. Biol.* **2010**, *36*, 1973–1980. [CrossRef] [PubMed]

23. Krogias, C.; Meves, S.H.; Hansen, C.; Mönnings, P.; Eyding, J. Ultrasound Perfusion Imaging of the brain–Routine and novel applications. Uncommon cases and review of the literature. *J. Neuroimaging* **2011**, *21*, 255–258. [CrossRef]

24. Herzberg, M.; Boy, S.; Hölscher, T.; Ertl, M.; Zimmermann, M.; Ittner, K.P.; Pemmerl, J.; Pels, H.; Bogdahn, U.; Schlachetzki, F. Prehospital stroke diagnostics based on neurological examination and transcranial ultrasound. *Crit. Ultrasound. J.* **2014**, *6*, 3. [CrossRef]

25. Lima, F.O.; Mont'Alverne, F.J.A.; Bandeira, D.; Nogueira, R.G. Pre-hospital assessment of large vessel occlusion strokes: Implications for modeling and planning stroke systems of care. *Front. Neurol.* **2019**, *10*, 955. [CrossRef] [PubMed]

26. Fuhrer, H.; Reinhard, M.; Niesen, W.D. Paradigm change? Cardiac output better associates with cerebral perfusion than blood pressure in ischemic stroke. *Front. Neurol.* **2017**, *8*, 706. [CrossRef]

27. Seidel, G.; Kaps, M.; Dorndorf, W. Transcranial color-coded duplex sonography of intracerebral hematomas in adults. *Stroke* **1993**, *24*, 1519–1527. [CrossRef]

28. Fainardi, E.; Borrelli, M.; Saletti, A.; Schivalocchi, R.; Azzini, C.; Cavallo, M.; Ceruti, S.; Tamarozzi, R.; Chieregato, A. CT perfusion mapping of hemodynamic disturbances associated to acute spontaneous intracerebral hemorrhage. *Neuroradiology* **2008**, *50*, 729–740. [CrossRef]

29. Kern, R.; Kablau, M.; Sallustio, F.; Fatar, M.; Stroick, M.; Hennerici, M.G.; Meairs, S. Improved detection of intracerebral hemorrhage with transcranial ultrasound perfusion imaging. *Cerebrovasc. Dis.* **2008**, *26*, 277–283. [CrossRef]

30. Niesen, W.; Schläger, A.; Reinhard, M.; Fuhrer, H. Transcranial sonography to differentiate primary intracerebral hemorrhage from cerebral infarction with hemorrhagic transformation. *J. Neuroimaging* **2018**, *28*, 370–373. [CrossRef]

31. Harrer, J.U.; Hornen, S.; Oertel, M.F.; Stracke, C.P.; Klötzsch, C. Comparison of perfusion harmonic imaging and perfusion mr imaging for the assessment of microvascular characteristics in brain tumors. *Ultraschall. Med.* **2008**, *29*, 45–52. [CrossRef] [PubMed]

32. Harrer, J.U.; Mayfrank, L.; Mull, M.; Klötzsch, C. Second harmonic imaging: A new ultrasound technique to assess human brain tumour perfusion. *J. Neurol. Neurosurg. Psychiatry* **2003**, *74*, 333–338. [CrossRef]

33. Harrer, J.U.; Möller-Hartmann, W.; Oertel, M.F.; Klötzsch, C. Perfusion imaging of high-grade gliomas: A comparison between contrast harmonic and magnetic resonance imaging. Technical note. *J. Neurosurg.* **2004**, *101*, 700–703. [CrossRef] [PubMed]

34. Wu, D.F.; He, W.; Lin, S.; Han, B.; Zee, C.S. Using Real-Time Fusion Imaging Constructed from Contrast-Enhanced Ultrasonography and Magnetic Resonance Imaging for High-Grade Glioma in Neurosurgery. *World Neurosurg.* **2019**, *125*, e98–e109. [CrossRef] [PubMed]

35. Della Pepa, G.M.; Ius, T.; Menna, G.; La Rocca, G.; Battistella, C.; Rapisarda, A.; Mazzucchi, E.; Pignotti, F.; Alexandre, A.; Marchese, E.; et al. "Dark corridors" in 5-ALA resection of high-grade gliomas: Combining fluorescence-guided surgery and contrast-enhanced ultrasonography to better explore the surgical field. *J. Neurosurg. Sci.* **2019**, *63*, 688–696. [CrossRef]

36. Nagelhus Hernes, T.A.; Lindseth, F.; Selbekk, T.; Wollf, A.; Solberg, O.V.; Harg, E.; Rygh, O.M.; Tangen, G.A.; Rasmussen, I.; Augdal, S.; et al. Computer-assisted 3D ultrasound-guided neurosurgery: Technological contributions, including multimodal registration and advanced display, demonstrating future perspectives. *Int. J. Med. Robot* **2006**, *2*, 45–59. [CrossRef] [PubMed]

37. Rasmussen, I.A., Jr.; Lindseth, F.; Rygh, O.M.; Berntsen, E.M.; Selbekk, T.; Xu, J.; Nagelhus Hernes, T.A.; Harg, E.; Håberg, A.; Unsgaard, G. Functional neuronavigation combined with intra-operative 3D ultrasound: Initial experiences during surgical resections close to eloquent brain areas and future directions in automatic brain shift compensation of preoperative data. *Acta Neurochir. (Wien)* **2007**, *149*, 365–378. [CrossRef]

38. Lassau, N.; Chami, L.; Chebil, M.; Benatsou, B.; Bidault, S.; Girard, E.; Abboud, G.; Roche, A. Dynamic contrast-enhanced ultrasonography (DCE-US) and anti-angiogenic treatments. *Discov. Med.* **2011**, *11*, 18–24.

39. Solbiati, L.; Ierace, T.; Tonolini, M.; Cova, L. Guidance and monitoring of radiofrequency liver tumor ablation with contrast-enhanced ultrasound. *Eur. J. Radiol.* **2004**, *51*, S19–S23. [CrossRef]

40. Prada, F.; Perin, A.; Martegani, A.; Aiani, L.; Solbiati, L.; Lamperti, M.; Casali, C.; Legnani, F.; Mattei, L.; Saladino, A.; et al. Intraoperative contrast-enhanced ultrasound for brain tumor surgery. *Neurosurgery* **2014**, *74*, 542–552. [CrossRef]

41. Engelhardt, M.; Hansen, C.; Eyding, J.; Wilkening, W.; Brenke, C.; Krogias, C.; Scholz, M.; Harders, A.; Ermert, H.; Schmieder, K. Feasibility of contrast-enhanced sonography during resection of cerebral tumours: Initial results of a prospective study. *Ultrasound. Med. Biol.* **2007**, *33*, 571–575. [CrossRef] [PubMed]

42. Vicenzini, E.; Delfini, R.; Magri, F.; Puccinelli, F.; Altieri, M.; Santoro, A.; Giannoni, M.F.; Bozzao, L.; Di Piero, V.; Lenzi, G.L. Semiquantitative human cerebral perfusion assessment with ultrasound in brain space-occupying lesions: Preliminary data. *J. Ultrasound. Med.* **2008**, *27*, 685–692. [CrossRef] [PubMed]

43. Daffertshofer, M.; Gass, A.; Ringleb, P.; Sitzer, M.; Sliwka, U.; Els, T.; Sedlaczek, O.; Koroshetz, W.J.; Hennerici, M.G. Transcranial lowfrequency ultrasound-mediated thrombolysis in brain ischemia: Increased risk of hemorrhage with combined ultrasound and tissue plasminogen activator: Results of a phase II clinical trial. *Stroke* **2005**, *36*, 1441–1446. [CrossRef] [PubMed]

44. Reinhard, M.; Hetzel, A.; Kruger, S.; Kretzer, S.; Talazko, J.; Ziyeh, S.; Weber, J.; Els, T. Blood-brain barrier disruption by low-frequency ultrasound. *Stroke* **2006**, *37*, 1546–1548. [CrossRef]

45. Jungehulsing, G.J.; Brunecker, P.; Nolte, C.H.; Fiebach, J.B.; Kunze, C.; Doepp, F.; Villringer, A.; Schreiber, S.J. Diagnostic transcranial ultrasound perfusion-imaging at 2.5 MHz does not affect the blood–brain barrier. *Ultrasound Med. Biol.* **2008**, *34*, 147–150. [CrossRef]

46. Harrer, J.U.; Eyding, J.; Ritter, M.; Schminke, U.; Schulte-Altedorneburg, G.; Köhrmann, M.; Nedelmann, M.; Schlachetzki, F. The potential of neurosonography in neurological emergency and intensive care medicine: Basic principles, vascular stroke diagnostics, and monitoring of stroke-specific therapy-part 1. *Ultraschall. Med.* **2012**, *33*, 218–235.

14

To Treat or Not to Treat: Importance of Functional Dependence in Deciding Intravenous Thrombolysis of "Mild Stroke" Patients

Giovanni Merlino [1],[*],[†], Carmelo Smeralda [2],[3],[†], Simone Lorenzut [1], Gian Luigi Gigli [2],[4], Andrea Surcinelli [2],[3] and Mariarosaria Valente [2],[3]

[1] Stroke Unit, Department of Neuroscience, Udine University Hospital, Piazzale S. Maria della Misericordia 15, 33100 Udine, Italy; simone.lorenzut@asufc.sanita.fvg.it
[2] Clinical Neurology, Udine University Hospital, 33100 Udine, Italy; carmelosmeralda@gmail.com (C.S.); gigli@uniud.it (G.L.G.); andsurcinelli@gmail.com (A.S.); mariarosaria.valente@uniud.it (M.V.)
[3] Department of Medical Area (DAME), University of Udine, 33100 Udine, Italy
[4] Department of Mathematics, Informatics and Physics (DMIF), University of Udine, 33100 Udine, Italy
[*] Correspondence: giovanni.merlino@asufc.sanita.fvg.it
[†] Drs. Merlino and Smeralda contributed equally as authors.

Abstract: Intravenous thrombolysis (IVT) in patients with a low National Institutes of Health Stroke Scale (NIHSS) score of 0–5 remains controversial. IVT should be used in patients with mild but nevertheless disabling symptoms. We hypothesize that response to IVT of patients with "mild stroke" may depend on their level of functional dependence (FD) at hospital admission. The aims of our study were to investigate the effect of IVT and to explore the role of FD in influencing the response to IVT. This study was a retrospective analysis of a prospectively collected database, including 389 patients stratified into patients receiving IVT (IVT$^+$) and not receiving IVT (IVT$^-$) just because of mild symptoms. Barthel index (BI) at admission was used to assess FD, dividing subjects with BI score < 80 (FD$^+$) and with BI score ≥ 80 (FD$^-$). The efficacy endpoints were the rate of positive disability outcome (DO$^+$) (3-month mRS score of 0 or 1), and the rate of positive functional outcome (FO$^+$) (mRS score of zero or one, plus BI score of 95 or 100 at 3 months). At the multivariate analysis, IVT treatment was an independent predictor of DO$^+$ (OR 3.12, 95% CI 1.34–7.27, $p = 0.008$) and FO$^+$ (OR: 4.70, 95% CI 2.38–9.26, $p = 0.001$). However, FD$^+$ IVT$^+$ patients had a significantly higher prevalence of DO$^+$ and FO$^+$ than those FD$^+$ IVT$^-$. Differently, IVT treatment did not influence DO$^+$ and FO$^+$ in FD$^-$ patients. In FD$^+$ patients, IVT treatment represented the strongest independent predictor of DO$^+$ (OR 6.01, 95% CI 2.59–13.92, $p = 0.001$) and FO$^+$ (OR 4.73, 95% CI 2.29–9.76, $p = 0.001$). In conclusion, alteplase seems to improve functional outcome in patients with "mild stroke". However, in our experience, this beneficial effect is strongly influenced by FD at admission.

Keywords: intravenous thrombolysis; NIHSS; Barthel index; functional dependence

1. Introduction

Many patients with acute ischemic strokes (AIS) have a low National Institutes of Health Stroke Scale (NIHSS) score at presentation [1,2]. Although the presence of these mild symptoms represents the most common reason for renouncing intravenous thrombolysis (IVT) [3], only 68% of these patients can be discharged home without a residual disability [4]. Thus, there is increasing interest in the use of IVT in AIS patients with a low NIHSS score at admission. Results coming from clinical studies on this topic are conflicting, since functional outcome results, as assessed by the modified Rankin scale (mRS) sometimes improve, and at other times, are not modified by IVT treatment [5–10].

Previous American Heart Association/American Stroke Association guidelines suggested to use IVT treatment in persons with a *wide spectrum* of neurological deficits (1996) and with *measurable* neurological deficits (2007) [11,12]. This concept has been updated in the most version of the guidelines, recommending that IVT should also be used in patients with mild, but nevertheless disabling symptoms [13]. However, the NIHSS is not able to assess severity of disability. For instance, it cannot be used to accurately assess posterior circulation disease, which may cause very disabling symptoms. In fact, already in 2013, Wendt et al. reported that language impairment, distal paresis, and gait disorder were common disabling deficits in patients with low NIHSS scores. The authors suggest that the judgment of whether a stroke is disabling should not be based on the NIHSS score, but on the assessment of individual neurologic deficits and their impact on functional impairment [14].

To date, only a trial has been performed to compare the efficacy of alteplase versus aspirin for AIS patients with minor and non-disabling neurological deficits (the PRISMS trial). The authors observed that alteplase did not increase the likelihood of favorable outcome compared to aspirin [15,16]. Although the PRISMS was a prospective, double-blind, and placebo-controlled trial, it suffered from two significant limitations. In fact, the study was terminated early because patient recruitment was below target and it adopted a definition of "not clearly disabling" that was subjective and required interpretation by individual clinicians. Thus, conclusions of the PRISMS trial cannot be generalized.

A possible reason for the uncertain effectiveness of alteplase in minor strokes is that patients with a low NIHSS score at admission may respond to IVT treatment in different ways, depending on their level of functional dependence (FD) at admission. In addition, we suggest that the severity of FD should be assessed by a standard measure, such as the Barthel index (BI), instead of using a subjective selection based on the judgment of each physician. The aims of our study were: (1) to investigate the effects of IVT in patients with "mild stroke", defined as a NIHSS score of 0–5 at presentation; (2) to explore the role of FD in influencing response to IVT in AIS patients with "mild stroke".

2. Materials and Methods

2.1. Patients

This study was based on a retrospective analysis of a prospectively-collected database of consecutive patients admitted to the Udine University Hospital for AIS from January 2015 to December 2018. Inclusion criteria were: age 18 years or older and NIHSS score of 0 to 5. Exclusion criteria were: presence of a pre-stroke mRS score > 1, large vessel occlusion on cranial CT-angiography, and time interval > 4.5 h from symptoms onset. Out of 1636 patients admitted for AIS, 389 were considered suitable for the study after considering inclusion and exclusion criteria. The study sample was stratified into 2 groups: AIS patients who received IVT (IVT$^+$) and patients to whom IVT was denied because of mild symptoms (IVT$^-$).

2.2. Data Collection

The following variables were collected: age, sex, vascular risk factors such as previous transient ischemic attack or previous stroke, ischemic heart disease, peripheral artery disease, obesity defined as a BMI $\geq$ 30, atrial fibrillation, hypertension, diabetes mellitus, hypercholesterolemia, current smoking status, and pharmacological treatment. Stroke severity was determined with the NIHSS at admission. Presence of intracranial hemorrhage (ICH) was detected. Definition of symptomatic ICH (sICH) was based on the European Cooperative Acute Stroke Study (ECASS) III protocol [17]. Functional outcome was assessed by means of the mRS score 3 months after the stroke, and of the BI score, calculated at admission and recalculated at 3-months. The mRS and the BI scores after discharge were recorded at the patients' routine clinical visit during a face-to-face examination.

2.3. Outcome Measures

Our efficacy endpoints were: (1) rate of positive disability outcome (DO$^+$), defined as a 3-month mRS score of 0 or 1; (2) rate of positive functional outcome (FO$^+$), defined as an mRS score of 0 or 1 *plus* a BI score of 95 or 100 at 3 months. The safety endpoints were: (1) rate of mortality at 3 months; (2) presence of sICH.

2.4. Statistical Analysis

Baseline characteristics and outcomes of the two patient groups (IVT$^+$ versus IVT$^-$) were compared by means of the chi-square test (Fisher's exact test) for categorical variables and the Student's *t*-test for independent samples when the continuous variables had a normal distribution.

The Mann–Whitney U test was used when the continuous variables had an abnormal distribution and for ordinal variables. Binary logistic regression was used to explore variables associated with outcome measures.

In order to explore whether there was a significant interaction between the types of presenting symptoms (according to the Barthel index) and the efficacy of thrombolysis, both patients treated and not treated with IVT were differentiated as: (1) patients without FD; (2) patients with FD predominantly due to weakness; (3) patients with FD predominantly due to imbalance; (4) patients with FD predominantly due to neglect and/or hemianopsia; (5) patients with FD predominantly due to other neurological symptoms, e.g., aphasia and confusion.

With the aim to verify if the level of FD at admission might influence response to IVT in AIS patients with "mild stroke", we divided our sample into subjects with a BI score < 80 (FD$^+$) and those with a BI score ≥ 80 (FD$^-$). We tested this hypothesis comparing the efficacy endpoints between FD$^+$ and FD$^-$ patients, treated and not treated with IVT.

Data are displayed in tables as means and standard deviations (SD), if not otherwise specified. All probability values are two-tailed. A *p* value of < 0.05 was considered to be statistically significant. Statistical analysis was carried out using the SPSS Statistics, Version 20.0 for Windows (Chicago, IL, USA).

3. Results

Our sample of 389 patients was composed of 235 males (60.4%) with a mean age of 68.5 ± 13.6 years, a median NIHSS score of 2 (IQR 1–3), and a median BI score of 75 (IQR 60-90). Almost one-half (51.7%) of our patients with "mild stroke" had a BI score < 80 at admission (FD$^+$ patients). Figure 1 shows the distribution of the BI score at admission in our sample.

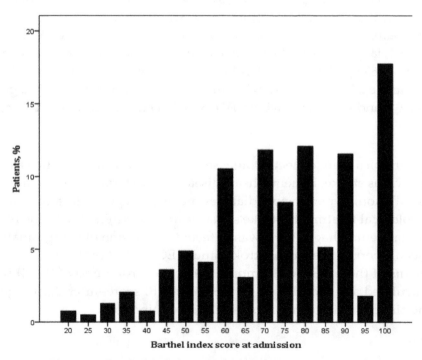

Figure 1. Barthel index score distribution in our sample.

Of the 389 enrolled patients with "mild stroke", 113 (29%) were treated with IVT (IVT$^+$), whereas in 276 (71%), IVT was denied because of mild symptoms (IVT$^-$). Baseline characteristics in IVT$^+$ and IVT$^-$ patients are summarized in Table 1. The two groups differed only in median NIHSS score and use of anticoagulants.

Table 1. Baseline characteristics.

	IVT$^+$ (n = 113)	IVT$^-$ (n = 276)	p
Demographic data and baseline clinical characteristics			
Age, years	68.2 ± 12.0	68.7 ± 14.2	0.7
Males, n (%)	67 (59.3)	168 (60.9)	0.8
NIHSS score at admission, median (IQR)	3 (2–4)	2 (1–3)	0.001
BI score at admission, median (IQR)	60 (75–90)	60 (75–90)	0.5
Medications prior to onset, n (%)			
Antiplatelet agents	39 (34.5)	79 (28.6)	0.2
Anticoagulant agents	1 (0.9)	25 (9.1)	0.003
Glucose level, mg/dl	126.4 ± 35.3	134.2 ± 64.7	0.3
Vascular risk factors			
Previous transient ischemic attack/stroke, n (%)	15 (13.3)	45 (16.3)	0.4
Ischemic heart disease, n (%)	19 (18.3)	27 (10.8)	0.06
Peripheral artery disease, n (%)	2 (1.9)	2 (0.8)	0.6
Obesity, n (%)	9 (8.7)	22 (8.8)	0.9
Atrial fibrillation, n (%)	19 (16.8)	67 (24.3)	0.1
Hypertension, n (%)	68 (60.2)	184 (66.7)	0.2
Diabetes mellitus, n (%)	17 (15.0)	63 (22.8)	0.08
Hypercholesterolemia, n (%)	43 (38.1)	102 (37.0)	0.8
Current smoking, n (%)	29 (26.1)	53 (21.1)	0.3

IVT = intravenous thrombolysis; NIHSS = National Institute of Health Stroke scale; BI = Barthel index.

At 3-months, IVT treatment improved both measures of outcome (DO$^+$ and FO$^+$). Although IVT$^+$ patients showed higher rates of sICH than those IVT$^-$, the prevalence of 3-month mortality did not differ between the two groups (see Table 2).

Table 2. Efficacy and safety endpoints in patients treated and not treated with IVT.

	IVT$^+$ (n = 113)	IVT$^-$ (n = 276)	p
Efficacy endpoints			
DO$^+$, n (%)	98 (86.7)	195 (70.7)	0.001
FO$^+$, n (%)	94 (83.9)	179 (65.6)	0.001
Safety endpoints			
Mortality at 3-months, n (%)	1 (0.9)	3 (1.1)	0.8
sICH, n (%)	5 (4.4)	3 (1.1)	0.03

IVT = intravenous thrombolysis; DO$^+$ (3-month mRS score of 0 or 1) = positive disability outcome; FO$^+$ (mRS score of 0 or 1, *plus* BI score of 95 or 100 at 3-months) = positive functional outcome; sICH = symptomatic intracranial hemorrhage.

By univariate analysis, apart from IVT treatment, a positive disability outcome (DO$^+$) was also associated with younger age (OR for 1-year increment in age 0.98, 95% CI 0.96–0.99, p = 0.02), lower NIHSS score at admission (OR 0.72 for 1-point increase in the scale, 95% CI 0.60–0.85, p = 0.001), higher BI score at admission (OR 1.06, 95% CI 1.05–1.08, p = 0.001), lower serum glucose at admission (OR 0.98 for each mg/dl increase in glucose, 95% CI 0.97–0.99, p = 0.01), a history of previous transient ischemic attack/stroke (OR 0.42, 95% CI 0.24–0.75, p = 0.003), obesity (OR 0.41, 95% CI 0.19–0.91, p = 0.02), and of diabetes mellitus (OR 0.45, 95% CI 0.27–0.77, p = 0.003). Regarding instead positive functional outcome (FO$^+$), younger age (OR for 1-year increment in age 0.98, 95% CI 0.96–0.99, p = 0.008), lower NIHSS score at admission (OR 0.72 for 1-point increase in the scale, 95% CI 0.61–0.85, p = 0.001), higher BI score at admission (OR 1.06, 95% CI 1.04–1.07, p = 0.001), a history of previous transient ischemic attack/stroke (OR 0.45, 95% CI 0.26–0.80, p = 0.005), hypertension (OR 0.61, 95% CI 0.38–0.98, p = 0.04), and diabetes mellitus (OR 0.52, 95% CI 0.31–0.87, p = 0.01) were related to FO$^+$ at 3 months.

By multivariate analysis, after controlling for variables significantly associated with the two efficacy endpoints at the univariate analysis, IVT treatment remained an independent predictor of DO$^+$ and FO$^+$ in patients with "mild stroke" (see Table 3).

Table 3. Multivariable analyses showing independent predictors of positive disability outcome and positive functional outcome.

DO$^+$	OR	95% CI	p
IVT treatment			
No	1.00		
Yes	3.12	1.34–7.27	0.008
Age	0.95	0.92–0.98	0.003
BI score at admission	1.06	1.04–1.09	0.001
FO$^+$	**OR**	**95% CI**	**p**
IVT treatment			
No	1.00		
Yes	4.70	2.38–9.26	0.001
Age	0.98	0.96–0.99	0.02
NIHSS score at admission	0.77	0.61–0.97	0.03
BI score at admission	1.06	1.04–1.07	0.001
Diabetes mellitus			
No	1.00		
Yes	0.53	0.29–0.98	0.04

DO$^+$ (3-month mRS score of 0 or 1) = positive disability outcome; FO$^+$ (mRS score of 0 or 1 *plus* BI score of 95 or 100 at 3-months) = positive functional outcome; IVT = intravenous thrombolysis; NIHSS = National Institute of Health Stroke scale; BI = Barthel index.

A beneficial effect of IVT was observed only in patients with FD predominantly due to weakness who significantly improved after treatment (DO$^+$: OR 4.88, 95% CI 2.01–11.83, p = 0.001; FO$^+$: OR 5.03, 95% CI 2.23–11.32, p = 0.001), different from patients without FD, or with other types of presenting symptoms (data not shown).

As shown in Figure 2, the prevalence of DO$^+$ was significantly higher in FD$^+$ IVT$^+$ patients than in those FD$^+$ IVT$^-$ (FD$^+$ IVT$^+$: 83.9% vs. FD$^+$ IVT$^-$: 52.5%, p = 0.001); differently, IVT treatment did not influence DO$^+$ in FD$^-$ patients (FD$^-$ IVT$^+$: 90.2% vs. FD$^-$ IVT$^-$: 89.1%, p = 0.8). Similarly, for functional outcome, FO$^+$ was significantly more common in FD$^+$ IVT$^+$ patients than in those FD$^+$ IVT$^-$ (FD$^+$ IVT$^+$: 77.4% vs. FD$^+$ IVT$^-$: 44.6%, p = 0.001), whereas rates of FO$^+$ were similar in FD$^-$ IVT$^+$ and FD$^-$ IVT$^-$ patients (90.2% vs. 85.4%, p = 0.4) (see Figure 3).

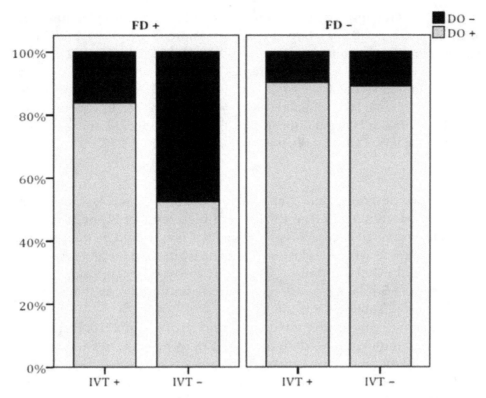

Figure 2. Effect of IVT on disability outcome rates in groups of patients with different levels of functional dependence at admission. DO = disability outcome; FD = functional dependence; IVT = intravenous thrombolysis.

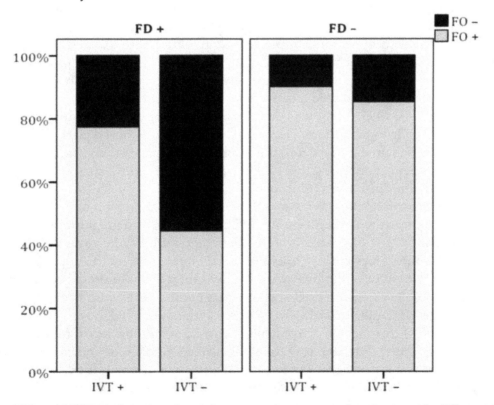

Figure 3. Effect of IVT on functional outcome rates in groups of patients with different levels of functional dependence at admission. FO= functional outcome; FD = functional dependence; IVT = intravenous thrombolysis.

In FD$^+$ patients, the following variables were independent predictors of outcome: IVT treatment (OR 6.01, 95% CI 2.59–13.92, $p = 0.001$), BI score at admission (OR 1.07, 95% CI 1.04–1.10, $p = 0.001$), a history of previous transient ischemic attack/stroke (OR 0.41, 95% CI 0.18–0.92, $p = 0.03$), and diabetes mellitus (OR 0.42, 95% CI 0.18–0.94, $p = 0.04$) for DO$^+$; IVT treatment (OR 4.73, 95% CI 2.29–9.76, $p = 0.001$), BI score at admission (OR 1.04, 95% CI 1.02–1.07, $p = 0.001$), and a history of previous transient ischemic attack/stroke (OR 0.44, 95% CI 0.20–0.96, $p = 0.04$) for FO$^+$. In contrast, IVT treatment did not affect functional outcome in FD$^-$ patients; in fact, BI score at admission was the only independent predictor of DO$^+$ (OR 1.22, 95% CI 1.07–1.39, $p = 0.002$), and FO$^+$ (OR 1.13, 95% CI 1.05–1.21, $p = 0.001$).

4. Discussion

For the first time we demonstrated that patients with "mild stroke", as defined as a NIHSS score of 0–5, should be selected for IVT on the basis of their level of FD at admission. In particular, subjects with moderate or severe FD, as assessed by the BI score, should be treated with IVT as soon as possible. In contrast, treatment with alteplase seems to be ineffective on patients who are functionally independent or with slight FD at admission. Thus, our study gives support to the latest American Heart Association/American Stroke Association guidelines recommending that IVT should be used for patients with mild but also disabling symptoms [13].

There is ongoing debate concerning what is a "mild stroke". In 2010, Fisher et al. explored the relationship of 6 different "minor stroke" definitions and outcomes. Since patients with a NIHSS score ≤ 3 had the best short- and medium-term outcome, the authors suggested to use this easily-applicable definition [18]. Although this definition has been used in some studies [19,20], a recent review of this topic reported that the NIHSS—with a score ranging from 0 to 5—is the most commonly used tool to define a "mild stroke" [21]. Similarly, we utilized an NIHSS score of 0 to 5 for identifying patients with supposed "mild" symptoms; our patients had a median NIHSS score of 2. However, despite their low NIHSS, several of them were affected by severe FD at admission; in fact, we observed a median BI score of 75, and 51.7% of the sample had a BI score < 80. This discrepancy may be due to the fact that the NIHSS is not able to detect symptoms of posterior circulation stroke, such as postural instability, gait disturbance, and dysphagia that can cause very severe disability. Thus, we think that patients with a low NIHSS score at presentation should be carefully evaluated regarding the presence of possible disabling symptoms before being labeled as affected by "mild stroke".

Originally published in 1965, the BI was developed to give physicians a suitable standard tool to assess and measure FD [22]. In fact, the BI covers all activities considered part of any assessment of activities of daily living, has an excellent reliability and validity, is easy to use, and only takes a few minutes [23]. Thus, we suggest adopting this tool in patients with "mild stroke", in order to correctly recognize patients with non-disabling symptoms.

Obviously, the exact distinction between stroke with disabling or non-disabling symptoms becomes extremely important when patients are affected by AIS and are suitable for IVT treatment. In our sample, more than 70% of AIS patients were not treated with IVT because they were deemed too good to be treated. This rate is perfectly in line with previous studies on this topic [6,9,10]. As shown in Table 1, the decision to treat or not to treat with IVT was merely based on the NIHSS score, whereas the level of FD was absolutely neglected. Use of anticoagulant agents was, as expected, significantly higher in AIS patients with "mild stroke" who were not treated, than in those who received IVT.

Previous studies on IVT treatment in AIS patients with mild symptoms report conflicting results [5–10]. In 2012 Huisa et al. investigated 133 patients with minor ischemic strokes, defined as an admission NIHSS score ≤ 5, and observed similar outcomes between patients treated and not treated with alteplase [5]. An Italian study of 128 patients with mild ischemic stroke confirmed that alteplase did not improve functional outcome [6]. Of 276 patients with mild ischemic stroke symptoms that were analyzed by Spokoyny et al., 83 were IVT treated. Treated and untreated patients had similar baseline characteristics except that the treated group had higher baseline NIHSS. Prevalence of mRS 2–6 at 90 days was 37.4% in the treated group and 31.1% in the untreated group ($p = 0.44$) [9]. In contrast, Urra et al. reported that IVT was associated with a greater proportion of patients with mild stroke who shifted down on the mRS score at 3 months (OR 2.66; 95% CI 1.49–4.74, $p = 0.001$) [7]. In a case-control study of 890 Austrian patients with a NIHSS score 0–5 at admission, IVT was associated with a better outcome after 3 months (OR 1.49, 95% CI 1.17–1.89, $p < 0.001$) [8]. More recently, Haeberlin et al. compared 3-month functional outcomes in 370 consecutive AIS patients with a NIHSS score ≤ 6. Although patients with mild AIS had a high chance of favorable outcomes irrespective of treatment type, subjects receiving IVT more often achieved complete remission of symptoms (mRS score = 0) (OR 3.33, $p < 0.0001$) [10]. Similarly to Urra et al. [7] and Haeberlin et al. [10], we observed a major beneficial effect of IVT on the outcome measures. Interestingly, it would seem that IVT efficacy is more pronounced in AIS patients affected by "mild stroke" than in those enrolled in regulatory randomized controlled trials, in which patients with minor symptoms were largely underrepresented [24]. We think that this discrepancy may be due to different study design between observational studies and randomized controlled trials. In fact, more often, non-interventional studies tend to overestimate the effects of the treatment and show more variability in estimates of the effects because of residual confounding, errors, and bias.

Discording results of IVT efficacy in "mild strokes" may be explained by differences in clinical characteristics among patients with minor symptoms. In particular, our patients who underwent IVT had a better 3-month functional outcome than those IVT$^-$, but presence of neurological symptoms due to weakness and level of FD at admission played a major role in influencing this association. If patients with "mild stroke" *plus* disabling symptoms (FD$^+$) were treated with alteplase, there was a significant improvement in functional outcome compared to those which were not treated. Indeed, more than 50% of patients with a BI score < 80 for whom IVT was denied did not achieve functional independence 3 months after stroke. In patients with "mild stroke" *plus* disabling symptoms, IVT represented the strongest predictor of DO$^+$ (OR: 6.01) and FO$^+$ (OR: 4.73). On the other hand, rates of favorable outcomes were very high in patients without disability, regardless of treatment type. In these patients, BI score at admission was the only independent predictor of DO$^+$ and FO$^+$, while IVT treatment did not influence functional outcomes. In contrast, Urra et al. report that IVT was associated with a greater proportion of patients with non-disabling minor strokes who shifted down on the mRS score at 3-months [7].

To date, only the PRISMS trial has been designed to assess the efficacy of IVT for the treatment of AIS with NIHSS 0–5, and without clearly disabling deficits. The authors designed a multicenter, randomized, double-blind, placebo-controlled trial with a sample size of 948 subjects [15]. Unfortunately, the study was terminated early because of low patient recruitment. Results of the 313 patients enrolled failed to demonstrate more favorable functional outcomes in patients treated with alteplase, as compared to those receiving only aspirin. However, the trial's early termination precludes any definitive conclusions on this topic. Moreover, definition of "not clearly disabling" was left to the subjective interpretation of individual clinicians [16].

Regarding safety endpoints, in our sample, alteplase treatment significantly increased the risk of sICH, even if rates of mortality were similar in patients IVT$^+$ and IVT$^-$. Bearing in mind that higher NIHSS scores predict a higher rate of sICH, it could be argued that our sICH rate in patients with "mild stroke" was high. However, a previous study performed in patients with minor stroke reported a sICH rate as high as 5% when IVT was administered [5].

Several limitations of this study need to be acknowledged. First, the retrospective design of our study was certainly a limit; however, all data were prospectively collected. Second, measures of outcome were obtained by physicians that were not blinded to IVT treatment, which may have influenced their rating. Third, information on intervals between stroke onset and IVT was not collected, thus we cannot exclude that elapsed time from symptoms onset may have influenced physicians' decisions to perform or not perform IVT treatment. Finally, since this was a hypothesis-generating study, further surveys are needed to test our preliminary hypotheses. In particular, interventional trials should be performed in order to exclude the presence of a bias by indication that could have affected our observational study.

In conclusion, alteplase seems to improve functional outcome in patients with a low NIHSS score. However, in our experience, this beneficial effect is strongly influenced by FD at admission. In patients with "mild stroke" *plus* disabling symptoms, IVT treatment should be administered as soon as possible; on the contrary, alteplase may not be used if minor and non-disabling deficits are diagnosed. In order to distinguish mild ischemic stroke patients with disabling or non-disabling symptoms, we suggest to use the BI. Our observational study brings further evidence to the results coming from a few other non-interventional studies and from one randomized trial interrupted before completion. Thus, further large interventional studies are needed to confirm our preliminary findings.

Author Contributions: Conceptualization, G.M. and C.S.; methodology, G.M. and C.S.; software, G.M. and C.S.; validation, S.L., G.L.G. and M.V.; formal analysis, G.M.; investigation, C.S., S.L. and A.S.; resources, C.S., S.L. and A.S.; data curation, G.M.; writing—original draft preparation, G.M.; writing—review and editing, G.M.; visualization, G.L.G; supervision, M.V. All authors have read and agreed to the published version of the manuscript.

References

1. Reeves, M.; Khoury, J.; Alwell, K.; Moomaw, C.; Flaherty, M.; Woo, D.; Khatri, P.; Adeoye, O.; Ferioli, S.; Kissela, N.; et al. Distribution of national institutes of health stroke scale in the Cincinnati/Northern Kentucky stroke study. *Stroke* **2013**, *44*, 3211–3213. [CrossRef]
2. Dhamoon, M.S.; Moon, Y.P.; Paik, M.C.; Boden-Albala, B.; Rundek, T.; Sacco, R.L.; Elkind, M.S. Long-term functional recovery after first ischemic stroke. *Stroke* **2009**, *40*, 2805–2811. [CrossRef]
3. Messé, S.R.; Khatri, P.; Reeves, M.J.; Smith, E.E.; Saver, J.L.; Bhatt, D.L.; Grau-Sepulveda, M.V.; Cox, M.; Peterson, E.D.; Fonarow, G.C.; et al. Why are acute ischemic stroke patients not receiving IV tPA? Results from a national registry. *Neurology* **2016**, *87*, 1565–1574. [CrossRef]
4. Barber, P.A.; Zhang, J.; Demchuk, A.M.; Hill, M.D.; Buchan, A.M. Why are stroke patients excluded from TPA therapy? An analysis of patient eligibility. *Neurology* **2001**, *56*, 1015–1020. [CrossRef] [PubMed]
5. Huisa, B.N.; Raman, R.; Neil, W.; Ernstrom, K.; Hemmen, T. Intravenous tissue plasminogen activator for patients with minor ischemic stroke. *J. Stroke Cerebrovasc. Dis.* **2012**, *21*, 732–736. [CrossRef] [PubMed]
6. Nesi, M.; Lucente, G.; Nencini, P.; Fancellu, L.; Inzitari, D. Aphasia predicts unfavorable outcome in mild ischemic stroke patients and prompts thrombolytic treatment. *J. Stroke Cerebrovasc. Dis.* **2014**, *23*, 204–208. [CrossRef] [PubMed]
7. Urra, X.; Ariño, H.; Llull, L.; Amaro, S.; Obach, V.; Cervera, A.; Chamorro, A. The outcome of patients with mild stroke improves after treatment with systemic thrombolysis. *PLoS ONE* **2013**, *8*, e59420. [CrossRef] [PubMed]
8. Greisenegger, S.; Seyfang, L.; Kiechl, S.; Lang, W.; Ferrari, J. Austrian Stroke Unit Registry Collaborators. Thrombolysis in patients with mild stroke: Results from the Austrian Stroke Unit Registry. *Stroke* **2014**, *45*, 765–769. [CrossRef]
9. Spokoyny, I.; Raman, R.; Ernstrom, K.; Khatri, P.; Meyer, D.M.; Hemmen, T.M.; Meyer, B.C. Defining mild stroke: Outcomes analysis of treated and untreated mild stroke patients. *J. Stroke Cerebrovasc. Dis.* **2015**, *24*, 1276–1281. [CrossRef]
10. Haeberlin, M.I.; Held, U.; Baumgartner, R.W.; Georgiadis, D.; Valko, P.O. Impact of intravenous thrombolysis on functional outcome in patients with mild ischemic stroke without large vessel occlusion or rapidly improving symptoms. *Int. J. Stroke* **2019**. [CrossRef]
11. Adams, H.P., Jr.; Brott, T.G.; Furlan, A.J.; Gomez, C.R.; Grotta, J.; Helgason, C.M.; Kwiatkowski, T.; Lyden, P.D.; Marler, J.R.; Torner, J.; et al. Guidelines for thrombolytic therapy for acute stroke: A supplement to the guidelines for the management of patients with acute ischemic stroke. A statement for healthcare professionals from a special writing group of the Stroke Council, American Heart Association. *Stroke* **1996**, *27*, 1711–1718. [PubMed]

12. Adams, H.O., Jr.; del Zoppo, G.; Alberts, M.J.; Bhatt, D.L.; Brass, L.; Furlan, A.; Grubb, R.L.; Higashida, R.T.; Jauch, E.C.; Kidwell, C.; et al. American Heart Association, American Stroke Association Stroke Council, Clinical Cardiology Council, Cardiovascular Radiology and Intervention Council, Atherosclerotic Peripheral Vascular Disease and Quality of Care Outcomes in Research Interdisciplinary Working Groups. Guidelines for the early management of adults with ischemic stroke: A guideline from the American Heart Association/American Stroke Association Stroke Council, Clinical Cardiology Council, Cardiovascular Radiology and Intervention Council, and the Atherosclerotic Peripheral Vascular Disease and Quality of Care Outcomes in Research Interdisciplinary Working Groups: The American Academy of Neurology Affirms the Value of This Guideline as an Educational Tool for Neurologists. *Stroke* **2007**, *38*, 1655–1711. [PubMed]

13. Powers, W.J.; Rabinstein, A.A.; Ackerson, T.; Adeoye, O.M.; Bambakidis, N.C.; Becker, K.; Biller, J.; Brown, M.; Demaerschalk, B.M.; David, L.; et al. American Heart Association Stroke Council. 2018 guidelines for the early management of patients with acute ischemic stroke: A guideline for healthcare professionals from the American Heart Association/American Stroke Association. *Stroke* **2018**, *49*, e46–e110. [CrossRef] [PubMed]

14. Wendt, M.; Tutuncu, S.; Fiebach, J.B.; Scheitz, J.F.; Audebert, H.J.; Nolte, C.H. Preclusion of ischemic stroke patients from intravenous tissue plasminogen activator treatment for mild symptoms should not be based on low National Institutes of Health Stroke Scale scores. *J. Stroke Cerebrovasc. Dis.* **2013**, *22*, 550–553. [CrossRef] [PubMed]

15. Yeatts, S.D.; Broderick, J.P.; Chatterjee, A.; Jauch, E.C.; Levine, S.R.; Romano, J.G.; Saver, J.L.; Vagal, A.; Purdon, B.; Devenport, J.; et al. Alteplase for the treatment of acute ischemic stroke in patients with low National Institutes of Health Stroke Scale and not clearly disabling deficits (Potential of rtPA for Ischemic Strokes with Mild Symptoms PRISMS): Rationale and design. *Int. J. Stroke* **2018**, *13*, 654–661. [CrossRef] [PubMed]

16. Khatri, P.; Kleindorfer, D.O.; Devlin, T.; Sawyer, R.N.; Starr, M.; Mejilla, J.; Broderick, J.; Chatterjee, A.; Jauch, E.C.; Levine, S.R.; et al. Effect of alteplase vs. aspirin on functional outcome for patients with acute ischemic stroke and minor nondisabling neur logic deficits: The PRISMS randomized clinical trial. *JAMA* **2018**, *320*, 156–166. [CrossRef]

17. Hacke, W.; Kaste, M.; Bluhmki, E.; Brozman, M.; Davalos, A.; Guidetti, D.; Larrue, V.; Lees, K.R.; Medeghri, Z.; Machnig, T.; et al. Thrombolysis with alteplase 3 to 4.5 h after acute ischemic stroke. *N. Engl. J. Med.* **2008**, *359*, 1317–1329. [CrossRef]

18. Fischer, U.; Baumgartner, A.; Arnold, M.; Nedeltchev, K.; Gralla, J.; Marco De Marchis, G.; Kappeler, L.; Mono, M.-L.; Brekenfeld, C.; Schroth, G.; et al. What is a minor stroke? *Stroke* **2010**, *41*, 661–666. [CrossRef]

19. Luengo-Fernandez, R.; Gray, A.M.; Rothwell, P.M. Effect of urgent treatment for transient ischaemic attack and minor stroke on disability and hospital costs (EXPRESS study): A prospective population-based sequential comparison. *Lancet Neurol.* **2009**, *8*, 218–219. [CrossRef]

20. Coutts, S.B.; Hill, M.D.; Campos, C.R.; Choi, Y.B.; Subramaniam, S.; Kosior, J.C.; Demchuk, A.M. Recurrent events in transient ischemic attack and minor stroke. *Stroke* **2008**, *39*, 2461–2466. [CrossRef]

21. Schwartz, J.K.; Capo-Lugo, C.E.; Akinwuntan, A.E.; Roberts, P.; Krishnan, S.; Belagaje, S.R.; Lovic, M.; Burns, S.P.; Hu, X.; Danzl, M.; et al. Classification of mild stroke: A mapping review. *Pm&r* **2019**, *11*, 996–1003.

22. Mahoney, F.I.; Barthel, D.W. Functional evaluation: The Barthel index. *Md. State Med. J.* **1965**, *14*, 61–65. [PubMed]

23. Barak, S.; Duncan, P.W. Issues in selecting outcome measures to assess functional recovery after stroke. *NeuroRx* **2006**, *3*, 505–524. [CrossRef] [PubMed]

24. Wardlaw Wardlaw, J.M.; Murray, V.; Berge, E.; del Zoppo, G.J. Thrombolysis for acute ischemic stroke. *Cochrane Database Syst. Rev.* **2014**, *7*, CD000213.

15

Impact of the Total Number of Carotid Plaques on the Outcome of Ischemic Stroke Patients with Atrial Fibrillation

Hyungjong Park [1,2], Minho Han [1], Young Dae Kim [1], Joonsang Yoo [2], Hye Sun Lee [3], Jin Kyo Choi [1], Ji Hoe Heo [1] and Hyo Suk Nam [1,*]

[1] Department of Neurology, Yonsei University College of Medicine, Seoul 03722, Korea;
    hjpark209042@gmail.com (H.P.); UMSTHOL18@yuhs.ac (M.H.); neuro05@yuhs.ac (Y.D.K.);
    JKSNAIL85@yuhs.ac (J.K.C.); jhheo@yuhs.ac (J.H.H.)
[2] Department of Neurology, Keimyung University School of Medicine, Daegu 42601, Korea;
    quarksea@gmail.com
[3] Biostatistics Collaboration Unit, Yonsei University College of Medicine, university, Seoul 03722, Korea;
    HSLEE1@yuhs.ac
* Correspondence: hsnam@yuhs.ac

Abstract: Background: Atrial fibrillation (AF) shares several risk factors with atherosclerosis. We investigated the association between total carotid plaque number (TPN) and long-term prognosis in ischemic stroke patients with AF. Methods: A total of 392 ischemic stroke patients with AF who underwent carotid ultrasonography were enrolled. TPN was assessed using B-mode ultrasound. The patients were categorized into two groups according to best cutoff values for TPN (TPN ≤ 4 vs. TPN ≥ 5). The long-term risk of major adverse cardiovascular events (MACE) and mortality according to TPN was investigated using a Cox hazard model. Results: After a mean follow-up of 2.42 years, 113 patients (28.8%) had developed MACE and 88 patients (22.4%) had died. MACE occurred more frequently in the TPN ≥ 5 group than in the TPN ≤ 4 group (adjusted hazard ratio [HR], 1.50; 95% confidence interval [CI], 1.01–2.21; $p < 0.05$). Moreover, the TPN ≥ 5 group showed an increased risk of all-cause mortality (adjusted HR, 2.69; 95% CI, 1.40–5.17; $p < 0.05$). TPN along with maximal plaque thickness and intima media thickness showed improved prognostic utility when added to the variables of the $CHAD_2DS_2$-VASc score. Conclusion: TPN can predict the long-term outcome of ischemic stroke patients with AF. Adding TPN to the $CHAD_2DS_2$-VASc score increases the predictability of outcome after stroke.

Keywords: atrial fibrillation; cerebral infarction; carotid stenosis; ultrasonography; outcomes

1. Introduction

Atrial fibrillation (AF) is the most common cause of cardioembolic stroke and is associated with poor prognosis in survivors after ischemic stroke. AF was reported to increase the annual risk of cardiovascular events by 5-fold [1,2]. In efforts to prevent cardiovascular events due to AF, researchers have focused on the identification of patients at high risk of developing cardiovascular events [3]. Several studies have suggested that atherosclerosis is associated with both the development and the outcome of AF [4]. For example, among the components of the $CHAD_2DS_2$-VASc score, age, hypertension, diabetes, history of stroke/transient ischemic attack, and vascular disease are known to be the important risk factors for atherosclerosis [5,6].

Carotid atherosclerosis $\geq 50\%$ in patients with AF is well known to be an independent risk factor for future ischemic stroke and vascular events [7–9]. However, the prognostic implication of carotid atherosclerosis < 50% is not well known. Carotid ultrasonography can easily detect mild carotid atherosclerosis through measurements of the carotid intima media thickness (IMT) and carotid plaque thickness [8–10]. However, little is known about the prognostic impact of the number of carotid plaques on the outcome of patients with AF. In this regard, we evaluated the association between the total carotid plaque number (TPN) and long-term prognosis in ischemic stroke patients with AF.

2. Materials and Methods

2.1. Study Population

This is a hospital-based observational study in ischemic stroke patients who were prospectively registered to a stroke registry from January 2007 to December 2013 in Severance Hospital, Seoul, South Korea. [11]. The registry enrolled consecutive patients with acute ischemic stroke within 7 days of onset. During admission, all patients were evaluated with brain magnetic resonance imaging and/or computed tomography, as well as cerebral angiography (magnetic resonance angiography, computed tomography angiography, or digital subtraction angiography). Systemic evaluation included 12-lead electrocardiography (ECG), chest radiography, standard blood tests, lipid profile, and continuous ECG monitoring during stay in the stroke unit. Specific evaluation for finding the cardioembolic source, such as transthoracic echocardiography, transesophageal echocardiography, and 24-h Holter monitoring was done.

The stroke subtypes according to the Trial of ORG 10172 in Acute Stroke Treatment (TOAST) classification [12] and the presence of angiographic abnormalities were prospectively determined using neuroradiologist reports and the consensus of stroke specialists in weekly stroke conferences, and prospectively entered into a computerized database.

This study was approved by the institutional review board of Severance Hospital, Yonsei University Health System, which waived the requirement for informed consent from patients owing to the retrospective nature of the analysis.

2.2. Clinical Variables

We collected data on demographics and risk factors of stroke including hypertension, diabetes, hyperlipidemia, coronary artery disease, peripheral artery disease, history of stroke, transient ischemic accident or thromboembolism, and smoking habit. Hypertension was defined as a systolic blood pressure of ≥ 140 mmHg or a diastolic blood pressure of ≥ 90 mmHg, or any history of anti-hypertensive agent use. Diabetes was defined as fasting glucose level ≥ 7.0 mmol/L, random blood glucose level ≥ 11.0 mmol/L, glycated hemoglobin ≥ 6.5%, or a history of oral hypoglycemic agent or insulin use. Hyperlipidemia was defined as serum total cholesterol ≥ 6.21 mmol/L, low-density lipoprotein cholesterol ≥ 4.14 mmol/L, or any history of use of lipid-lowering agents after a diagnosis of hyperlipidemia. AF was diagnosed on the basis of the findings of routine ECG, Holter monitoring, or continuous ECG monitoring on the current admission or before admission. Paroxysmal AF was also considered the presence of AF. Congestive heart failure was determined from the history of heart failure diagnosis, treatment with loop diuretics, and ejection fraction ≤35% on echocardiography. Coronary artery occlusive disease (CAOD) was defined as any history of unstable angina, myocardial infarction, and CAOD. Peripheral artery occlusive disease was defined as any history of a diagnosis of peripheral artery disease at any hospital regardless of the presence or absence of intervention or medication for peripheral artery disease. Patients were considered current smokers if they had smoked any cigarettes within 1 year before admission. Medication history including anti-coagulant, anti-platelet, anti-hypertensive, and lipid-lowering agent use was collected. Laboratory data were also obtained for complete blood count, lipid profile, blood urea nitrogen level, and creatinine level. The severity of stroke was determined using the National Institute Health Stroke Scale (NIHSS) score at admission.

2.3. Carotid Artery Assessment

Carotid artery plaques were assessed using B-mode ultrasound (iU22 ultrasound system; Philips, Bothell, WA, USA) with a 3-9-MHz multifrequency linear array transducer. All measurements were done in a semi-dark room by two trained ultrasonographers. Bilateral longitudinal and transverse images of the common carotid arteries (CCAs) and internal carotid arteries (ICAs) were always obtained and the presence of plaque was decided after comparison of longitudinal and transverse images. The IMT in the CCAs was defined as the distance of the interface between the lumen-intima and the media-adventitia. The far wall of the carotid artery was visualized bilaterally in the CCAs (20–50 mm proximal to the bifurcation of blood flow), carotid bulb (0–20 mm proximal to the bifurcation of blood flow), and internal and external carotid arteries (0–20 mm distal to the bifurcation of blood flow). At 20, 25, and 30 mm proximal to the bifurcation of blood flow, IMT was bilaterally measured at the far wall of the CCAs during end-diastole, and calculated as the mean value for each patient. According to the Mannheim criteria [13], carotid plaque was defined as a focal structure encroaching into the arterial lumen by at least 0.5 mm, > 50% of surrounding IMT values, or thickness $\geq$ 1.5 mm above the distance of the interface between the lumen-intima and the media-adventitia.

The thickness of each plaque in the carotid arteries in the whole scanned area was also bilaterally measured. The TPN was determined by simply counting (bilaterally) the number of plaques in proximal ICAs and CCAs. The best cutoff values for TPN were determined using the Contal and O'Quigley method, which calculates the maximum hazard ratio (HR) based on log-rank statistics [14].

2.4. Follow-Up and Outcomes

After discharge, each patient was followed up with regularly at 3 months, 1 year, and yearly thereafter. At each follow-up visit, medical information including occurrence of any cardiovascular events, newly detected vascular risk factors, lifestyle modification after stroke, and re-admission to another hospital was obtained via face-to-face interviews with neurologists or through clinical research associates in the outpatient clinic. When the patients missed a scheduled visit, we obtained the information from the patients or their proxy through a telephone interview with a structured questionnaire [15]. In addition, we also obtained mortality data based on death certificates from the Korean National Statistical Office (http://www.kostat.go.kr).

The primary end point was major adverse cardiovascular events (MACE; cardiovascular mortality, non-cardiovascular mortality, and occurrence of non-fatal stroke or myocardial infarction). Cardiovascular mortality was defined as any mortality due to stroke, myocardial infarction, other cardiac disease, or unobserved sudden death. The secondary outcome was all-cause mortality. The censoring date was December 31, 2013.

2.5. Statistical Analysis

The data were presented as mean $\pm$ standard deviation or medians (interquartile range [IQR]), as appropriate. Differences between the two groups were compared with the chi-square test, Fisher's exact test, Student's t-test, and the Mann–Whitney U-test, as appropriate. Survival analysis was conducted, and survival curves were plotted using Kaplan–Meier analysis. The difference of survival time between groups was analyzed using a log-rank test. To determine the independent predictor of MACE and all-cause mortality, Cox proportional hazard regression analysis was used, and HR and 95% confidence interval (CI) values were summarized. Cox proportional hazard regression analysis was conducted with adjustments for age, sex, initial NIHSS score, and variables with $p < 0.1$ in the univariate analysis.

To evaluate the added value of carotid plaque burden for the prognosis of ischemic stroke caused by AF, we constructed the model incorporating variables in the $CHA_2DS_2\text{-}VAS_c$ score and other variables associated with carotid plaque burden such as IMT, maximal carotid plaque thickness, and TPN. We compared the following five models: (1) $CHA_2DS_2\text{-}VAS_c$ score variables alone; (2) addition of IMT; (3) addition of maximal carotid plaque thickness; (4) addition of TPN; and (5) addition of IMT, maximal carotid plaque thickness, and TPN. For internal validation of the newly developed model, time-dependent receiver-operating characteristic curves and areas under the curve (AUCs) were determined based on Heagerty's incident / dynamic AUCs during the median follow-up time [16]. A boot strapping method with 1000 re-samplings for calculating the 95% CI and the difference between the c-indices of each model was applied [17]. All tests were two-sided, and $p < 0.05$ was considered statistically significant. Statistical analysis was performed using R software, version 3.1.3 (R Foundation of Statistical Computing, Vienna, Austria).

3. Results

3.1. Patients' Characteristics

A total of 3727 consecutive ischemic stroke/transient ischemic attack patients were enrolled during the study period. After the exclusion of 2896 patients without AF, a total of 831 patients with AF remained. Among them, 150 patients without carotid ultrasonography and 76 patients with valvular heart disease were excluded. Patients who had > 50% stenosis in the intracranial or extracranial arteries ($n = 143$), complex aortic atheroma (≥ 4 mm or mobile atheroma) ($n = 6$), lacunar infarction ($n = 50$), and other rare etiologies ($n = 14$) according to the TOAST classification were also excluded. Finally, a total of 392 patients were analyzed (Figure 1).

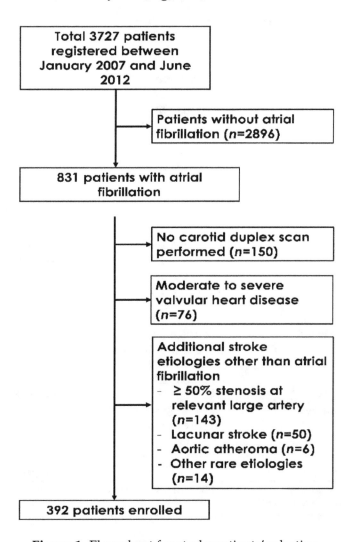

Figure 1. Flow sheet for study patients' selection.

The baseline characteristics of the enrolled patients are summarized in Table 1. The mean age of the total enrolled patients was 69.2 ± 10.3 years, and 225 (57.5%) patients were men. The median NIHSS score at admission was 5.5 (IQR 2–13). Before admission, 88 (22.4%) patients were taking oral anticoagulants. Carotid plaques were found in 343 (87.5%) patients. The median TPN was 3 (IQR 2–6). The median IMT and plaque thickness was 0.8 (IQR 0.7–0.9) and 2.1 (IQR 1.7–2.9), respectively. The inter-rater reliability based on the intraclass correlation coefficient (ICC) between ultrasonographers for carotid duplex sonography parameters was excellent, as follows: TPN (ICC: 0.983, $p < 0.001$), IMT (ICC: 0.966, $p < 0.001$), and maximal plaque thickness (ICC: 0.892, $p = 0.001$). In case of disagreement between ultrasonographers regarding parameters of the carotid duplex sonography, any disagreement was resolved by consensus. Following the Contal and O'Quigley method, the patients were categorized into two groups according to the best cutoff values for TPN (TPN ≤ 4 vs. TPN ≥ 5). The TPN ≤ 4 group consisted of 239 (71.0%) patients, and the TPN ≥ 5 group comprised 153 (39.0%) patients. Patients in the TPN ≥ 5 group were older and more likely to have hypertension, CAOD, statin use, or anti-hypertensive drug use. In addition, the TPN ≥ 5 group had higher IMT (0.9 ± 0.2 vs. 0.8 ± 0.2, $p < 0.001$) and larger maximal plaque thickness (3.0 ± 0.9 vs. 1.7 ± 1.1, $p < 0.001$) than the TPN ≤ 4 group.

Table 1. Clinical characteristics of study patients according to the total carotid plaque number (TPN).

	TPN ≤ 4 (N = 239)	TPN ≥ 5 (N = 153)	P Value
Demographics			
Age, years	66.4 ± 10.5	73.5 ± 8.4	< 0.001
Sex, men	134 (56.1)	91 (59.5)	0.575
Initial NIHSS score	5 (2–13)	6 (2–13)	0.639
Risk factors			
Hypertension	155 (64.9)	126 (82.4)	< 0.001
Diabetes mellitus	53 (22.2)	46 (30.1)	0.102
Smoking	38 (15.9)	23 (15.0)	0.930
Hyperlipidemia	38 (15.9)	37 (24.2)	0.057
PAOD	5 (2.1)	7 (4.6)	0.275
CAOD	47 (19.7)	50 (32.7)	0.005
CHF	33 (13.8)	21 (13.7)	1.000
Laboratory findings			
Hemoglobin, g/dL	14.1 ± 2.1	13.5 ± 1.5	0.001
White blood cell, × 10^9/L	8202.7 ± 2827.0	7830.1 ± 2939.5	0.211
Platelet, × 10^9/L	225.6 ± 69.9	224.6 ± 70.0	0.885
Blood urea nitrogen, mmol/L	17.4 ± 6.3	18.8 ± 9.6	0.190
Creatinine, μmol/L	1.0 ± 0.8	1.3 ± 1.6	0.128
Total cholesterol, mmol/L	170.8 ± 35.8	167.2 ± 39.4	0.361
Triglyceride, mmol/L	96.2 ± 50.2	89.5 ± 45.3	0.184
HDL-cholesterol, mmol/L	45.0 ± 11.5	44.8 ± 11.9	0.865
LDL-cholesterol, mmol/L	106.5 ± 32.3	103.6 ± 35.7	0.399
Premorbid medication			
Antiplatelet agent	98 (41.0)	76 (49.7)	0.114
Anticoagulants	60 (25.1)	28 (18.3)	0.147
Statin	36 (15.1)	44 (28.8)	0.002
Antihypertensive agent	93 (38.9)	81 (52.9)	0.009
Carotid duplex measurement			
IMT, mm	0.8 ± 0.2	0.9 ± 0.2	< 0.001
Maximal plaque thickness, mm	1.7 ± 1.1	3.0 ± 0.9	< 0.001
Total plaque number, n	2 (1–3)	7 (5–10.5)	< 0.001

Data are shown as n (%), mean ± SD, or median (IQR). SD, standard deviation; IQR, interquartile range; NIHSS, National Institute of Health Stroke Scale; PAOD, peripheral artery occlusive disease; CAOD, coronary artery occlusive disease; CHF, congestive heart failure;; HDL, high density lipoprotein; LDL, low density lipoprotein; IMT, intimal medial thickness.

3.2. Outcome

The mean follow-up period was 2.42 ± 1.83 years. During the follow-up, a total of 113 (28.8%) MACE occurred in 60 (25.1%) patients of the TPN ≤ 4 group and in 53 (34.6%) patients of the TPN ≥ 5 group. In Kaplan–Meier analysis, the TPN ≥ 5 group showed a higher MACE rate than the TPN ≤ 4 group (log-rank test, $p < 0.001$) (Figure 2A). Multivariate Cox proportional regression analysis showed that the TPN ≥ 5 group had a significantly higher MACE rate than the TPN ≤ 4 group after adjusting for age, sex, and variables with $p < 0.1$ in univariate analysis (adjusted hazard ratio [HR], 1.50; 95% CI, 1.01–2.21; $p < 0.05$) (Table 2).

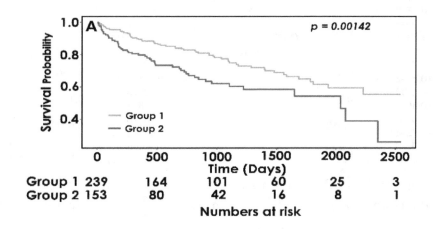

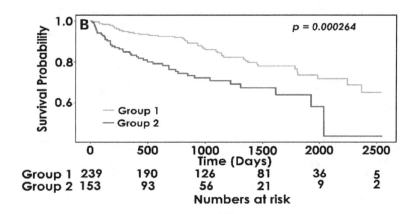

Figure 2. Kaplan–Meier analysis for (**A**) major adverse cardiovascular event (MACE); (**B**) all-cause mortality according to the total carotid plaque number (TPN).

In terms of all-cause mortality, 88 (22.4%) patients had died during the follow up period. In Kaplan–Meier curve analysis, the TPN ≥ 5 group showed a higher mortality rate than the TPN ≤ 4 group (log-rank test, $p < 0.001$) (Figure 2B). In multivariate Cox proportional regression analysis after adjusting for age, sex, and variables with $p < 0.10$ in univariate analysis, patients in the TPN ≥ 5 group showed an increased risk of all-cause mortality (adjusted HR, 2.69; 95% CI, 1.40–5.17; $p < 0.05$) compared with patients in the TPN ≤ 4 group (Table 2).

Table 2. Unadjusted and adjusted hazard ratio for MACE and all-cause mortality according to the total carotid number of plaque.

	MACE				All-Cause Mortality			
	Univariate Analysis		Multivariate Analysis		Univariate Analysis		Multivariate Analysis	
	HR (95% CI)	P Value	HR (95% CI)	P Value	HR (95% CI)	P Value	HR (95% CI)	P Value
Demographics								
Age	1.05 (1.03–1.07)	0.000	1.04 (1.01–1.06)	0.002	1.07 (1.05–1.10)	0.000	1.05 (1.02–1.08)	0.003
Sex	0.66 (0.45–0.95)	0.027	1.03 (0.67–1.59)	0.887	0.66 (0.43–1.00)	0.051	0.95 (0.49–1.84)	0.874
Initial NIHSS score	1.06 (1.03–1.08)	0.000	1.05 (1.02–1.08)	0.001	1.07 (1.04–1.00)	0.446	1.07 (1.03–1.11)	0.000
Risk factors								
Hypertension	1.32 (0.86–2.04)	0.208			1.21 (0.74–1.96)	0.446		
Diabetes mellitus	1.02 (0.66–1.56)	0.933			1.10 (0.68–1.78)	0.106		
Smoking	1.18 (0.72–1.93)	0.512			1.16 (0.66–2.02)	0.603		
PAOD	1.70 (0.69–4.18)	0.247			2.68 (1.08–6.65)	0.033	1.25 (0.36–4.41)	0.727
CAOD	1.51 (1.01–2.26)	0.046	1.14 (0.75–1.75)	0.532	1.74 (1.11–2.73)	0.016	1.18 (0.64–2.16)	0.588
CHF	1.66(1.05–2.61)	0.029	1.22 (0.76–1.97)	0.411	2.31 (1.43–3.72)	0.001	1.72 (0.83–3.57)	0.148
Laboratory findings								
Hemoglobin	0.88 (0.80–0.95)	0.002	0.91 (0.82–1.01)	0.909	0.86 (0.79–0.94)	0.001	0.94 (0.79–1.11)	0.466
White blood cell	1.00 (1.00–1.00)	0.831			1.00 (1.00–1.00)	0.836		
Platelet	1.00 (1.00–1.00)	0.361			1.00 (0.99–1.00)	0.040	1.00 (0.99–1.00)	0.998
BUN	1.02 (0.99–1.05)	0.157			1.03 (1.01–1.06)	0.018	1.01 (0.98–1.05)	0.590
Creatinine	1.05 (0.88–1.24)	0.600			1.08 (0.91–1.28)	0.371		
Total cholesterol	1.00 (0.99–1.00)	0.089			0.99 (0.99–1.00)	0.067		
Triglyceride	1.00 (1.00–1.00)	0.929	1.00 (0.99–1.01)	0.184	1.00 (1.00–1.00)	0.974		
HDL–cholesterol	1.00 (0.98–1.01)	0.844			1.00 (0.98–1.02)	0.987		
LDL–cholesterol	0.99 (0.99–1.00)	0.071	1.00 (0.99–1.00)	0.234	0.99 (0.99–1.00)	0.051		
Premorbid medication								
Antiplatelet agent	1.03 (0.71–1.49)	0.867			1.02 (0.67–1.56)	0.916		
Anticoagulants	0.78 (0.49–1.23)	0.288			0.83(0.50–1.40)	0.494		
Statin	1.41 (0.92–2.16)	0.117			1.28 (0.78–2.11)	0.330		
Antihypertensive agent	1.45 (0.99–2.13)	0.056			1.75 (1.13–2.70)	0.011	1.73 (0.89–3.38)	0.106
Total plaque number								
TPN ≤ 4 (reference)	1		1		1		1	
TPN ≥ 5	1.82 (1.25–2.64)	0.002	1.50 (1.01–2.21)	0.044	2.16 (1.41–3.29)	< 0.001	2.69 (1.40–5.17)	0.003

MACE, major adverse cardiovascular events; HR, hazard ratio; CI, confidential interval; National Institute of Health Stroke Scale; PAOD, peripheral artery occlusive disease; CAOD, coronary artery occlusive disease; CHF, congestive heart failure; BUN, blood urea nitrogen; HDL, high density lipoprotein; LDL, low density lipoprotein; IMT, intimal medial thickness.

3.3. Prognostic Utility of Carotid Plaque Burden on Ischemic Stroke Caused by AF

During the median follow-up period, the c-indices of Heagerty's incident/dynamic AUC of each model were calculated (Table 3 and Supplementary Figure S1). The baseline model consisted of age, sex, congestive heart failure, diabetes mellitus, CAOD, and peripheral artery occlusive disease, which are the same variables of the $CHAD_2DS_2$-VASc score. The c-index for the baseline model was 0.651 (95% CI, 0.605–0.705) in MACE and 0.712 (95% CI, 0.658–0.766) in all-cause mortality. In model 5, including of all parameters of carotid plaque burden including TPN, maximal plaque thickness, and IMT improved prognostic utility that with the $CHAD_2DS_2$-VASc score alone in MACE (c-index, 0.686, 95% CI, 0.638–0.737, $p = 0.045$) and all-cause mortality (c-index, 0.734, 95% CI (0.686–0.786, $p = 0.025$).

Table 3. C-indices of Heagerty's incident/dynamic AUC for predicting MACE and all-cause mortality

	MACE			All–Cause Mortality		
	c–Index (95% CI)	Difference	P–Value	c–Index	Difference	P–Value
Model 1 *	0.651 (0.605–0.705)	Reference		0.696 (0.647–0.753)	Reference	
Model 2 †	0.661 (0.613–0.714)	0.010 (−0.005–0.033)	0.267	0.712 (0.658–0.766)	0.016 (−0.005–0.046)	0.218
Model 3 ‡	0.672 (0.626–0.726)	0.020 (0.001–0.049)	0.214	0.716 (0.670–0.769)	0.019 (0.001–0.045)	0.113
Model 4 §	0.657 (0.609–0.710)	0.006 (0–0.022)	0.317	0.701 (0.651–0.756)	0.005 (−0.001–0.021)	0.405
Model 5 ‖	0.686 (0.638–0.737)	0.034 (0.006–0.071)	0.045	0.734 (0.686–0.786)	0.038 (0.006–0.075)	0.025

AUC, area under the curve; MACE, major adverse cardiovascular events; CI, confidence interval. * Model 1: CHA_2DS_2-VAS$_c$ variables (age, sex, hypertension, diabetes mellitus, congestive heart failure, coronary artery occlusive disease, peripheral artery occlusive disease) † Model 2: Model 1 plus carotid intima medial thickness; ‡ Model 3: Model 1 plus total number of plaque; § Model 4: Model 1 plus maximal thickness of plaque; ‖ Model 5: Model 1 plus carotid intima medial thickness plus maximal plaque thickness plus total number of plaque.

4. Discussion

The present study revealed that carotid plaque burden of < 50% carotid stenosis was a strong prognostic marker in patients with AF. Among the parameters of carotid plaque burden, TPN is easily counted during carotid ultrasonography examination. It showed an impact on the outcome of ischemic stroke patients with AF. Moreover, the carotid plaque burden improved the predictive value of the $CHAD_2DS_2$-VASc score in predicting cardiovascular events and mortality in ischemic stroke patients with AF.

AF is the most common cause of cardioembolic stroke. Patients with AF had markedly reduced survival compared with those without AF. In the Framingham Heart Study, the risk factor-adjusted odds ratio for death was 1.5 and 1.9 in men and women, respectively [18]. Patients with AF frequently have concomitant cerebral atherosclerosis (20–50% of cases) [19,20]. It is well known that atherosclerosis is a systemic disorder that plays an important role in the prognosis of patients with AF [4]. It can be assumed that patients with AF are more likely to have additional atherosclerotic burden and may have poor prognosis. We previously reported that patients who have both large artery atherosclerosis (>50% atherosclerotic stenosis in the relevant artery) and cardioembolism showed higher cardiovascular mortality than patients with a single cause of either large artery atherosclerosis or cardioembolism [21]. Thus, it can be inferred that concomitant carotid atherosclerosis with AF is associated with the development of cardiovascular events despite the presence of < 50% stenosis.

To date, little is known about the impact of < 50% atherosclerotic stenosis of the carotid artery on the outcome of ischemic stroke patients with AF. The presence of large artery atherosclerosis can be screened using luminography including computed tomography angiography, magnetic resonance angiography, or digital subtraction angiography. However, arterial wall changes including small plaques or increased IMT in the carotid artery cannot be detected using luminography. Carotid ultrasonography is a noninvasive imaging examination that can easily and accurately evaluate carotid plaques and IMT in the arterial lumen.

We found that the TPN ≥ 5 group had a 1.5-fold higher MACE rate than the TPN ≤ 4 group after adjustments. Moreover, considering all parameters of carotid plaque burden, including TPN, maximal plaque thickness, and IMT, contributed to the improvement of the risk stratification of ischemic stroke patients with AF over that with the $CHAD_2DS_2$-VASc risk score alone. The components of the $CHAD_2DS_2$-VASc score are clinical variables including old age, hypertension, diabetes, and vascular disease. These variables are also well-known risk factors for atherosclerosis [6]. Therefore, adding the carotid plaque burden to the model improves the risk prediction.

In line with our findings, cohort studies including non-stroke patients also reported similar results. In ARAPACIS (Atrial Fibrillation Registry for Ankle-brachial Index Prevalence Assessment: Collaborative Italian Study), a prospective nationwide observational cohort study in patients with non-valvular AF, the investigators reported that carotid plaque detection improves the predictive value of the $CHAD_2DS_2$-VASc score in patients with AF [22]. The ARIC (Atherosclerosis Risk in Communities) study investigators also reported that carotid IMT and the presence of carotid plaque are associated with an increased risk of ischemic stroke in patients with AF. The addition of carotid IMT and carotid plaque to the model provided an incremental predictive value for the risk of stroke over the $CHAD_2DS_2$-VASc score alone in adults with AF who had no prior ischemic stroke. Although we reached similar findings, a difference of the present study from the two cohort studies is that we enrolled only ischemic stroke patients with AF. Another difference is that we adopted TPN because this variable can be easily and acutely measured on routine carotid ultrasonography [10].

Currently, the method for the secondary prevention of ischemic stroke caused by AF is anticoagulation with a vitamin K antagonist or a direct oral anticoagulant (DOAC) [23]. However, vitamin K antagonists can prevent only 67% of future ischemic stroke events and DOAC did not show superiority over vitamin K antagonists [24,25]. Identification of high-risk patients for future events despite anticoagulation treatment is important. Carotid atherosclerosis and atherosclerotic burden can be easily detected using carotid duplex ultrasonography. Although TPN is less accurate and operator-dependent method than quantification measurement of carotid plaque such as total plaque area [26,27], TPN can be easily counted and may be helpful in identifying high risk patients in daily clinical practice. Our study has several limitations. First, unstable plaque morphology and hypoechoic plaque are associated with an increased risk of ischemic stroke; however, we did not analyze the characteristics of individual plaques. Nevertheless, unstable carotid plaque is known to be prevalent in advanced carotid atherosclerosis, and our study did not include patients with >50% stenosis in an intracranial or extracranial artery. Thus, the influence of the morphologic feature of carotid plaques may be little. Second, carotid duplex ultrasonography was conducted by two ultrasonographers; however, the measurement agreement between them was high. Third, potential selection bias may exist. To minimize selection bias, we recruited consecutive ischemic stroke patients with AF.

5. Conclusions

In conclusion, TPN is an important risk predictor in ischemic stroke patients with AF. In addition, considering all parameters of carotid plaque burden including TPN, maximal plaque thickness, and IMT may contribute to improving the risk prediction in ischemic stroke patients with AF, compared with the prediction with the clinical variables of $CHAD_2DS_2$-VASc score alone. These findings suggest that carotid ultrasonography may be useful in reclassifying these patients.

Author Contributions: Conceptualization, H.P. and H.S.N.; Methodology, Y.D.K., and J.Y.; Formal analysis, M.H., H.S.L., and J.K.C.; Investigation, H.P., Y.D.K., and J.Y.; Writing—original draft preparation, H.P and H.S.N.; Writing—review and editing, H.P., J.H.H., and H.S.N.; Supervision, H.P., M.H., Y.D.K., J.Y., H.S.L., J.K.C., J.H.H., and H.S.N. Read and approved the final manuscript, all authors.

Acknowledgments: We thank Junghye Choi, BS, for her efforts in data collection.

References

1. Schnabel, R.B.; Yin, X.; Gona, P.; Larson, M.G.; Beiser, A.S.; McManus, D.D.; Newton-Chen, C.; Lubitz, S.A.; Magnani, J.W.; Ellinor, P.T.; et al. 50 year trends in atrial fibrillation prevalence, incidence, risk factors, and mortality in the framingham heart study: A cohort study. *Lancet* **2015**, *386*, 154–162. [CrossRef]
2. Wolf, P.A.; Mitchell, J.B.; Baker, C.S.; Kannel, W.B.; D'Agostino, R.B. Impact of atrial fibrillation on mortality, stroke, and medical costs. *Arch. Intern. Med.* **1998**, *158*, 229–234. [CrossRef]
3. Lau, D.H.; Nattel, S.; Kalman, J.M.; Sanders, P. Modifiable risk factors and atrial fibrillation. *Circulation* **2017**, *136*, 583–596. [CrossRef]
4. Bekwelem, W.; Jensen, P.N.; Norby, F.L.; Soliman, E.Z.; Agarwal, S.K.; Lip, G.Y.; Pan, W.; Folsom, A.R.; Longstreth, W.T., Jr.; Alonso, A.; et al. Carotid atherosclerosis and stroke in atrial fibrillation: The atherosclerosis risk in communities study. *Stroke* **2016**, *47*, 1643–1646. [CrossRef] [PubMed]
5. European Heart Rhythm Association; European Association for Cardio-Thoracic Surgery; Camm, A.J.; Kirchhof, P.; Lip, G.Y.; Schotten, U.; Savelieva, I.; Ernst, S.; van Gelder, I.C.; Al-Attar, N.; et al. Guidelines for the management of atrial fibrillation: The task force for the management of atrial fibrillation of the European Society of Cardiology (ESC). *Eur. Heart J.* **2010**, *31*, 2369–2429. [PubMed]
6. Cha, M.J.; Kim, Y.D.; Nam, H.S.; Kim, J.; Lee, D.H.; Heo, J.H. Stroke mechanism in patients with non-valvular atrial fibrillation according to the CHADS$_2$ and CHAD$_2$DS$_2$-VASc score. *Eur. J. Neurol.* **2012**, *19*, 473–479. [CrossRef]
7. Nagai, Y.; Kitagawa, K.; Sakaguchi, M.; Shimizu, Y.; Hashimoto, H.; Yamagami, H.; Narita, M.; Ohtsuki, T.; Hori, M.; Matsumoto, M. Significance of earlier carotid atherosclerosis for stroke subtypes. *Stroke* **2001**, *32*, 1780–1785. [CrossRef]
8. Steinvil, A.; Sadeh, B.; Bornstein, N.M.; Havakuk, O.; Greenberg, S.; Arbel, Y.; Konigstein, M.; Finkelstein, A.; Banai, S.; Halkin, A. Impact of carotid atherosclerosis on the risk of adverse cardiac events in patients with and without coronary disease. *Stroke* **2014**, *45*, 2311–2317. [CrossRef] [PubMed]
9. Störk, S.; van den Beld, A.W.; von Schacky, C.; Angermann, C.E.; Lamberts, S.W.; Grobbee, D.E.; Bots, M.L. Carotid artery plaque burden, stiffness, and mortality risk in elderly men: A prospective, population-based cohort study. *Circulation* **2004**, *110*, 344–348. [CrossRef] [PubMed]
10. Maeda, S.; Sawayama, Y.; Furusyo, N.; Shigematsu, M.; Hayashi, J. The association between fatal vascular events and risk factors for carotid atherosclerosis in patients on maintenance hemodialysis: Plaque number of dialytic atherosclerosis study. *Atherosclerosis* **2009**, *204*, 549–555. [CrossRef] [PubMed]
11. Lee, B.I.; Nam, H.S.; Heo, J.H.; Kim, D.I. Yonsei stroke registry. Analysis of 1,000 patients with acute cerebral infarctions. *Cerebrovasc. Dis.* **2001**, *12*, 145–151. [CrossRef] [PubMed]
12. Adams, H.P., Jr.; Bendixen, B.H.; Kappelle, L.J.; Biller, J.; Love, B.B.; Gordon, D.L.; Marsh, E.E. Classification of subtype of acute ischemic stroke. Definitions for use in a multicenter clinical trial. Toast. Trial of org 10172 in acute stroke treatment. *Stroke* **1993**, *24*, 35–41. [CrossRef] [PubMed]
13. Touboul, P.J.; Hennerici, M.G.; Meairs, S.; Adams, H.; Amarenco, P.; Bornstein, N.; Csiba, L.; Desvarieux, M.; Ebrahim, S.; Hernadez, R.H.; et al. Mannheim carotid intima-media thickness and plaque consensus (2004–2006–2011). An update on behalf of the advisory board of the 3rd, 4th and 5th watching the risk symposia, at the 13th, 15th and 20th european stroke conferences, Mannheim, Germany, 2004, Brussels, Belgium, 2006, and Hamburg, Germany, 2011. *Cerebrovasc. Dis.* **2012**, *34*, 290–296. [PubMed]
14. Contal, C.; O'Quigley, J. An application of changepoint methods in studying the effect of age on survival in breast cancer. *Comput. Stat. Data Anal.* **1999**, *30*, 253–270. [CrossRef]
15. Yoo, J.; Song, D.; Baek, J.H.; Kim, K.; Kim, J.; Song, T.J.; Lee, H.S.; Choi, D.; Kim, Y.D.; Nam, H.S.; et al. Poor long-term outcomes in stroke patients with asymptomatic coronary artery disease in heart CT. *Atherosclerosi* **2017**, *265*, 7–13. [CrossRef]

16. Heagerty, P.J.; Zheng, Y. Survival model predictive accuracy and ROC curves. *Biometrics* **2005**, *61*, 92–105. [CrossRef]

17. Uno, H.; Cai, T.; Pencina, M.J.; D'Agostino, R.B.; Wei, L. On the C-statistics for evaluating overall adequacy of risk prediction procedures with censored survival data. *Stat. Med.* **2011**, *30*, 1105–1117. [CrossRef] [PubMed]

18. Benjamin, E.J.; Wolf, P.A.; D'Agostino, R.B.; Silbershatz, H.; Kannel, W.B.; Levy, D. Impact of atrial fibrillation on the risk of death: The framingham heart study. *Circulation* **1998**, *98*, 946–952. [CrossRef] [PubMed]

19. Chang, Y.J.; Ryu, S.J.; Lin, S.K. Carotid artery stenosis in ischemic stroke patients with nonvalvular atrial fibrillation. *Cerebrovasc. Dis.* **2002**, *13*, 16–20. [CrossRef]

20. Kanter, M.C.; Tegeler, C.H.; Pearce, L.A.; Weinberger, J.; Feinberg, W.M.; Anderson, D.C.; Gomez, C.R.; Rothrock, J.F.; Helgason, C.M.; Hart, R.G.; et al. Carotid stenosis in patients with atrial fibrillation. Prevalence, risk factors, and relationship to stroke in the Stroke Prevention in Atrial Fibrillation Study. *Arch. Intern. Med.* **1994**, *154*, 1372–1377. [CrossRef] [PubMed]

21. Kim, Y.D.; Cha, M.J.; Kim, J.; Lee, D.H.; Lee, H.S.; Nam, C.M.; Nam, H.S.; Heo, J.H. Long-term mortality in patients with coexisting potential causes of ischemic stroke. *Int. J. Stroke* **2015**, *10*, 541–546. [CrossRef] [PubMed]

22. Basili, S.; Loffredo, L.; Pastori, D.; Proietti, M.; Farcomeni, A.; Vestri, A.R.; Pignatelli, P.; Davì, G.; Hiatt, W.R.; Lip, G.Y.H.; et al. Carotid plaque detection improves the predictive value of cha2ds2-vasc score in patients with non-valvular atrial fibrillation: The ARAPACIS study. *Int. J. Cardiol.* **2017**, *231*, 143–149. [CrossRef] [PubMed]

23. Kirchhof, P.; Benussi, S.; Kotecha, D.; Ahlsson, A.; Atar, D.; Casadei, B.; Castella, M.; Diener, H.-C.; Heidbuchel, H.; Hendriks, J.; et al. 2016 ESC guidelines for the management of atrial fibrillation developed in collaboration with EACTS. *Eur. Heart J.* **2016**, *37*, 2893–2962. [CrossRef] [PubMed]

24. Hart, R.G.; Pearce, L.A.; Aguilar, M.I. Meta-analysis: Antithrombotic therapy to prevent stroke in patients who have nonvalvular atrial fibrillation. *Ann. Intern. Med.* **2007**, *146*, 857–867. [CrossRef] [PubMed]

25. Lip, G.Y.; Lane, D.A. Stroke prevention in atrial fibrillation: A systematic review. *JAMA* **2015**, *313*, 1950–1962. [CrossRef]

26. Mitchel, C.; Korcarz, C.E.; Genper, A.D.; Kaufman, J.D.; Post, W.; Tracy, R.; Gassett, A.J.; Ma, N.; McClelland, R.L.; Stein, J.H. Ultrasound carotid plaque features, cardiovascular disease risk factors and events: The Multi-Ethnic Study of Atherosclerosis. *Atheroslcerosis* **2018**, *276*, 195–202. [CrossRef]

27. López-Melgar, B.; Fernández-Friera, L.; Sánchez-González, J.; Vilchez, J.P.; Cecconi, A.; Mateo, J.; Penālvo, J.L.; Oliva, B.; García-Ruiz, J.M.; Kauffman, S.; et al. Accurate quantification of atherosclerotic plaque volume by 3D vascular ultrasound using the volumetric linear array method. *Atherosclerosis* **2016**, *248*, 230–237. [CrossRef]

16

Endothelial Progenitor Cells as a Marker of Vascular Damage But not a Predictor in Acute Microangiopathy-Associated Stroke

Adam Wiśniewski [1,*], Joanna Boinska [2], Katarzyna Ziołkowska [2], Adam Lemanowicz [3], Karolina Filipska [4], Zbigniew Serafin [3], Robert Ślusarz [4], Danuta Rość [2] and Grzegorz Kozera [5]

[1] Department of Neurology, Collegium Medicum in Bydgoszcz, Nicolaus Copernicus University in Toruń, Skłodowskiej 9 Street, 85-094 Bydgoszcz, Poland

[2] Department of Pathophysiology, Collegium Medicum in Bydgoszcz, Nicolaus Copernicus University in Toruń, Skłodowskiej 9 Street, 85-094 Bydgoszcz, Poland; joanna_boinska@cm.umk.pl (J.B.); katarzyna_stankowska@cm.umk.pl (K.Z.); drosc@cm.umk.pl (D.R.)

[3] Department of Radiology, Collegium Medicum in Bydgoszcz, Nicolaus Copernicus University in Toruń, Skłodowskiej 9 Street, 85-094 Bydgoszcz, Poland; adam.lemanowicz@cm.umk.pl (A.L.); serafin@cm.umk.pl (Z.S.)

[4] Department of Neurological and Neurosurgical Nursing, Collegium Medicum in Bydgoszcz, Nicolaus Copernicus University in Toruń, Łukasiewicza 1 Street, 85-821 Bydgoszcz, Poland; karolinafilipskakf@gmail.com (K.F.); robert_slu_cmumk@wp.pl (R.Ś.)

[5] Medical Simulation Centre, Medical University of Gdańsk, Faculty of Medicine, Dębowa 17 Street, 80-208 Gdańsk, Poland; gkozera1@wp.pl

* Correspondence: adam.lek@wp.pl

Abstract: Background: The aim of the study was to assess the number of endothelial progenitor cells (EPCs) in patients with acute stroke due to cerebral microangiopathy and evaluate whether there is a relationship between their number and clinical status, radiological findings, risk factors, selected biochemical parameters, and prognosis, both in ischemic and hemorrhagic stroke. Methods: In total, 66 patients with lacunar ischemic stroke, 38 patients with typical location hemorrhagic stroke, and 22 subjects from the control group without acute cerebrovascular incidents were included in the prospective observational study. The number of EPCs was determined in serum on the first and eighth day after stroke onset using flow cytometry and identified with the immune-phenotype classification determinant (CD)45−, CD34+, CD133+. Results: We demonstrated a significantly higher number of EPCs on the first day of stroke compared to the control group (med. 17.75 cells/μL (0–488 cells/μL) vs. 5.24 cells/μL (0–95 cells/μL); $p = 0.0006$). We did not find a relationship between the number of EPCs in the acute phase of stroke and the biochemical parameters, vascular risk factors, or clinical condition. In females, the higher number of EPCs on the first day of stroke is related to a favorable functional outcome on the eighth day after the stroke onset compared to males ($p = 0.0355$). We found that a higher volume of the hemorrhagic focus on the first day was correlated with a lower number of EPCs on the first day (correlation coefficient (R) = -0.3378, $p = 0.0471$), and a higher number of EPCs on the first day of the hemorrhagic stroke was correlated with a lower degree of regression of the hemorrhagic focus (R = -0.3896, $p = 0.0367$). Conclusion: The study showed that endothelial progenitor cells are an early marker in acute microangiopathy-associated stroke regardless of etiology and may affect the radiological findings in hemorrhagic stroke. Nevertheless, their prognostic value remains doubtful in stroke patients.

Keywords: endothelial progenitor cells; ischemic stroke; hemorrhage; prognosis; clinical outcome

1. Introduction

Stroke is an important social and medical problem in the 21st century, as it is one of the main causes of morbidity and long-term disability and the second most frequent cause of death in the world [1]. Ischemic stroke associated with disturbances of the blood flow to the brain tissue, leading to necrosis of the part of the brain covered by ischemia (80–85%), is the most common. Hemorrhagic stroke (15–20%) associated with extravasation of blood to the brain is less common but has greater mortality [2]. Stroke may be the result of endothelial dysfunction (in the course of cerebral microangiopathy), as well as the cause of vascular endothelial damage. Stroke due to small vessel disease, i.e., lacunar stroke, is associated with pathological changes (classical atherosclerosis, fibrosis, enamel, and calcification) of small cerebral vessels (diameter below 600 μm), and accounts for approximately 20–25% of all ischemic strokes [3]. Among hemorrhagic strokes, the most common, typical location (deep) intracerebral hemorrhage, seems to have been most related to microangiopathy. It results from blood extravasation from stabbing branches (most often lenticular-striatum arteries) supplying the basal ganglia and thalamus. It is related to pathological changes of the vessel's walls (including cells of the endothelium) in the course of improperly treated hypertension [4].

Endothelial progenitor cells (EPCs) are a recognized marker of both the degree of endothelial damage and the ability to regenerate the endothelium. Due to their multiplication potential, they can differentiate into many cells, but most often, they proliferate into mature circulating endothelial cells. Thanks to mediators, such as VEGF (vascular endothelial growth factor), SDF-1 (stromal-derived factor), and G-CSF (granulocyte colony-stimulating factor), they migrate to damaged areas of the brain affected by ischemia. They play an important role in the regeneration of the nervous tissue, glial cell nutrition, reduction of neuronal apoptosis, and blood–brain barrier stabilization. They are associated with postnatal angiogenesis, especially in neovascularization of blood vessels damaged by ischemia [5–7]. This is particularly important in patients with stroke. As a result, they are increasingly considered as a potential treatment method for stroke patients, especially with ischemic stroke, and the initial results of their use in studies on mice and rats seem encouraging [8–12]. However, the role and importance of these cells in stroke patients is still the subject of controversy, and reports on this subject are scarce and often ambiguous. It is believed that a large number of EPCs, due to their regenerative and repairing properties, may affect the size of the ischemic focus and even the clinical and functional status of the patients, and thus, the prognosis [13]. Therefore, the aim of this study was to assess the number of EPCs in the blood serum and their potential relationship with the clinical condition, radiological image, and prognosis in patients in the acute phase of stroke caused by cerebral microangiopathy.

2. Material and Methods

2.1. Study Design and Participants

The study was conducted in accordance with the Declaration of Helsinki and the protocol was approved by the Bioethics Committee of Nicolaus Copernicus University in Torun at Collegium Medicum of Ludwik Rydygier in Bydgoszcz (KB No. 769/2014). The study included subjects who, having read the study protocol, signed the informed consent to participate in the study. The researchers explained all stages of the study to the subjects and presented all potential risks associated with the research.

The definition of stroke, updated in 2013 by the American Heart Association/American Stroke Association (AHA/ASA), was used, which is an episode of a sudden neurological disorder caused by focal cerebral, spinal, or retinal ischemia lasting over 24 h or corresponding to the morphological features of ischemia of the central nervous system [14].

The study was conducted from February 2015 to December 2017 in the Department of Neurology at Collegium Medicum in Bydgoszcz of Nicolaus Copernicus University in Torun in the University Hospital No. 1 in Bydgoszcz. This prospective and observational study included stroke patients with cerebral microangiopathy: 66 patients with lacunar ischemic stroke, 38 patients with typical location intracerebral hemorrhage, and 22 people from the control group.

The group of patients with lacunar stroke included patients with no significant hemodynamic stenoses of large pre-skull vessels or cardiogenic-embolic background, and the performed neuroimaging confirmed the presence of a lacunar focus and/or revealed chronic vascular changes with a typical location and morphology (subcortical lesions, periventricular lesions, leukoaraiosis features) [15]. The typical location intracerebral hemorrhage was diagnosed based on the results of a computed tomography scan performed during the patient's admission. Patients with symptomatic cerebral hemorrhage in the course of taking oral anticoagulants and patients with extensive lobal hemorrhage during amyloid angiopathy were excluded. We included only stroke subjects admitted to the hospital with a duration of stroke symptoms no longer than 12 h. The control group consisted of people of similar age and vascular risk factors hospitalized in the Department of Neurology for reasons other than acute cerebrovascular disease and did not represent cerebrovascular incidents in the last 3 years.

Exclusion criteria included lack of the patient's consent to participate in the study or inability to express it consciously (stroke with aphasia or quantitative disturbances of consciousness); patients with documented oncological history; patients with chronic inflammatory processes, e.g., chronic venous thrombosis of the lower limbs or chronic ischemia of the lower limbs; patients with a stroke or TIA during the last 3 years; and patients with severe bleeding in the last 2 years, e.g., gastrointestinal bleeding, level of hemoglobin < 9 g/dL, hematocrit value < 35%; and duration of stroke symptoms more than 12 h before hospital admission.

Routine laboratory tests were performed at the Laboratory Diagnostics Department of the University Hospital No. 1 in Bydgoszcz in the morning within 24 h from the onset of stroke symptoms. About 6 mL of blood were collected from the veins of the forearm from patients to determine the following biochemical parameters in the blood serum: C reactive protein (CRP), fibrinogen, and homocysteine (Atellica Solution, Siemens Healthcare, Erlangen, Germany).

In all patients, computed tomography without contrast was performed at the time of admission to the hospital in the Hospital Emergency Department of A. Jurasz University Hospital No. 1 in Bydgoszcz using a 64-row Brilliance computer CT scanner (Phillips, Eindhoven, The Netherlands). In subjects with hemorrhagic stroke, the volume of hemorrhagic focus was assessed in mL on the 1st and 8th day of the stroke using the special Philips software. The degree of hemorrhagic focus regression was the volume difference between the 1st and 8th day.

2.2. Flow Cytometry

Determination of EPCs in blood in stroke subjects was performed on admission, within the first 24 h (1st day), and on the 8th day of the disease, using flow cytometry. In the control group, cell determinations were made on the 1st day of the hospital stay. The method for the determination of the level of circulating EPCs was based on previous reports [16,17]. Fresh blood (4.5 mL) with minimal stasis was collected into cooled tubes (Becton Dickinson Vacutainer® System, Plymouth, UK) containing potassium ethylenediaminetetraacetic acid (K2EDTA) and analyzed within 2 h. The samples were obtained in the morning between 8 and 10 a.m., after a 12-h period of overnight fasting. The approach of the current study was to use three concurrent markers of classification determinant (CD)45−, CD34+, CD133+, to increase the accuracy of endothelial progenitor detection. Cells were further confirmed by a fluorescent-activated cell sorting (FACS) Calibur flow cytometer (Becton Dickinson, San Diego, USA) using monoclonal antibodies directed against antigens specific for circulating endothelial progenitor cells (Figure 1). The data acquired was analyzed by using CellQuest software (Becton Dickinson). Circulating EPC counts were assessed by flow cytometry according to the procedure provided by Mancuso et al. [16]. Fresh peripheral blood (50 μL) was incubated with Peridinin-Chlorophyll-Protein–Cyanine (PerCP-Cy5.5)-conjugated anti-CD45 (concentration 25 μg/mL), as well as allophycocyanin (APC)-conjugated anti-CD34 antibodies (concentration 25 μg/mL) (all BD Biosciences, Pharmingen, San Diego, CA, USA), and phycoerythrin (PE)-conjugated anti-CD133 (concentration 50 µg/mL) (Miltenyi Biotec, Bergisch Gladbach, Germany). EPCs were defined as negative for hematopoietic marker CD45, positive for endothelial progenitor marker CD133, and positive for endothelial cell marker CD34, showing expression on early hematopoietic and vascular-associated tissue. At least 100,000 events were measured in each sample. The total cell count was calculated by TruCount tubes (BD Biosciences, San Jose, CA, USA) containing a calibrated number of fluorescent beads, and 'lyse-no-wash' procedures were used in the present study to improve the sensitivity [17]. Absolute EPCs numbers (cells/µL) were calculated based on the following pattern: Number of measured EPCs/number of fluorescent beads counted × number of beads/µL.

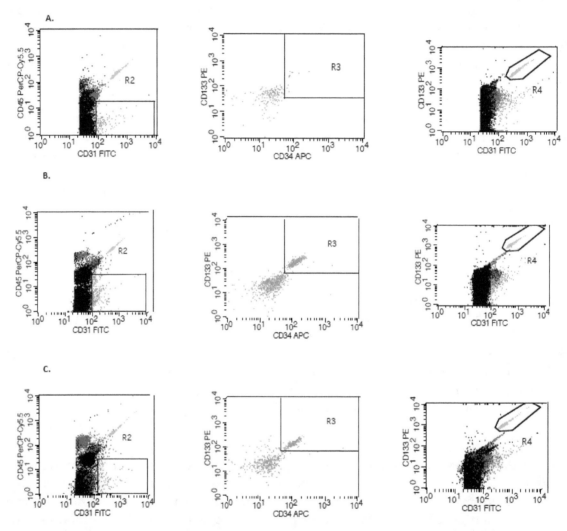

Figure 1. Sample of selected flow cytometric plots for the identification of circulating endothelial. progenitor cells in the control group (**A**), in patients with ischemic stroke (**B**), and hemorrhagic stroke (**C**). Peridinin-Chlorophyll-Protein–Cyanine-conjugated anti-CD45 (CD45 PerCP-Cy5.5), allophycocyanin-conjugated anti-CD34 antibodies (CD34 APC), phycoerythrin-conjugated anti-CD133 (CD133 PE), fluorescin isothiocyanate anti-CD31 (CD31 FITC). R2,R3,R4—regions defined in flow-cytometric dot plots for the detection of relevant surface markers of mononuclear cells, R2—gate for CD45 PerCP-Cy5.5/CD31 FITC; R3—gate for CD133 PE/CD34 APC; R4—gate for CD133 PE/CD31 FITC.

2.3. Clinical Outcome

Both the clinical and functional condition were assessed by means of standardized research tools: the National Institute of Health Stroke Scale (NIHSS) and the Modified Rankin Scale (mRS) [18,19], within the first 24 h after admission to the hospital (1st day) and on the 8th day of hospitalization. Two subgroups of stroke patients were identified based on the stroke severity: A subgroup with a mild and moderate neurological deficit (0–10 points on the NIHSS scale), and a subgroup with a severe neurological deficit (>10 points on the NIHSS scale). Due to the functional condition, two subgroups of patients with stroke were identified: Those with a favorable prognosis (0–2 points on the mRS scale) and those with an unfavorable prognosis (3–5 points on the mRS scale).

2.4. Statistical Analysis

The statistical analysis of collected data was performed with the help of the statistical program STATISTICA—version 13.1 (Dell Inc., Round Rock, TX, USA). Due to the unfulfilled assumptions related to the possibility of using parametric tests (Shapiro–Wilk for normality and Levene's for homogeneity of variance), non-parametric tests were used in the analysis, namely the Mann–Whitney U test, Wilcoxon test, Kruskal–Wallis test, Spearman's rank correlation test, and independence chi-square test. Variables not characterized by normal distribution were described using the median (median value), quartile distribution, and range. Multivariate regression analysis (MANOVA) was conducted to estimate relations between EPCs and clinical or functional condition. The significance level $p < 0.05$ was considered statistically significant.

3. Results

The general characteristics and comparison of the population of the studied patients are presented in Table 1. Patients with hemorrhagic stroke were in a significantly worse functional condition (mRS) on the first day compared to ischemic stroke subjects.

Table 1. Comparison of selected anthropometric, biochemical parameters, risk factors, and clinical status in patients with ischemic stroke, hemorrhagic stroke, and in the control group.

Parameter	Ischemic Stroke	Hemorrhage	Control Group	p-Values
Sex, male, (%) [1]	62.1	55.3	36.4	0.1088
Sex, female, (%) [1]	37.9	44.7	63.6	0.1267
Age (median, range) [3]	69 (45–88)	73.5 (45–91)	63.5 (50–82)	0.1034
Smoking, (%) [1]	32.6	28.9	24.5	0.3457
Hypertension, (%) [1]	90.9	94.7	81.8	0.2555
Hyperlipidemia, (%) [1]	60.6	50	54.5	0.566
Diabetes, (%) [1]	37.9	21.8	27.3	0.186
CRP (mg/L), (median, range) [2]	4.50 (0.39–58.12)	5.79 (0.38–70.1)	-	0.2117
Homocystein (µg/mL) (median, range) [2]	11.05 (3.52–30.92)	9.22 (2.65–42.8)	-	0.6341
Fibrinogen (g/L), (median, range) [2]	284 (59–590)	315.5 (157–463)	-	0.2985
NIHSS 1st day (points) (median, range) [2]	6 (2–21)	6 (1–21)	-	0.6103
NIHSS 8th day (points) (median, range) [2]	3 (0–15)	3 (0–14)	-	0.7086
mRS 1st day (points) (median, range) [2]	4 (2–5)	5 (3–5)	-	0.0001 *
mRS 8th day (points) (median, range) [2]	2 (0–5)	3 (0–4)	-	0.2377

[1] chi square test, [2] Mann–Whitney U test, [3] Kruskal–Wallis test, * statistical significance, CRP, C-reactive protein; NIHSS, National Institute of Health Stroke Scale; mRS, modified Rankin Scale.

There was a significantly higher number of EPCs in the blood on the first day of stroke (regardless of etiology) compared to the control group (respectively, med. 17.75 cells/µL (0–488 cells/µL) vs. 5.24 cells/µL (0–95 cells/µL); $p = 0.0006$). There was a significantly higher number of EPCs in the blood serum on the first day of ischemic stroke compared to the control group (med. 18.65 cells/µL (0–278 cells/µL) vs. 5.24 cells/µL (0–95 cells/µL); $p = 0.0011$) and on the first day of hemorrhagic stroke compared to the control group (med. 17.17 cells/µL (0–488 cells/µL) vs. 5.24 cells/µL (0–95 cells/µL); $p = 0.0034$) (Figure 2).

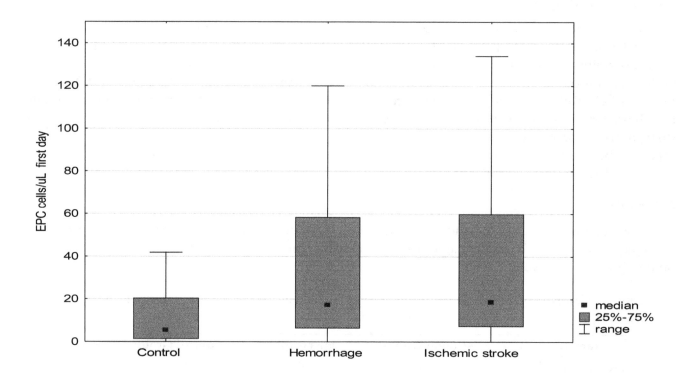

Figure 2. Comparison of the number of endothelial progenitor cells (EPCs) on the first day between the patients with ischemic stroke, hemorrhagic stroke, and the control group.

There were no significant differences in the number of EPCs between patients with ischemic and hemorrhagic stroke both on the first day and on the eighth day of the disease. Prospective analysis did not show significant changes in the number of EPCs in the blood of patients with stroke (regardless of etiology) between the first and eighth day of the disease.

The number of EPCs did not differ significantly in men and women, both in the whole population and in the group with stroke (regardless of etiology) on the first day or in the group with stroke on the eight day of the disease. There were no significant correlations between the age and the number of EPCs on the first day in the whole population (R = 0.0370, $p = 0.6809$), and in patients with hemorrhagic stroke on the first (R = 0.0783, $p = 0.6402$) and eighth day (R = −0.0762, $p = 0.6489$) and ischemic stroke on the first (R = −0.0326, $p = 0.7949$) and eighth day (R = 0.0939, $p = 0.4529$).

There were no significant relationships between the number of EPCs on the first and eighth day after a stroke event with hypertension, hyperlipidemia, smoking, and diabetes in ischemic stroke (Table 2), as well as in hemorrhagic stroke (Table 3).

Table 2. Comparison of the number of endothelial progenitor cells (EPCs) on the first and eighth day of ischemic stroke between patients with present and absent vascular risk factors.

Parameter	EPCs/μL 1st Day			EPCs/μL 8th Day		
	Present	Absent	p-Values *	Present	Absent	p-Values *
Hypertension	17.14 (0–278.11)	23.24 (2.77–112.21)	0.8847	24.45 (0.46–316.89)	62.47 (18–323.29)	0.0536
Hyperlipidemia	14.69 (0–178.86)	25.55 (4.12–278.11)	0.1785	25.02 (0.40–316.89)	25.72 (2.03–323.29)	0.4724
Diabetes	14.47 (0–178.86)	25.12 (1.01–278.11)	0.0701	31.16 (0.40–323.29)	24.51 (0.46–316.89)	0.7014
Smoking	16.32 (0–178.86)	22.13 (2.77–112.21)	0.1654	27.85 (0.40–323.29)	31.69 (2.03–323.29)	0.1324

* Mann–Whitney U test. Results are median (range) in cells/μL.

Table 3. Comparison of the number of endothelial progenitor cells (EPCs) on the first and eighth day of hemorrhagic stroke between patients with present and absent vascular risk factors.

Parameter	EPCs/μL 1st Day			EPCs/μL 8th Day		
	Present	Absent	p-Values *	Present	Absent	p-Values *
Hypertension	17.75 (0–488.41)	4.43 (3.75–5.11)	0.0722	17.93 (0–325.43)	22.44 (0.10–44.78)	0.4522
Hyperlipidemia	31.23 (0.62–338.00)	15.51 (0–488.41)	0,7042	37.62 (1.21–325.43)	11.64 (0–233.20)	0.1443
Diabetes	17.48 (6.36–58.38)	16.47 (0–488.41)	0.7608	17.15 (3.01–10020)	17.93 (0–325.43)	0.7608
Smoking	25.67 (0.62–338.00)	21.98 (0–488.41)	0.6983	23.68 (1.21–325.43)	17.44 (0.10–233.20)	0.6684

* Mann–Whitney U test Results are median (range) in cells/uL.

There were no significant correlations between EPCs on the first and eighth day after a stroke event with the selected biochemical parameters, both in ischemic and hemorrhagic stroke (Table 4).

Table 4. Correlations between the number of endothelial progenitor cells (EPCs) on the first and eighth day of ischemic and hemorrhagic stroke and the selected biochemical parameters.

	EPCs/μL 1st Day				EPCs/μL 8th Day			
	Ischemic Stroke		Hemorrhage		Ischemic Stroke		Hemorrhage	
	R	p	R	p	R	p	R	p
CRP	0.1630	0.1909	−0.0242	0.8854	0.0986	0.4308	−0.1526	0.3602
fibrinogen	−0.1731	0.1644	0.1135	0.4974	0.1095	0.3816	−0.0459	0.7840
homocystein	−0.0879	0.4827	0.0578	0.7309	−0.0376	0.7639	0.2465	0.1356

Spearman's rank correlation, CRP, C-reactive protein, R, correlation coefficient.

There were no significant correlations between the number of EPCs on the first day of stroke (regardless of etiology) and the clinical condition (NIHSS scale) on the first day ($R = 0.0128; p = 0.8790$) and on the eighth day ($R = 0.1300; p = 0.1882$), as well as between the number of EPCs on the eighth day of stroke and the clinical condition on the first day ($R = 0.1846; p = 0.0607$) and on the eighth day ($R = 0.1243; p = 0.2085$). There were no significant relationships between the number of EPCs on the first day of stroke (regardless of etiology) and the functional condition (mRS scale) on the first day ($R = 0.0318; p = 0.7480$), and on the eighth day ($R = -0.1239; p = 0.2099$), as well as between the number of EPCs on the eighth day of stroke and the functional condition on the first day ($R = 0.0049; p = 0.9606$) and on the eighth day ($R = 0.0672; p = 0.4973$). Considering the etiology of stroke, there were no significant correlations between the number of EPCs on the first and eighth day of the disease and the clinical or functional condition, both in ischemic and hemorrhagic stroke (Table 5).

Table 5. Correlations between the number of endothelial progenitor cells (EPCs) on the first and eighth day of ischemic and hemorrhagic stroke and the clinical and functional status on the first and eighth day of stroke.

	EPCs/µL 1st Day				EPCs/µL 8th Day			
	Ischemic Stroke		Hemorrhagic Stroke		Ischemic Stroke		Hemorrhagic Stroke	
	R	p	R	p	R	p	R	p
NIHSS 1st day	−0.0469	0.7084	0.0932	0.5778	0.1842	0.1387	0.2108	0.2038
NIHSS 8th day	−0.1469	0.2388	−0.0888	0.5959	0.1446	0.2465	0.0857	0.6085
mRS 1st day	0.1359	0.2765	−0.1228	0.4624	0.0230	0.8544	0.0837	0.6171
mRS 8th day	−0.1355	0.2766	0.1300	0.1882	0.0858	0.4933	0.0648	

Spearman's rank correlation, NIHSS, National Institute of Health Stroke Scale, mRS, modified Rankin Scale. R, correlation coefficient.

There were no significant differences between patients with severe and mild neurological deficit on the first day of stroke in relation to the number of EPCs on the first day (total $p = 0.4802$; ischemic stroke $p = 0.7837$; hemorrhagic stroke $p = 0.4166$) and on the eighth day (total $p = 0.1794$; ischemic stroke $p = 0.2969$; hemorrhagic stroke $p = 0.4457$). Similarly, there were no significant differences between patients with severe and mild neurological deficit on the eighth day of stroke in relation to the number of EPCs on the first day (total $p = 0.4545$; ischemic stroke $p = 0.3248$; hemorrhagic stroke $p = 0.9568$) and on the eighth day (total $p = 0.6479$; ischemic stroke $p = 0.2069$; hemorrhagic stroke $p = 0.5335$). There were no significant differences between patients with favorable and unfavorable prognosis on the first day of stroke in relation to the number of EPCs on the first day (total $p = 0.9383$; ischemic stroke $p = 0.8786$; hemorrhagic stroke $p = 0.8903$) and on the eighth day (total $p = 0.9072$; ischemic stroke $p = 0.9264$; hemorrhagic stroke $p = 0.9278$). Similarly, there were no significant differences between patients with a favorable and unfavorable prognosis on the eighth day of stroke in relation to the number of EPCs on the first day (total $p = 0.1470$; ischemic stroke $p = 0.2369$; hemorrhagic stroke $p = 0.4559$) and on the eighth day (total $p = 0.6969$; ischemic stroke $p = 0.9485$; hemorrhagic stroke $p = 0.4559$).

In the multivariate model of regression adjusted for sex, type of stroke, and clinical or functional condition, we demonstrated that in females, a higher number of EPCs on the first day of stroke is related to a favorable outcome on the eighth day after the stroke onset compared to males ($p = 0.0355$) (Figure 3). There were no significant correlations regarding the other analyzed dependencies.

There was a negative but significant correlation between the volume of hemorrhagic focus on the first day of hemorrhage and the number of EPCs on the first day of hemorrhagic stroke (R = −0.3378, $p = 0.0471$) (Figure 4).

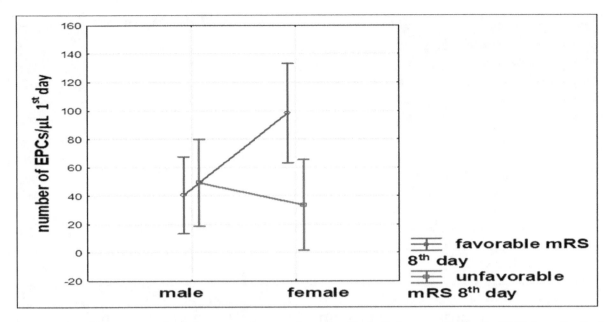

Figure 3. Multivariate analysis between the number of endothelial progenitor cells (EPCs) on the first day of stroke, sex, and functional outcome on the eighth day in the modified Rankin scale (mRS).

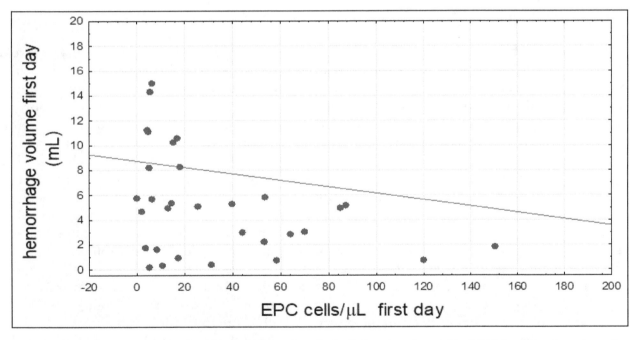

Figure 4. Correlation between the number of endothelial progenitor cells (EPCs) on the first day of hemorrhagic stroke and the volume of hemorrhagic focus on the first day of stroke.

There were no significant correlations between the number of EPCs on the eighth day of hemorrhagic stroke with the volume of hemorrhagic focus on the first day ($R = -0.0791$, $p = 0.6513$) and on the eighth day ($R = -0.0002$, $p = 0.9897$), as well as between the number of EPCs on the first day and the volume of hemorrhagic focus on the eighth day ($R = -0.1294$, $p = 0.4803$). A negative correlation between the number of EPCs on the first day of hemorrhagic stroke and the degree of regression of the hemorrhagic focus was demonstrated ($R = -0.3896$, $p = 0.0367$) (Figure 5).

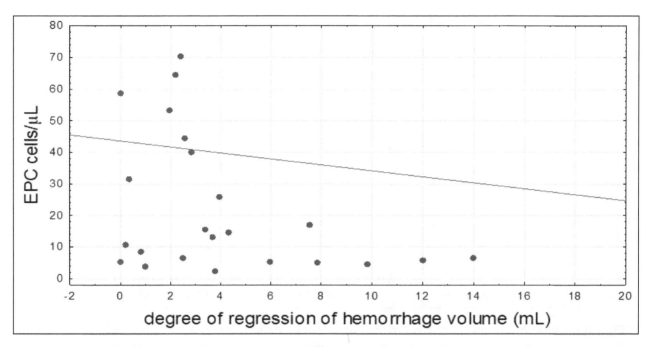

Figure 5. Correlation between the number of endothelial progenitor cells (EPCs) on the first day of hemorrhagic stroke and the degree of regression of the hemorrhagic focus.

4. Discussion

The results of this study showed that, in the acute phase of ischemic and hemorrhagic stroke, a significantly higher number of EPCs were observed than in the control group. This confirms that damage to the cerebral endothelium, whether in the course of acute ischemia or mechanical damage to the vascular wall, leads to significant mobilization and proliferation of EPCs. This is probably the mechanism of differentiation into mature endothelial cells, which, due to the production of numerous cytokines, are actively involved in the repair and neovascularization of damaged brain tissues [7]. Similar conclusions were drawn by Yip et al., Meamar et al., and Regueiro et al. [20–22], who, assessing patients in the acute phase of ischemic stroke, also found a significantly higher number of EPCs than in control. Similarly, Paczkowska et al. [23] obtained a higher number of EPCs in the acute stage of hemorrhagic stroke in comparison to the control group. The results of our research and the above show that regardless of the etiology, it is the state of sudden damage to vascular endothelium (similar to acute myocardial infarction and acute limb ischemia) that clearly activates EPCs' proliferation, where EPCs are the main repair and regenerative element of the damaged endothelial cells [24,25]. It is worth noting that Ghani et al. and Deng Y et al. [26,27] in their studies obtained different results and a lower number of EPCs in the acute phase of ischemic stroke than those in the control group, and Zhou et al. [28] noted a lower number of EPCs in patients with both acute ischemic and hemorrhagic stroke, compared to the control group. The differences in the results of the above studies could have resulted from a different population of patients and a different configuration of superficial antigens used in flow cytometry to detect EPCs.

The data in the literature show that, in acute cerebrovascular incidents, EPCs are activated within the first 24 h, reach their maximum blood level around the 7th day, and gradually decrease after 21–28 days. Most authors assessed only patients with ischemic stroke [27,29,30] and only a few assessed patients with either ischemic or hemorrhagic stroke [28]. Taguchi et al. and Marti-Fabregas et al. [29,30] showed statistically significantly more EPCs after 7 days of acute ischemic stroke than during the first 24 h. Zhou et al. [28] also obtained similar results but in both ischemic and hemorrhagic stroke. In this work, although in both types of stroke the number of cells was higher on the eighth day of the disease than on the first day, these differences did not reach statistical significance. Nevertheless, the results of this study confirmed that mobilization of EPCs occurs within a few hours after the onset of symptoms of stroke; within 24 h, the number of EPCs in the blood serum reaches a very high level, and the state of high activation persists for at least the first week of the disease. Due to the fact that the area of interest was the acute phase of cerebrovascular incidents, the number of EPCs on day 21–28 was not assessed. In addition, in this study, the number of EPCs did not differ significantly in patients with ischemic and hemorrhagic stroke (similar results were presented by Zhou et al.), both on the first and on the eighth day, which suggests that acute brain endothelial damage, and not its etiopathogenesis, plays a leading role in the activation of EPCs.

In this research, no significant correlations were found between the number of EPCs and the selected biochemical parameters of blood (CRP, homocysteine, fibrinogen), as well as risk factors of vascular diseases, which suggests their potential lack of influence on the number of activated EPCs. It is suggested that the above factors may affect the chronic number of EPCs in the blood, without affecting their mobilization and activation capacity in acute endothelial damage, such as in stroke.

In the present study, it was not shown that the number of EPCs in the acute phase of stroke significantly affected the clinical and functional status of the patients or was associated with early prognosis. There were no significant correlations between the number of EPCs on the first and eighth day of the stroke and the score on the mRS or NIHSS scale on the first and eighth day, both in ischemic and hemorrhagic stroke. In addition, the division of patients into groups with a favorable and unfavorable prognosis and with a mild and severe neurological deficit did not differentiate both types of strokes based on the number of EPCs. Zhou et al. also did not demonstrate the effect of the number of EPCs on the clinical state and prognosis of patients (both in ischemic and hemorrhagic stroke) and Marti-Fabregas et al. did not find a significant correlation in ischemic stroke [28,30]. In contrast, Sobrino et al. [31] noted that a large number of EPCs on the seventh day of ischemic stroke is associated with a better clinical condition, expressed by a lower score of the NIHSS scale. However, it should be noted that they were only evaluating patients with non-lacunar stroke, while the analysis of this work is related only to patients with lacunar stroke. On the other hand, Yip et al. [20] noted that a small number of EPCs on the second day of ischemic stroke is associated with a worse clinical deficit, expressed by a higher score on the NIHSS scale. However, they took into account all patients with ischemic stroke, regardless of the etiopathogenesis, i.e., both patients with lacunar and non-lacunar strokes. Pias-Peleteiro et al. [32] analyzed the relationships between the number of EPCs and the functional condition and prognosis in patients with hemorrhagic stroke and showed that a higher number of EPCs on the seventh day is associated with a better distant prognosis expressed by a small number of points on the mRS scale on the 12th month from the hemorrhage. Conversely, Sobrino et al. [33] noted that a large number of EPCs on the seventh day of hemorrhagic stroke is associated with a better prognosis and functional state of patients in the third month from the hemorrhage, also expressed by lower scores on the mRS scale. Nevertheless, ambiguous and often contradictory results of studies on the impact of EPCs on the prognosis of stroke patients suggest further research in this subject.

Multivariate analysis showed that the relation between the number of EPCs and functional condition may depend on the sex. In females, a higher number of EPCs is related with a favorable functional status. This preliminary finding reported in this study underlines the potential impact of sex hormones for a possible role of EPCs in stroke prognosis. More research is required to improve these initial findings.

The results of this study showed that a large number of EPCs on the first day of hemorrhagic stroke is associated with a smaller volume of the hemorrhagic focus. Zhou et al. [26] also analyzed similar relationships but found no significant association between the number of EPCs in the acute stage of hemorrhagic stroke and the volume of the hemorrhagic focus. In contrast, Pias-Peleteiro et al. and Sobrino et al. [32,33] showed a similar significant negative correlation between the number of EPCs on the seventh day of hemorrhagic stroke and the volume of the residual hemorrhagic focus, respectively, on the third and sixth month after the hemorrhage. Other authors analyzed the volume of the ischemic focus and showed that a large number of EPCs in the acute phase of ischemic stroke is associated with a relatively smaller volume of the ischemic focus in the diffusion sequence (DWI) [31,34]. In the present study, the relationship between the number of EPCs and the volume of the ischemic focus was not analyzed.

To our best knowledge, this is the first study analyzing the relationship between the number of EPCs and the degree of regression of the hemorrhagic focus. The significant negative correlation obtained in this research is a novelty in this field and is in contradiction to the well-known repair and regenerative function of EPCs suggested by most authors. Subjects with a higher number of EPCs on the first day presented with the lowest regression level of the hematoma volume. The results reported in this study may shed new light on the role of EPCs in hemorrhagic stroke and significantly undermine and raise doubt to their repair properties. Most of the recent pre-clinical studies in animal models demonstrated a protective and regenerative function of EPCs after cerebrovascular insult [12,35–38]. Several mechanisms of possible action were reported, especially by suppressing oxidative stress, apoptosis, mitochondrial impairment, and inflammation processes [35–37]. The essential role of EPCs in increasing brain angiogenesis has been highlighted in animal models of stroke [12,38]. However, the lack of references in the literature and the small number of patients with hemorrhagic stroke in this study suggest that verification of the obtained data and further research in this area in multi-center randomized trials is needed.

This study has its limitations. The effect of the number of EPCs on the distant prognosis in patients with stroke was not analyzed. The moderate number of patients and small control group is also a limitation. However, these numbers seemed sufficient to draw conclusions. Conversely, for formal reasons (conscious consent for the study for the bioethics committee), the analysis did not include patients with a severe neurological deficit, e.g., patients with consciousness disorders, so the study did not include the actual cross-section of patients with stroke but only patients with a milder clinical condition. Determination of EPCs by only one measurement at different times within the first 24 h of stroke is also a main limitation and could have a great impact on the results. The authors are aware that for the dynamic changes in the function and number of EPCs under ischemic or inflammatory conditions, the use of microbeads and Q-dot-based nanoparticles is superior to conventional flow cytometry. Most statistical analyses were univariate, which could have reduced the reliability of the results.

5. Conclusions

The study showed that endothelial progenitor cells are an early marker of cerebral vascular damage, both in ischemic and hemorrhagic stroke. The research highlights, for the first time, a negative correlation between the level of EPCs and the degree of regression of a hemorrhagic focus and that this relation between the number of EPCs and functional condition may depend on the sex. However, the prognostic value of EPCs for the clinical condition and early prognosis of stroke patients remains doubtful.

Author Contributions: Conceptualization, A.W.; methodology, A.W., G.K., J.B., K.Z.; software, J.B., K.Z. validation, G.K., D.R.; formal Analysis, A.W., K.F., and G.K.; investigation, A.W.; resources, D.R., Z.S.; data curation, J.B., A.L.; writing—original draft preparation, A.W. and K.F.; writing—review and editing, A.W.; visualization, A.W.; supervision, G.K., D.R., R.Ś.; project administration, A.W. and G.K. All authors have read and agreed to the published version of the manuscript.

References

1.   Naghavi, M.; Wang, H.; Lozano, R.; Davis, A.; Liang, X.; Zhou, M.; Vollset, S.E.; Ozgoren, A.A.; Abdalla, S.; Abd-Allah, F.; et al. Global, regional, and national age-sex specific all-cause and cause-specific mortality for 240 causes of death, 1990-2013: A systematic analysis for the Global Burden of Disease Study 2013. *Lancet* **2015**, *385*, 117–171.

2.   Mozaffarian, D.; Benjamin, E.J.; Go, A.S.; Arnett, D.K.; Blaha, M.J.; Cushman, M.; de Ferranti, S.; Despres, J.P.; Fullerton, H.J.; Howard, W.J.; et al. Heart disease and stroke statistics—2015 update: A report from the American Heart Association. *Circulation* **2015**, *131*, 434–441. [CrossRef]

3.   Giwa, M.O.; Williams, J.; Elderfield, K.; Jiwa, N.S.; Bridges, L.R.; Kalaria, R.N.; Markus, H.S.; Esiri, M.M.; Hainsworth, A.H. Neuropathologic evidence of endothelial changes in cerebral small vessel disease. *Neurology* **2011**, *78*, 167–174. [CrossRef] [PubMed]

4.   Grysiewicz, R.A.; Thomas, K.; Pandey, D.K. Epidemiology of Ischemic and Hemorrhagic Stroke: Incidence, Prevalence, Mortality, and Risk Factors. *Neurol. Clin.* **2008**, *26*, 871–895. [CrossRef]

5.   Li, Y.-F.; Ren, L.-N.; Guo, G.; Cannella, L.A.; Chernaya, V.; Samuel, S.; Liu, S.-X.; Wang, H.; Yang, X. Endothelial progenitor cells in ischemic stroke: An exploration from hypothesis to therapy. *J. Hematol. Oncol.* **2015**, *8*, 33. [CrossRef]

6.   Du, F.; Zhou, J.; Gong, R.; Huang, X.; Pansuria, M.; Virtue, A.; Li, X.; Wang, H.; Yang, X.F. Endothelial progenitor cells in atherosclerosis. *Front. Biosci.* **2012**, *17*, 2327–2349. [CrossRef] [PubMed]

7.   Chu, K.; Jung, K.-H.; Lee, S.-T.; Park, H.-K.; Sinn, D.-I.; Kim, J.-M.; Kim, N.-H.; Kim, J.-H.; Kim, S.-J.; Song, E.-C.; et al. Circulating endothelial progenitor cells as a new marker of endothelial dysfunction or repair in acute stroke. *Stroke* **2008**, *39*, 1441–1447. [CrossRef]

8.   Gutiérrez-Fernández, M.; Otero-Ortega, L.; Ramos-Cejudo, J.; Rodríguez-Frutos, B.; Fuentes, B.; Tejedor, E.D. Adipose tissue-derived mesenchymal stem cells as a strategy to improve recovery after stroke. *Expert Opin. Boil. Ther.* **2015**, *15*, 873–881. [CrossRef]

9.   Moubarik, C.; Guillet, B.; Youssef, B.; Codaccioni, J.L.; Pierchecci, M.D.; Sebatier, F.; Lionel, P.; Dou, L.; Foucault-Bertaud, A.; Velly, L.; et al. Transplanted late outgrowth endothelial progenitor cells as cel therapy product for stroke. *Stem Cell Rev.* **2011**, *7*, 208–220. [CrossRef]

10.   Nakamura, K.; Tsurushima, H.; Marushima, A.; Nagano, M.; Yamashita, T.; Suzuki, K.; Ohneda, O.; Matsumura, A. A subpopulation of endothelial progenitor cells with low aldehyde dehydrogenase activity attenuates acute ischemic brain injury in rats. *Biochem. Biophys. Res. Commun.* **2012**, *418*, 87–92. [CrossRef]

11.   Fan, Y.; Shen, F.; Frenzel, T.; Zhu, W.; Ye, J.; Liu, J.; Chen, Y.; Su, H.; Young, W.L.; Yang, G.-Y. Endothelial progenitor cell transplantation improves long-term stroke outcome in mice. *Ann. Neurol.* **2009**, *67*, 488–497. [CrossRef] [PubMed]

12.   Rosell, A.; Morancho, A.; Navarro-Sobrino, M.; Martinez-Saez, E.; Guillamon, M.M.H.; Lope-Piedrafita, S.; Barceló, V.; Borrás, F.; Penalba, A.; Garcia-Bonilla, L.; et al. Factors Secreted by Endothelial Progenitor Cells Enhance Neurorepair Responses after Cerebral Ischemia in Mice. *PLoS ONE* **2013**, *8*, e73244. [CrossRef] [PubMed]

13.   Liao, S.; Luo, C.; Cao, B.; Hu, H.; Wang, S.; Yue, H.; Chen, L.; Zhou, Z. Endothelial Progenitor Cells for Ischemic Stroke: Update on Basic Research and Application. *Stem Cells Int.* **2017**, *2017*. [CrossRef] [PubMed]

14.   Sacco, R.L.; Kasner, S.E.; Broderick, J.P.; Caplan, L.R.; Connors, J.J.; Culebras, A.; Elkind, M.S.; George, M.G.; Hamdan, A.D.; Higashida, R.T.; et al. An updated definition of stroke for the 21st century: A statement for healthcare professionals from the American Heart Association/American Stroke Association. *Stroke* **2013**, *44*, 2064–2089. [CrossRef]

15.   Wardlaw, J.M.; Smith, E.E.; Biessels, G.J.; Cordonnier, C.; Fazekas, F.; Frayne, R.; Lindley, R.I.; O'Brien, J.; Barkhof, F.; Benavente, O.R.; et al. Neuroimaging standards for research into small vessel disease and its contribution to ageing and neurodegeneration. *Lancet Neurol.* **2013**, *12*, 822–838. [CrossRef]

16.   Mancuso, P.; Antoniotti, P.; Quarna, J.; Calleri, A.; Rabascio, C.; Tacchetti, C.; Braidotti, P.; Wu, H.-K.; Zurita, A.J.; Saronni, L.; et al. Validation of a Standardized Method for Enumerating Circulating Endothelial Cells and Progenitors: Flow Cytometry and Molecular and Ultrastructural Analyses. *Clin. Cancer Res.* **2009**, *15*, 267–273. [CrossRef]

17.   Ruszkowska-Ciastek, B.; Sokup, A.; Leszcz, M.; Drela, E.; Stankowska, K.; Boinska, J.; Haor, B.; Ślusarz, R.; Lisewska, B.; Gadomska, G.; et al. The number of circulating endothelial progenitor cells in healthy individuals—Effect of some anthropometric and environmental factors (a pilot study). *Adv. Med. Sci.* **2015**, *60*, 58–63. [CrossRef]

18.   Lyden, P. Using the National Institutes of Health Stroke Scale. *Stroke* **2017**, *48*, 513–519. [CrossRef]

19.   Quinn, T.J.; Dawson, J.; Walters, M.R.; Lees, K.R. Variability in modified Rankin scoring across a large cohort of international observers. *Stroke* **2008**, *39*, 2975–2979. [CrossRef]

20. Yip, H.-K.; Chang, L.-T.; Chang, W.-N.; Lu, C.-H.; Liou, C.-W.; Lan, M.-Y.; Liu, J.S.; Youssef, A.A.; Chang, H.-W. Level and Value of Circulating Endothelial Progenitor Cells in Patients After Acute Ischemic Stroke. *Stroke* **2008**, *39*, 69–74. [CrossRef] [PubMed]

21. Meamar, R.; Nikyar, H.; Dehghani, L.; Talebi, M.; Dehghani, M.; Ghasemi, M.; Ansari, B.; Saadatnia, M. The role of endothelial progenitor cells in transient ischemic attack patients for future cerebrovascular events. *J. Res. Med. Sci.* **2016**, *21*, 47. [CrossRef] [PubMed]

22. Regueiro, A.; Cuadrado-Godia, E.; Bueno-Betí, C.; Diaz-Ricart, M.; Oliveras, A.; Novella, S.; Gené, G.G.; Jung, C.; Subirana, I.; Ortiz-Pérez, J.T.; et al. Mobilization of endothelial progenitor cells in acute cardiovascular events in the PROCELL study: Time-course after acute myocardial infarction and stroke. *J. Mol. Cell. Cardiol.* **2015**, *80*, 146–155. [CrossRef]

23. Paczkowska, E.; Gołąb-Janowska, M.; Bajer-Czajkowska, A.; Machalinska, A.; Ustianowski, P.; Rybicka, M.; Kłos, P.; Dziedziejko, V.; Safranow, K.; Nowacki, P.; et al. Increased circulating endothelial progenitor cells in patients with haemorrhagic and ischaemic stroke: The role of Endothelin-1. *J. Neurol. Sci.* **2013**, *325*, 90–99. [CrossRef]

24. Leone, A.M.; Rutella, S.; Bonanno, G.; Abbate, A.; Rebuzzi, A.G.; Giovannini, S.; Lombardi, M.; Galiuto, L.; Liuzzo, G.; Andreotti, F.; et al. Mobilization of bone marrow-derived stem cells after myocardial infarction and left ventricular function. *Eur. Hear. J.* **2005**, *26*, 1196–1204. [CrossRef]

25. Roberts, N.; Jahangiri, M.; Xu, Q. Progenitor cells in vascular disease. *J. Cell. Mol. Med.* **2005**, *9*, 583–591. [CrossRef]

26. Ghani, U.; Shuaib, A.; Salam, A.; Nasir, A.; Shuaib, U.; Jeerakathil, T.; Sher, F.; O'Rourke, F.; Nasser, A.M.; Schwindt, B.; et al. Endothelial Progenitor Cells During Cerebrovascular Disease. *Stroke* **2005**, *36*, 151–153. [CrossRef] [PubMed]

27. Deng, Y.; Wang, J.; He, G.; Qu, F.; Zheng, M. Mobilization of endothelial progenitor cell in patients with acute ischemic stroke. *Neurol. Sci.* **2017**, *39*, 437–443. [CrossRef] [PubMed]

28. Zhou, W.-J.; Zhu, D.-L.; Yang, G.-Y.; Zhang, Y.; Wang, H.-Y.; Ji, K.-D.; Lu, Y.-M.; Gao, P.-J.; Zhou, D.-L.Z.W.-J. Circulating endothelial progenitor cells in Chinese patients with acute stroke. *Hypertens. Res.* **2009**, *32*, 306–310. [CrossRef] [PubMed]

29. Taguchi, A.; Matsuyama, T.; Moriwaki, H.; Hayashi, T.; Hayashida, K.; Nagatsuka, K.; Todo, K.; Mori, K.; Stern, D.M.; Soma, T.; et al. Circulating CD34-Positive Cells Provide an Index of Cerebrovascular Function. *Circulation* **2004**, *109*, 2972–2975. [CrossRef] [PubMed]

30. Martí-Fàbregas, J.; Crespo, J.; Delgado-Mederos, R.; Martínez-Ramírez, S.; Peña, E.; Marín, R.; Dinia, L.; Jiménez-Xarrié, E.; Fernández-Arcos, A.; Pérez-Pérez, J.; et al. Endothelial progenitor cells in acute ischemic stroke. *Brain Behav.* **2013**, *3*, 649–655. [CrossRef] [PubMed]

31. Sobrino, T.; Hurtado, O.; Moro, M.A.; Rodríguez-Yáñez, M.; Castellanos, M.; Brea, D.; Moldes, O.; Blanco, M.; Arenillas, J.F.; Leira, R.; et al. The increase of circulating endothelial progenitor cells after acute ischemic stroke is associated with good outcome. *Stroke* **2007**, *38*, 2759–2764. [CrossRef] [PubMed]

32. Pías-Peleteiro, J.; Pérez-Mato, M.; López-Arias, E.; Rodríguez-Yáñez, M.; Blanco, M.; Campos, F.; Castillo, J.; Sobrino, T. Increased Endothelial Progenitor Cell Levels are Associated with Good Outcome in Intracerebral Hemorrhage. *Sci. Rep.* **2016**, *6*, 28724. [CrossRef]

33. Sobrino, T.; Arias, S.; Pérez-Mato, M.; Agulla, J.; Brea, D.; Rodríguez-Yáñez, M.; Castillo, J. Cd34+progenitor cells likely are involved in the good functional recovery after intracerebral hemorrhage in humans. *J. Neurosci. Res.* **2011**, *89*, 979–985. [CrossRef] [PubMed]

34. Bogoslovsky, T.; Chaudhry, A.; Latour, L.; Maric, D.; Luby, M.; Spatz, M.; Frank, J.; Warach, S. Endothelial progenitor cells correlate with lesion volume and growth in acute stroke. *Neurology* **2010**, *75*, 2059–2062. [CrossRef]

35. Park, D.-H.; Eve, D.J.; Musso, J.; Klasko, S.K.; Cruz, E.; Borlongan, C.V.; Sanberg, P.R. Inflammation and Stem Cell Migration to the Injured Brain in Higher Organisms. *Stem Cells Dev.* **2009**, *18*, 693–702. [CrossRef] [PubMed]

36. Tajiri, N.; Duncan, K.; Antoine, A.; Pabon, M.; Acosta, S.A.; De La Peña, I.C.; Hernadez-Ontiveros, D.G.; Shinozuka, K.; Ishikawa, H.; Kaneko, Y.; et al. Stem cell-paved biobridge facilitates neural repair in traumatic brain injury. *Front. Syst. Neurosci.* **2014**, *8*, 116. [CrossRef]

37. Chen, J.; Chopp, M. Neurorestorative treatment of stroke: Cell and pharmacological approaches. *NeuroRX* **2006**, *3*, 466–473. [CrossRef]

38. Morancho, A.; Ma, F.; Barcelo, V.; Giralt, D.; Montaner, J.; Rosell, A. Impaired vascular remodeling after endothelial progenitor cell transplantation in MMP9-deficient mice suffering cortical cerebral ischemia. *J. Cereb. Blood Flow Metab.* **2015**, *35*, 1547–1551. [CrossRef]

17

Timing of Transfusion, not Hemoglobin Variability, is Associated with 3-Month Outcomes in Acute Ischemic Stroke

Chulho Kim [1,2,*], Sang-Hwa Lee [1], Jae-Sung Lim [3], Mi Sun Oh [3], Kyung-Ho Yu [3], Yerim Kim [4], Ju-Hun Lee [4], Min Uk Jang [5], San Jung [6] and Byung-Chul Lee [3,*]

[1] Department of Neurology, Chuncheon Sacred Heart Hospital, Chuncheon 24253, Korea; neurolsh@hallym.or.kr
[2] Chuncheon Translational Research Center, Hallym University College of Medicine, Chuncheon 24252, Korea
[3] Department of Neurology, Hallym University Sacred Heart Hospital, Anyang 14068, Korea; jaesunglim@hallym.or.kr (J.-S.L.); iyyar@hallym.or.kr (M.S.O.); ykh1030@hallym.or.kr (K.-H.Y.)
[4] Department of Neurology, Kangdong Sacred Heart Hospital, Seoul 05355, Korea; brainyrk@kdh.or.kr (Y.K.); leejuhun@kdh.or.kr (J.-H.L.)
[5] Department of Neurology, Dongtan Sacred Heart Hospital, Hwaseong 18450, Korea; mujang@hallym.or.kr
[6] Department of Neurology, Kangnam Sacred Heart Hospital, Seoul 07440, Korea; neurojs@hallym.or.kr
* Correspondence: gumdol52@hallym.or.kr (C.K.); ssbrain@hallym.ac.kr (B.-C.L.);

Abstract: Objectives: This study aimed to investigate whether transfusions and hemoglobin variability affects the outcome of stroke after an acute ischemic stroke (AIS). Methods: We studied consecutive patients with AIS admitted in three tertiary hospitals who received red blood cell (RBC) transfusion (RBCT) during admission. Hemoglobin variability was assessed by minimum, maximum, range, median absolute deviation, and mean absolute change in hemoglobin level. Timing of RBCT was grouped into two categories: admission to 48 h (early) or more than 48 h (late) after hospitalization. Late RBCT was entered into multivariable logistic regression model. Poor outcome at three months was defined as a modified Rankin Scale score ≥3. Results: Of 2698 patients, 132 patients (4.9%) received a median of 400 mL (interquartile range: 400–840 mL) of packed RBCs. One-hundred-and-two patients (77.3%) had poor outcomes. The most common cause of RBCT was gastrointestinal bleeding (27.3%). The type of anemia was not associated with the timing of RBCT. Late RBCT was associated with poor outcome (odd ratio (OR), 3.55; 95% confidence interval (CI), 1.43–8.79; p-value = 0.006) in the univariable model. After adjusting for age, sex, Charlson comorbidity index, and stroke severity, late RBCT was a significant predictor (OR, 3.37; 95% CI, 1.14–9.99; p-value = 0.028) of poor outcome at three months. In the area under the receiver operating characteristics curve comparison, addition of hemoglobin variability indices did not improve the performance of the multivariable logistic model. Conclusion: Late RBCT, rather than hemoglobin variability indices, is a predictor for poor outcome in patients with AIS.

Keywords: anemia; cerebral infarction; blood transfusion; red blood cells; outcome assessment

1. Introduction

Anemia is an independent predictor for mortality and cardiovascular disease in the general population [1]. The incidence of anemia in acute ischemic stroke (AIS) is 20–30%, and both extreme of admission hemoglobin has a U-shaped association with poor clinical outcomes [1,2]. Cerebral autoregulation enables the brain to maintain sufficient oxygenation in the blood when the cerebral perfusion pressure decreases [3]. However, this autoregulatory response to brain ischemia is already impaired in ischemic penumbra. Thus, anemia can have harmful effects on infarct growth or poor outcome [4,5].

As the erythropoietin trial has failed to validate the efficacy of outcomes in patients with AIS [6], red blood cell transfusion (RBCT) is the only way to normalize hemoglobin in patients with anemia. However, RBCT is associated with increased blood viscosity and a proinflammatory/prothrombotic state related with stored RBC and its additives [7,8]. The impact of hemoglobin status and RBCT on acute ischemic stroke is controversial [1]. In several studies, low hemoglobin status was associated with poor outcomes in patients with AIS; however, these studies focused on admission hemoglobin level and did not assess whether RBCT was performed during the admission [1]. There are several reports on the association between RBCT and AIS outcome. Moman et al. have reported that RBCT is associated with a longer hospital stay in patients with AIS with no difference in mortality [9]. They used propensity score matching to evaluate the impact of transfusion; however, they did not assess the hemoglobin status in all participants. Kellert et al. studied the association between RBCT and mortality and 3-month outcomes in patients with AIS admitted to a neurologic intensive care unit [10]. They reported that RBCT was not associated with mortality or 3-month outcomes. Further, they did not show variation in hemoglobin levels based on RBCT. In addition, one systematic review has suggested that anemia increases the mortality rate in patients with acute stroke; however, the association between RBCT and change in hemoglobin level were not evaluated [1]. Optimal hemoglobin management in acute stroke care should not only consider admission hemoglobin levels, but also the change in hemoglobin levels and RBCT during the hospitalization. Therefore, our aim is to assess the effect of type of anemia, timing of RBCT, and hemoglobin variability index during admission on the 3-month outcomes in patients with AIS, who received RBCT.

2. Material and Methods

2.1. Study Population

This retrospective observational study included prospectively collected stroke registry patients. Three tertiary teaching hospitals, part of the Clinical Research Center to Stroke—5 database and all laboratory data and clinical outcomes were prospectively collected, and central queries were revised bimonthly [11]. This study was approved by the Hallym University Hospital IRB (No. 2017-43), and an informed consent for registry enrollment and prospective outcome capture was given by all participants or next of kin. Our stroke registry included information of consecutive patients admitted within 7 days of the onset of stroke symptom. We screened patients diagnosed with AIS between January 2015 and December 2017. AIS was diagnosed if focal neurologic deficits persisted for more than 24 h and relevant lesions were confirmed by diffusion MRI. Patients without prospective outcome capture or relevant laboratory and clinical variables were excluded from this study.

2.2. Data Collection

The prospective registry data contained only admission hemoglobin level; therefore, all sequential hemoglobin levels during the hospital admission were extracted using the clinical data warehouse. The hemoglobin level was monitored according to the 2013 American Heart Association/American Stroke Association guideline. We used hemoglobin variability index as minimum, maximum, range (maximum-minimum), standard deviation (SD), coefficient of variance (CoV), median absolute deviation (MAD), and mean absolute change (MAC). Of these variability indices, MAC reflects a more temporal variation of the parameter than other variability indices [12]. Anemia was defined as a hemoglobin level of <13.0 g/dL for men and <12.0 g/dL for women according to World Health Organization criteria.

Whether the patient received RBCT was validated by filtering of the clinical data warehouse and retrospective chart review. We did not assess the administration of other blood products such as platelet concentrate or fresh frozen plasma. The criteria for determining the RBCT might vary from case to case, but they are commonly performed when hemoglobin falls below 8 g/dL. The timing of RBCT was divided into two categories—admission to 48 h (early) and >48 h after admission (late) [13]. The reason for RBCT was classified into five categories—gastrointestinal (GI) bleeding, cancer-related anemia, iron-deficiency anemia (IDA)/anemia of chronic disorder (ACD), surgery/procedure-related anemia, and others. GI bleeding was defined as the bleeding from the GI tract with an evidence of bleeding on endoscopy [14]. IDA was defined as an anemia with biochemical evidence of iron deficiency. ACD was defined as an anemia associated with chronic inflammatory, infectious disease, or malignancies [15]. Anemia associated with chronic kidney disease was also classified into this category. Cancer-related anemia was defined as anemia accompanied by a newly diagnosed, active, or metastatic cancer [16]. The determination of IDA/ACD or cancer-related anemia was mutually exclusive. For example, when the patient being treated with active cancer showed the IDA/ACD pattern, it was defined as cancer-related anemia. Surgery/procedure-related anemia was defined as newly developed anemia within 24 h after surgery or procedure without evidence of the other cause [17]. Finally, anemia without obvious causes was classified as other types of anemia (Figure 1).

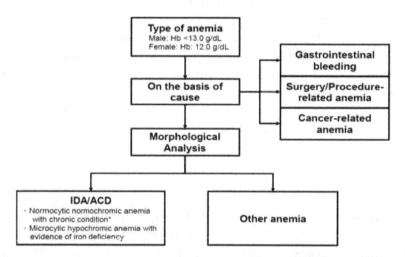

Figure 1. Type of anemia according to cause of anemia or morphological analysis of erythrocytes. * Patients with anemia of chronic disease were classified as cancer-related anemia when they had active cancer. Hb: hemoglobin; IDA: iron-deficiency anemia; ACD: anemia of chronic disease. We included the additional laboratory results that can affect the hemoglobin levels and anemia status: white blood cell (WBC) and platelet counts; blood urea nitrogen, creatinine, and blood glucose levels; international normalized ratio; and blood pressure. The functional outcome was assessed by modified Rankin Scale (mRS) score at 3 months [18], and stroke severity was measured using the National Institute of Health Stroke Scale (NIHSS) score at admission [19]. The primary outcome was poor outcome at 3 months, which was defined the mRS score of 3–6 [20]. Secondary analysis was performed to assess the significance of each hemoglobin variability parameters during admission in poor outcome prediction.

2.3. Statistical Analysis

We compared the baseline characteristics of patients who received early and late RBC transfusion. The patients were divided into the good (mRS 0–2) and poor (mRS 3–6) group according to the 3-month outcome. Baseline demographic and clinical characteristics were compared using the $\chi 2$ or t-test (Mann–Whitney U test) as appropriate. Univariable logistic regression analysis was performed to assess the predictors for poor outcome. The multivariable logistic regression model was used for independent variables with a p-value of <0.05 in the univariable model or with the clinical relevance. We used four different multivariable models: model 1 adjusting for age and sex; model 2 adjusting for age, sex, and the Charlson comorbidity index (CCI); model 3 adjusting for age, sex, CCI, and NIHSS; and model 4 adjusting for age, sex, CCI, NIHHS, WBC count, and fasting blood glucose. For assessing the significance of hemoglobin variability parameters, model performance for each multivariable logistic regression analysis was performed using the area under the receiver operating characteristics curve (AUROC). Significant statistical differences among independent variables were considered with a *p*-value of 0.05 in multivariable models. All statistical analyses were performed using R (Foundation for Statistical Computing, Vienna, Austria, http://www.R-project.org).

3. Results

3.1. Baseline Characteristics

Among the 2698 patients with AIS, 592 (21.9%) were anemic at the time of admission and 132 (4.9%) received RBCT during the admission (Table S1). Patients who received RBCT were older, more likely to be male, had history of previous stroke and smoking, and a higher stroke severity and cardioembolic cause of stroke than those who did not receive RBCT. The number of patients taking anticoagulants was higher in the RBCT group, but there was no difference in the previous use of antiplatelet agents before the index stroke between the two groups.

In total, 63 of 132 (47.7%) patients received early RBCT (Table 1). The mean age of patients who received RBCT during admission was the mean (± standard deviation) of 71.6 (±13.5) years, and 46.2% patients were men. Patients who received early RBCT were less likely to have previous strokes than those who received late RBCT. CCI and NIHSS score were not different between the early and late RBCT group. The proportion of patients with poor outcome (mRS >2) at 3 months was less in the early RBCT group than in the late RBCT group.

Table 1. Baseline characteristics of the participants.

Parameters	Early Transfusion (*n* = 63)	Late Transfusion (*n* = 69)	*p*
Age, years	68.6 ± 16.3	74.4.1 ± 9.7	0.450
Male	30 (47.6%)	31 (44.9%)	0.893
Past medical history			
Stroke	16 (25.4%)	30 (43.5%)	0.002
Hypertension	41 (65.1%)	52 (75.4%)	0.270
Diabetes	17 (27.0%)	23 (33.3%)	0.546
Hyperlipidemia	18 (28.6%)	20 (29.0%)	0.985
Current smoking	19 (30.2%)	12 (17.4%)	0.128
Charlson comorbidity index	5.0 (3.0–7.0)	5.0 (4.0–7.0)	0.221
Stroke subtype			0.116
Cardioembolic	14 (22.2%)	25 (36.2%)	
Non-cardioembolic	49 (77.8%)	44 (63.8%)	
NIHSS score	9.0 (2.5–16.0)	13.0 (6.0–18.0)	0.091
Thrombolysis	9 (14.3%)	6 (8.7%)	0.461
Onset to visit time, hour	3.7 (1.2–30.0)	4.9 (1.0–30.5)	0.879
Laboratory parameter			
WBC, $10^3/\mu L$	9.1 ± 4.5	9.4 ± 4.3	0.660
Platelet, $10^3/\mu L$	280 ± 152	234 ± 111	0.050
BUN, mg/dL	22.2 ± 15.6	22.5 ± 16.9	0.926
Creatinine, mg/dL	1.2 ± 1.3	1.3 ± 1.2	0.614
Total cholesterol, mg/dL	147.0 ± 49.7	160.0 ± 48.3	0.130
TG, mg/dL	95.5 ± 55.2	113.0 ± 55.5	0.078
HDL, mg/dL	45.6 ± 13.2	42.0 ± 11.8	0.108
LDL, mg/dL	90.3 ± 41.2	92.6 ± 42.9	0.759
FBS, mg/dL	133.0 ± 57.3	139.0 ± 55.9	0.574
INR	1.2 ± 0.7	1.3 ± 0.9	0.816
Systolic BP, mmHg	140 ± 25	140 ± 28	0.997
Diastolic BP, mmHg	81.8 ± 13.7	78.9 ± 17.3	0.284
History of antithrombotics usage	23 (36.5%)	34 (49.3%)	0.193
Poor outcome (mRS >2)	43 (68.3%)	61 (88.4%)	0.009

Categorical variables are represented by the number (column percent), and continuous variable are represented by mean (± standard deviation) or median (interquartile range) as appropriate. SD: standard deviation; iqr: interquartile range; NIHSS: National Institute of Health Stroke Scale; WBC: white blood cell, BUN: blood urea nitrogen; TG: triglycerides; HDL: high-density lipoprotein; LDL: low-density lipoprotein; FBS: fasting blood sugar; INR: international normalized ratio; BP: blood pressure; mRS: modified Rankin Scale.

Patients who had poor outcomes had more severe stroke, shorter onset to admission time, and had a higher WBC count and fasting blood glucose level than those with good outcomes. Patients who received intravenous thrombolysis and RBCT were in the poor outcome group (Table 2).

Table 2. The comparison of clinical and laboratory parameters between good and poor outcome group.

Parameters	Poor ($n = 104$)	Good ($n = 28$)	p
Age, years	70.1 ± 14.9	72.0.1 ± 13.2	0.514
Male	43 (41.3%)	18 (64.3%)	0.051
Past medical history			
Stroke	39 (37.5%)	7 (25.0%)	0.313
Hypertension	75 (72.1%)	18 (64.3%)	0.567
Diabetes	34 (32.7%)	6 (21.4%)	0.358
Hyperlipidemia	29 (27.9%)	9 (32.1%)	0.836
Current smoking	21 (20.2)	10 (35.7)	0.142
Stroke subtype			0.718
Cardioembolic	32 (30.8%)	7 (25.0%)	
Non-cardioembolic	70 (68.6%)	23 (76.7%)	
NIHSS, score	13.0 (7.0–18.0)	3.0 (1.0–4.5)	<0.001
Thrombolysis	15 (14.4%)	0 (0.0%)	0.072
onset to visit time, hour	3.2 (0.9–26.0)	12.9 (3.2–61.7)	0.012
Laboratory parameter			
WBC, $10^3/\mu L$	9.7 ± 4.6	7.4 ± 2.7	0.011
Platelet, $10^3/\mu L$	246 ± 127	292 ± 152	0.102
BUN, mg/dL	21.5 ± 14.8	25.8 ± 20.6	0.211
Creatinine, mg/dL	1.2 ± 1.3	1.3 ± 0.9	0.878
Total cholesterol, mg/dL	157.0 ± 50.2	142.0 ± 44.3	0.178
TG, mg/dL	103.0 ± 53.5	109.0 ± 63.4	0.558
HDL, mg/dL	44.5 ± 12.1	40.3 ± 13.7	0.120
LDL, mg/dL	93.6 ± 43.5	84.0 ± 35.5	0.290
FBS, mg/dL	143.0 ± 58.7	110.0 ± 37.5	0.006
INR	1.3 ± 0.9	1.1 ± 0.1	0.274
Systolic BP, mmHg	143.0 ± 26.6	132.0 ± 24.4	0.058
Diastolic BP, mmHg	81.2 ± 16.2	77.0 ± 13.4	0.211
History of antithrombotics usage	46 (44.2%)	11 (39.3%)	0.780
Number of Hb measure	13.0 (6.0–23.5)	8.0 (5.8–19.3)	0.309
Admission Hb, g/dL	9.7 ± 2.6	8.8 ± 2.5	0.129
Hb variability parameter			
Mean, g/dL	10.2 ± 1.5	9.4 ± 1.2	0.012
Median, g/dL	10.2 ± 1.5	9.5 ± 1.2	0.018
Minimum, g/dL	8.0 ± 1.8	7.2 ± 1.4	0.025
Maximum, g/dL	12.2 ± 1.9	11.3 ± 1.7	0.026
IQR, g/dL	1.6 ± 0.9	1.6 ± 0.9	0.806
Range, g/dL	4.2 ± 1.9	4.1 ± 1.6	0.889
SD, g/dL	1.3 ± 0.5	1.4 ± 0.5	0.640
MAD, g/dL	1.1 ± 0.7	1.2 ± 0.7	0.529
CoV, %	12.9 ± 4.8	14.4 ± 4.5	0.134
MAC, g/dL	0.7 ± 0.4	0.8 ± 0.2	0.165
Type of anemia			0.164
GI bleeding	24 (23.1)	12 (42.9)	
Cancer-related	18 (17.3)	2 (7.1)	
IDA or ACD	24 (23.1)	8 (28.6)	
Surgery/Procedure-related	23 (22.1)	4 (14.3)	
Others	15 (14.4)	2 (7.1)	
Transfusion amount, mL	400 (400–800)	800 (400–1140)	0.337
Timing of transfusion			0.009
Early (≤ 48 h)	43 (41.3%)	20 (71.4%)	
Late (> 48 h)	61 (58.7%)	8 (28.6%)	

Categorical variables are represented by the number (column percent) and continuous variable are represented by mean (± standard deviation) or median (interquartile range) as appropriate. NIHSS: National Institute of Health Stroke Scale; WBC: white blood cell; BUN: blood urea nitrogen; TG: triglycerides; HDL: high-density lipoprotein; LDL: low-density lipoprotein; FBS: fasting blood sugar; INR: international normalized ratio; BP: blood pressure; Hb: hemoglobin; IQR: interquartile range; SD: standard deviation; MAD: median absolute deviation; CoV: coefficient of variation; MAC: mean absolute change; GI: gastrointestinal; IDA: iron deficiency anemia; ACD: anemia of chronic disorder.

3.2. Type of Anemia, RBC Transfusion and Hemoglobin Variability

GI bleeding (27.3%) was the most common cause of RBCT, followed by IDA/ACD (24.2%), surgery/procedure-related anemia (20.5%), and cancer-related anemia (15.2%). Most RBCT was performed within seven days of hospitalization (Figure 2a). The type of anemia was not associated with poor outcomes ($p = 0.164$ for chi-square, Table 2) and the timing of RBCT (Figure 2b and Table 3). However, patients with poor outcomes were found to have received RBCT later than those with good outcomes ($p = 0.009$ for chi-square, Table 2). The amount of RBCT showed left-shifted distribution and was higher in the good outcome group than in the poor outcome group, but it was not statistically significant ($p = 0.337$ for Wilcoxon signed-rank test).

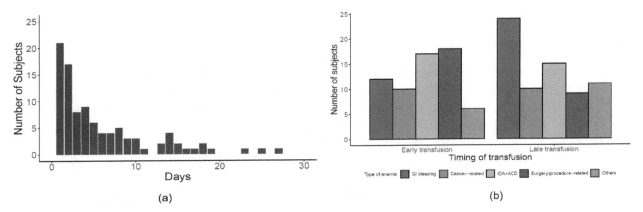

(a)   (b)

Figure 2. The timing of red blood cell transfusion and the relationship of type of anemia between early and late red blood cell transfusion: (**a**) The frequency of red blood cell transfusion performed after hospitalization (X-axis means the timing (days) of RBCT after admission; Y-axis means the number of subjects who received red blood cell transfusion). (**b**) The differences of proportion in type of anemia according to the timing of the red blood cell transfusion (early vs. late).

Table 3. The comparison of hemoglobin variability parameters and type of anemia between early and late transfusion group.

Parameters	Early Transfusion (n = 63)	Late Transfusion (n = 69)	Total (n =132)	p
Number of Hb measure, number	7.0 (4.0–14.0)	19.0 (10.0–30.0)	13.0 (6.0–23.0)	<0.001
Admission Hb, mg/dL	9.4 ± 2.7	9.6±2.5	9.5 ± 2.6	0.639
Hb variability parameter				
Mean, mg/dL	10.1 ± 1.8	9.9 ± 1.1	10.0 ± 1.5	0.391
Median, mg/dL	10.3 ± 1.9	9.9 ± 1.1	10.1 ± 1.5	0.109
Minimum, mg/dL	8.2 ± 2.1	7.6 ± 1.3	7.9 ± 1.7	0.065
Maximum, mg/dL	11.7 ± 1.9	12.3 ± 1.8	12.0 ± 1.9	0.052
IQR, mg/dL	1.3 ± 0.8	1.8 ± 1.0	1.9 ± 0.6	0.004
Range, mg/dL	3.5 ± 1.6	4.7 ± 1.8	4.1 ± 1.8	<0.001
SD, mg/dL	1.3 ± 0.5	1.4 ± 0.5	1.3 ± 0.5	0.292
MAD, mg/dL	1.0 ± 0.7	1.3 ± 0.7	0.5 ± 0.5	0.025
CoV, %	12.6 ± 4.8	13.7 ± 4.7	13.2 ± 4.8	0.212
MAC, mg/dL	0.8 ± 0.4	0.6 ± 0.3	0.4 ± 0.3	0.004
Type of anemia				0.080
GI bleeding	12 (19.0)	24 (34.8)	36 (27.3)	
Cancer-related	10 (15.9)	10 (14.5)	20 (15.2)	
IDA or ACD	17 (27.0)	15 (21.7)	32 (24.2)	
Surgery/Procedure-related	18 (28.6)	9 (13.0)	27 (20.5)	
Others	6 (9.5)	11 (16.0)	17 (12.9)	
Transfusion amount, mL	400 (400–800)	640 (400–1120)	400 (400–840)	0.448

Categorical variables are represented by the number (column percent) and continuous variable are represented by mean (± standard deviation) or median (interquartile range) as appropriate. Hb: hemoglobin; IQR: interquartile range; SD: standard deviation; MAD: median absolute deviation; CoV: coefficient of variation; MAC: mean absolute change; GI: gastrointestinal; IDA: iron deficiency anemia; ACD: anemia of chronic disorder.

During hospitalization, 2359 hemoglobin measurements were performed for the 132 patients receiving RBCT (Table 3). The median (interquartile range (IQR)) of hemoglobin measurements in each patient with RBCT was 13 (6–13) and the number of hemoglobin measurement was more frequent in the late RBCT group than in the early RBCT group (p <0.001). Among the hemoglobin variability parameters, IQR, range, and median absolute deviation (MAD) hemoglobin levels were lower and the mean absolute change (MAC) hemoglobin levels was higher in the early RBCT group than in the late RBCT group (Table 3). Mean, median, minimum, and maximum hemoglobin levels were higher in patients with poor outcomes than in those with good outcomes (Table 2). Other hemoglobin variability parameters including IQR, range, standard deviation (SD), MAD, coefficient of variation (CoV), and MAC hemoglobin were not different between the two groups.

3.3. Predictors for Poor Outcome

The proportion of patients with poor outcomes was 78.8% (104/132). In the univariable analysis, higher NIHSS score, late RBCT was associated with poor outcomes (odds ratio (OR), 3.55; 95% confidence interval (CI), 1.43–8.79) in univariable analysis. When we adjusted age, sex, CCI, NIHSS score, WBC count, and fasting blood sugar level, late RBCT was a significant predictor for poor outcomes (OR, 3.37; 95% CI, 1.14–9.99, Table 4).

Because of the high correlation between the hemoglobin variability parameters (Figure S1), the statistical significances of hemoglobin variability indices were compared to identify if the AUROC value indicating the model performance increased significantly when the hemoglobin variability parameters were added into the original logistic regression model. The performance of the original multivariable logistic regression was AUROC (0.883; 95% CI, 0.821–0.936, p <0.001). Figure 3 shows the model performance of each logistic regression model, which additionally included each hemoglobin variability parameter in the original model. However, there were no additional improvements in model performance when the hemoglobin variability indices were included in the original model.

Table 4. The predictors of poor outcome in multivariable logistic regression analysis according to the timing of the transfusion.

	Crude Model		Model 1		Model 2		Model 3		Model 4	
	OR (95% CI)	p	OR (95% CI)	p	OR (95% CI)	p	OR (95% CI)	p	OR (95% CI)	p
Late transfusion	3.55 (1.43–8.79)	0.006	3.61 (1.42–9.19)	0.007	3.65 (1.43–9.29)	0.007	3.21 (1.14–9.09)	0.028	3.37 (1.14–9.99)	0.028
Age			1.00 (0.97–1.03)	0.983	1.00 (0.96–1.03)	0.806	0.99 (0.95–1.04)	0.694	0.98 (0.93–1.03)	0.403
Male			0.38 (0.16–0.93)	0.035	0.38 (0.15–0.92)	0.033	0.43 (0.16–1.17)	0.099	0.42 (0.15–1.21)	0.109
CCI					1.04 (0.86–1.27)	0.677	1.06 (0.84–1.35)	0.629	1.07 (0.83–1.39)	0.592
NIHSS							1.22 (1.11–1.34)	<0.001	1.19 (1.08–1.31)	<0.001
WBC, $10^3/\mu L$									1.16 (0.98–1.37)	0.089
FBS, mg/dL									1.01 (1.00–1.02)	0.189

Model 1 adjusted for age and sex; Model 2 included variables in Model 1 plus Charlson comorbidity index; Model 3 included variables in Model 2 plus National Institute of Health Stroke Scale score; Model 4 included variables in Model 3 plus white blood cell count and fasting blood sugar. OR: odds ratio; CI: confidence interval; CCI: Charlson comorbidity index; NIHSS: National Institute of Health Stroke Scale; WBC: white blood cell; FBS: fasting blood sugar.

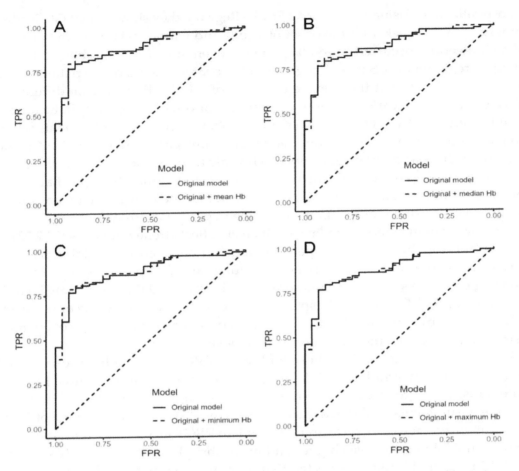

Figure 3. Receiver operating characteristics curve showing performances of original logistic regression model and the other models with hemoglobin variability parameter. The original model was the final logistic regression model in Table 4. The area under the curve of the Receiver Operating Characteristic (AUROC) of the original model was 0.883. AUROC of mean (**A**), median (**B**), minimum (**C**), and maximum (**D**) hemoglobin-adjusted models were 0.884, 0.885, 0.889, and 0.882, respectively. TPR: true positive rate; FPR: false positive rate; Hb: hemoglobin.

4. Discussion

In this study, 21.9% patients with AIS were anemic at admission and 4.9% had received RBCT during hospitalization. Approximately 79% patients who received RBCT had a poor outcome at three months. The mean, median, minimum, and maximum hemoglobin levels were higher in patients with poor outcomes than in those with good outcomes. However, differences in hemoglobin variability indices, including IQR, range, SD, CoV, MAD, and MAC, did not differ between the two groups. Late RBCT was a significant predictor for poor outcome in patients with AIS in the multivariable model. However, hemoglobin variability indices were not associated with functional outcome in patients with AIS and RBCT.

We found that 5% AIS had received RBCT during hospitalization, and more than two-thirds of those had a poor outcome at three months. Additionally, late transfusion, rather than hemoglobin variability indices during hospitalization, was a significant predictor for poor outcome. Our study included all hemoglobin measurements performed during the hospital stay and differs from previous studies as we only investigated patients with AIS who had received RBCT. When analyzing the effect of hemoglobin on the AIS outcome, RBCT should be stratified RBCT or by analyzing only patients who had received RBCT.

Limited studies have assessed the relationship between the type of anemia and the functional outcome in patients with AIS. Ogata et al. have investigated the effect of GI bleeding in patients with

AIS during hospitalization. Using the Fukuoka Stroke Registry, they showed that GI bleeding occurred most commonly within 1 week after the onset of stroke and was associated with poor outcome [21]. In our study, GI bleeding occurred in 38.8% patients, even after 7 days of hospitalization. As the antiplatelet agent regimen in AIS was changed and the characteristics of the patients varied in each study, there is a possibility that the prevalent period of GI bleeding may be different. However, RBCT performed to correct various causes of anemia not only during hospitalization but also at admission. In the retrospective observational study by Sharma et al., 28% of patients without anemia on admission developed anemia during admission [22]. In prospectively collected UK Regional Stroke Register data, hypochromic microcytic or normochromic normocytic anemia were associated with poor clinical outcomes in patients with AIS [23]. They concluded that the type of anemia is a salient indicator of comorbidity burden. Therefore, we suggest that the type of anemia or timing of RBCT could be an important predictor of functional outcome in patients with AIS.

In general, low or high hemoglobin levels adversely affect stroke outcomes [2,22,23]. The reason that our results did not show the U-shaped relationship between hemoglobin levels and stroke outcomes was due to the difference in patient population. The previous reports have assessed admission hemoglobin levels for all patients admitted with AIS, and this study only included patients with AIS who received RBCT during the hospital stay. Likewise, when analyzing only patients who had received RBCT, we can hypothesize that the other variables, including the type of anemia, had more impact on stroke outcome than the initial hemoglobin level.

RBCT had a poorer outcome than those with early RBCT due to admission hemoglobin level not differing between early and late RBCT group; however, the IQR and range hemoglobin were higher in late transfusion group than in early RBCT group in our report. Furthermore, the number of hemoglobin measurements performed during the hospital stay was an average of 7 times in early RBCT group, but an average of 19 measurements in late RBCT group. Based on these observations, the change in hemoglobin status was higher and more abrupt in the late transfusion group than in the early RBCT group, and it can be expected that more frequent hemoglobin measurements in late RBCT group were made to monitor this rapid change. The autoregulatory mechanism for maintaining cerebral blood flow is already lost in infarct core, and that mechanism is already maximized in the penumbral area [24]. Therefore, the rapid drop in hemoglobin may further exacerbate the oligemia and cause infarct growth in penumbral area. In a study by Bellwald et al., decreased hemoglobin level after hospital arrival was associated with the amount and velocity of infarct growth in patients with AIS [25]. We did not assess infarct growth of our participants; rapid alteration of hemoglobin status in the late RBCT group may have a worse effect on the cerebral autoregulatory mechanism, which can exacerbate stroke outcome. Second, although the type of anemia was not statistically different between early and late RBCT group ($p = 0.080$) in our data, different cause of RBCT may affect stroke outcome. Surgery/procedure-related anemia was higher in the early RBCT group, and GI bleeding was higher in the late RBCT group in our study. However, our study did not include a large number of patients who received RBCT (only 5% in total AIS population), it should be reassessed in a larger prospective study whether this type of anemia affected stroke outcome.

In general population, history of RBCT is associated with 1.6-fold increase in the risk of ischemic stroke [26]. This association is explained by the fact that stored RBC increases blood viscosity, and decreases nitric oxide concentration, vasoconstriction, and platelet activation [1]. On the other hand, low hemoglobin is inversely correlated with initial infarct volume or infarct growth, and the author suggested that RBCT would be beneficial for recovery of stroke [1]. However, restrictive transfusion strategy in patients of cardiovascular diseases was not inferior compared to liberal strategy in two systematic review [1]. In our data, transfusion amount did change between the good and poor outcome group, though those with good outcome had low mean, median, minimum, and maximum hemoglobin compared to those with poor outcome. Our study did not directly assess the exact transfusion strategy because the study design was retrospective in nature. However, we suggested that restrictive transfusion strategies can reduce the thrombotic complication and maximize the beneficial effect by RBCT compared to the liberal strategy in AIS patients.

In our study, hemoglobin variability indices did not affect the functional outcome in patients with AIS. In the previous report, minimum or maximum hemoglobin level was associated with worse outcome [1]. However, these hemoglobin parameters did not affect the stroke outcome in our study. Kellert et al. studied the impact of low hemoglobin level and transfusion in neurologic intensive care unit patients and found that hemoglobin parameters were not associated with in-hospital mortality or 90-day functional outcomes, but they were associated with length of intensive care unit length of stay and duration of mechanical ventilation [10]. The author suggested that the impact of hemoglobin parameters in neurologically severe patients might be reduced by the important predictors such as stroke severity. In our study, patients with RBCT had more severe stroke than those without RBCT (median NIHSS score 13 vs. 3). Our study also suggests that stroke severity, rather than hemoglobin parameters, is an important predictor for poor outcome in patients with severe ischemic stroke. However, as our study and Kellert's study had a small sample size, larger prospective studies are needed to confirm these associations.

Our study had some limitations. First, our study was a small sampled-sized retrospective observation, and therefore there is a chance of selection bias and residual confounding. However, the incidence of anemia and the proportion who had received RBCT during hospitalization were comparable to other studies on patients with AIS [1]. Second, the effect of RBCT on functional outcome was likely to be underestimated because we only collected RBCT data, which were performed only during hospitalization. However, anemia usually developed 2–11 days following admission in patients with AIS [27]. Therefore, only several patients would receive RBCT after discharge.

Despite these limitations, our study had several strengths. First, we minimized residual confounding by including information such as stroke severity, type of anemia, and timing and amount of RBCT. Second, the characteristics of patients with AIS who received RBCT differ significantly compared to those who did not receive RBCT. If the rare event (such as patients with RBCT; ~5% of all AIS patients) is evaluated with logistic regression method, the results may be vulnerable to biases [28]. We solved this problem by analyzing the binary outcome only in patients with RBCT and minimized the interaction between anemia and RBCT transfusion. Third, cerebral perfusion can be changed dynamically depending on the degree of anemia and whether the RBCT is performed or not. We evaluated all hemoglobin measurements during the hospitalization. In addition, we analyzed the overall hemoglobin parameters such as SD, CoV, and MAD, and temporal variation parameter such as MAC. In addition, we identified all bleeding events during hospitalization and reflected them in the type of anemia variable.

5. Conclusions

Late RBCT was associated with 3-month poor outcome in patients with AIS. To verify this, a larger prospective study is needed for assessing the type of anemia and cause of RBCT, and the fluctuation of hemoglobin status during the admission.

Author Contributions: Conceptualization, B.-C.L.; Data curation, M.U.J.; Formal analysis, C.K., S.-H.L., J.-S.L., and M.S.O.; Funding acquisition, C.K.; Methodology, S.-H.L., Y.K., and J.-H.L.; Resources, Y.K. and S.J.; Supervision, K.-H.Y., J.-H.L., and B.-C.L.; Visualization, J.-S.L. and M.U.J.; Writing—original draft, C.K. and B.-C.L.; Writing—review & editing, M.S.O., K.-H.Y., and S.J. All authors have read and agreed to the published version of the manuscript.

References

1. Sarnak, M.J.; Tighiouart, H.; Manjunath, G.; MacLeod, B.; Griffith, J.; Salem, D.; Levey, A.S. Anemia as a risk factor for cardiovascular disease in the atherosclerosis risk in communities (ARIC) study. *J. Am. Coll. Cardiol.* **2002**, *40*, 27–33.

2. Wei, C.C.; Zhang, S.T.; Tan, G.; Zhang, S.H.; Liu, M. Impact of anemia on in-hospital complications after ischemic stroke. *Eur. J. Neurol.* **2018**, *25*, 768–774.

3. Powers, W.J. Cerebral hemodynamics in ischemic cerebrovascular disease. *Ann. Neurol.* **1991**, *29*, 231–240.

4. Tsai, C.F.; Yip, P.K.; Chen, C.C.; Yeh, S.J.; Chung, S.T.; Jeng, J.S. Cerebral infarction in acute anemia. *J. Neurol.* **2010**, *257*, 2044–2051.

5. Kellert, L.; Herweh, C.; Sykora, M.; Gussmann, P.; Martin, E.; Ringleb, P.A.; Steiner, T.; Bösel, J. Loss of penumbra by impaired oxygen supply? Decreasing Hemoglobin levels predict infarct growth after acute ischemic stroke. *Cerebrovasc. Dis. Extra* **2012**, *2*, 99–107.

6. Ehrenreich, H.; Weissenborn, K.; Prange, H.; Schneider, D.; Weimar, C.; Wartenberg, K.; Schellinger, P.D.; Bohn, M.; Becker, H.; Wegrzyn, M.; et al. Recombinant human erythropoietin in the treatment of acute ischemic stroke. *Stroke* **2009**, *40*, e647–e656.

7. Goel, R.; Patel, E.U.; Cushing, M.M.; Frank, S.M.; Ness, P.M.; Takemoto, C.M.; Vasovic, L.V.; Sheth, S.; Nellis, M.E.; Shaz, B.; et al. Association of perioperative red blood cell transfusions with venous thromboembolism in a North American registry. *JAMA. Surg.* **2018**, *153*, 826–833.

8. Byrnes, J.R.; Wolberg, A.S. Red blood cells in thrombosis. *Blood* **2017**, *130*, 1795–1799.

9. Moman, R.N.; Kor, D.J.; Chandran, A.; Hanson, A.C.; Schroeder, D.R.; Rabinstein, A.A.; Warner, M.A. Red blood cell transfusion in acute brain injury subtypes: An observational cohort study. *J. Crit. Care* **2019**, *50*, 44–49.

10. Kellert, L.; Schrader, F.; Ringleb, P.; Steiner, T.; Bösel, J. The impact of low hemoglobin levels and transfusion on critical care patients with severe ischemic stroke STroke: Relevant impact of HemoGlobin, Hematocrit and Transfusion (STRAIGHT)—An observational study. *J. Crit. Care* **2014**, *29*, 236–240.

11. Kim, J.Y.; Kang, K.; Kang, J.; Koo, J.; Kim, D.H.; Kim, B.J.; Kim, W.J.; Kim, E.G.; Kim, J.G.; Kim, J.M.; et al. Executive summary of stroke statistics in Korea 2018: A report from the epidemiology research council of the Korean stroke society. *J. Stroke* **2019**, *21*, 42–59.

12. Kohnert, K.D.; Heinke, P.; Fritzsche, G.; Vogt, L.; Augstein, P.; Salzsieder, E. Evaluation of the mean absolute glucose change as a measure of glycemic variability using continuous glucose monitoring data. *Diabetes Technol. Ther.* **2013**, *15*, 448–454.

13. Chelemer, S.B.; Prato, B.S.; Cox Jr., P.M.; O'Connor, G.T.; Morton, J.R. Association of bacterial infection and red blood cell transfusion after coronary artery bypass surgery. *Ann. Thorac. Surg.* **2002**, *73*, 138–142.

14. Raju, G.S.; Gerson, L.; Das, A.; Lewis, B.; American Gastroenterological Association (AGA). Institute medical position statement on obscure gastrointestinal bleeding. *Gastroenterology* **2007**, *133*, 1694–1696.

15. Weiss, G.; Goodnough, L.T. Anemia of chronic disease. *N. Engl. J. Med.* **2005**, *352*, 1011–1023.

16. Ludwig, H.; Van, B.S.; Barrett-Lee, P.; Birgegård, G.; Bokemeyer, C.; Gascón, P.; Kosmidis, P.; Krzakowski, M.; Nortier, J.; Olmi, P.; et al. The European Cancer Anaemia Survey (ECAS): A large, multinational, prospective survey defining the prevalence, incidence, and treatment of anaemia in cancer patients. *Eur. J. Cancer* **2004**, *40*, 2293–2306.

17. Valeri, C.R.; Dennis, R.C.; Ragno, G.; Macgregor, H.; Menzoian, J.O.; Khuri, S.F. Limitations of the hematocrit level to assess the need for red blood cell transfusion in hypovolemic anemic patients. *Transfusion* **2006**, *46*, 365–371.

18. Sulter, G.; Steen, C.; De Keyser, J.D. Use of the Barthel index and modified Rankin Scale in acute stroke trials. *Stroke* **1999**, *30*, 1538–1541.

19. Wityk, R.J.; Pessin, M.S.; Kaplan, R.F.; Caplan, L.R. Serial assessment of acute stroke using the NIH Stroke Scale. *Stroke* **1994**, *25*, 362–365.

20. Jansen, I.G.; Mulder, M.J.; Goldhoorn, R.-J.B. Endovascular treatment for acute ischaemic stroke in routine clinical practice: Prospective, observational cohort study (MR CLEAN registry). *BMJ.* **2018**, *360*, k949.

21. Ogata, T.; Kamouchi, M.; Matsuo, R.; Kuroda, J.; Ago, T.; Sugimori, H.; Inoue, T.; Kitazono, T.; Fukuoka Stroke Registry. Gastrointestinal bleeding in acute ischemic stroke: Recent trends from the Fukuoka stroke registry. *Cerebrovasc. Dis. Extra* **2014**, *4*, 156–164.

22. Sharma, K.; Johnson, D.J.; Johnson, B.; Frank, S.M.; Stevens, R.D. Hemoglobin concentration does not impact 3-month outcome following acute ischemic stroke. *BMC. Neurol.* **2018**, *18*, 78.

23. Barlas, R.S.; McCall, S.J.; Bettencourt-Silva, J.H.; Clark, A.B.; Bowles, K.M.; Metcalf, A.K.; Mamas, M.A.; Potter, J.F.; Myint, P.K. Impact of anaemia on acute stroke outcomes depends on the type of anaemia: Evidence from a UK stroke register. *J. Neurol. Sci.* **2017**, *383*, 26–30.

24. Yamada, S.; Koizumi, A.; Iso, H.; Wada, Y.; Watanabe, Y.; Date, C.; Yamamoto, A.; Kikuchi, S.; Inaba, Y.; Kondo, T.; et al. History of blood transfusion before 1990 is a risk factor for stroke and cardiovascular diseases: The Japan collaborative cohort study (JACC study). *Cerebrovasc. Dis.* **2005**, *20*, 164–171.

25. Jordan, J.D.; Powers, W.J. Cerebral autoregulation and acute ischemic stroke. *Am. J. Hypertens.* **2012**, *25*, 946–950.

26. Bellwald, S.; Balasubramaniam, R.; Nagler, M.; Burri, M.S.; Fischer, S.D.A.; Hakim, A.; Dobrocky, T.; Yu, Y.; Scalzo, F.; Heldner, M.R.; et al. Association of anemia and hemoglobin decrease during acute stroke treatment with infarct growth and clinical outcome. *PLoS ONE* **2018**, *13*, e0203535.

27. Abe, A.; Sakamoto, Y.; Nishiyama, Y.; Suda, S.; Suzuki, K.; Aoki, J.; Kimura, K. Decline in Hemoglobin during hospitalization may be associated with poor outcome in acute stroke patients. *J. Stroke Cerebrovasc. Dis.* **2018**, *27*, 1646–1652.

28. Bradburn, M.J.; Deeks, J.J.; Berlin, J.A.; Russell Localio, A. Much ado about nothing: A comparison of the performance of meta-analytical methods with rare events. *Stat. Med.* **2007**, *26*, 53–77.

Permissions

All chapters in this book were first published by MDPI; hereby published with permission under the Creative Commons Attribution License or equivalent. Every chapter published in this book has been scrutinized by our experts. Their significance has been extensively debated. The topics covered herein carry significant findings which will fuel the growth of the discipline. They may even be implemented as practical applications or may be referred to as a beginning point for another development.

The contributors of this book come from diverse backgrounds, making this book a truly international effort. This book will bring forth new frontiers with its revolutionizing research information and detailed analysis of the nascent developments around the world.

We would like to thank all the contributing authors for lending their expertise to make the book truly unique. They have played a crucial role in the development of this book. Without their invaluable contributions this book wouldn't have been possible. They have made vital efforts to compile up to date information on the varied aspects of this subject to make this book a valuable addition to the collection of many professionals and students.

This book was conceptualized with the vision of imparting up-to-date information and advanced data in this field. To ensure the same, a matchless editorial board was set up. Every individual on the board went through rigorous rounds of assessment to prove their worth. After which they invested a large part of their time researching and compiling the most relevant data for our readers.

The editorial board has been involved in producing this book since its inception. They have spent rigorous hours researching and exploring the diverse topics which have resulted in the successful publishing of this book. They have passed on their knowledge of decades through this book. To expedite this challenging task, the publisher supported the team at every step. A small team of assistant editors was also appointed to further simplify the editing procedure and attain best results for the readers.

Apart from the editorial board, the designing team has also invested a significant amount of their time in understanding the subject and creating the most relevant covers. They scrutinized every image to scout for the most suitable representation of the subject and create an appropriate cover for the book.

The publishing team has been an ardent support to the editorial, designing and production team. Their endless efforts to recruit the best for this project, has resulted in the accomplishment of this book. They are a veteran in the field of academics and their pool of knowledge is as vast as their experience in printing. Their expertise and guidance has proved useful at every step. Their uncompromising quality standards have made this book an exceptional effort. Their encouragement from time to time has been an inspiration for everyone.

The publisher and the editorial board hope that this book will prove to be a valuable piece of knowledge for researchers, students, practitioners and scholars across the globe.

List of Contributors

Ann-Rong Yan and Mark Naunton
School of Health Sciences, Faculty of Health, University of Canberra, Canberra 2617, Australia

Gregory M. Peterson
School of Health Sciences, Faculty of Health, University of Canberra, Canberra 2617, Australia
School of Pharmacy and Pharmacology, University of Tasmania, Hobart 7000, Australia

Israel Fernandez-Cadenas
Stroke Pharmacogenomics and Genetics Group, Neurovascular Research Laboratory, Hospital de Sant Pau, 08041 Barcelona, Spain

Reza Mortazavi
School of Health Sciences, Faculty of Health, University of Canberra, Canberra 2617, Australia
Prehab Activity Cancer Exercise Survivorship Research Group, Faculty of Health, University of Canberra, Canberra 2617, Australia

Nikola Tułowiecka and Małgorzata Szczuko
Department of Human Nutrition and Metabolomics, Pomeranian Medical University in Szczecin, 71-460 Szczecin, Poland

Dariusz Kotlęga
Department of Neurology, Pomeranian Medical University in Szczecin, 71-252 Szczecin, Poland
Department of Applied and Clinical Physiology, Collegium Medicum University of Zielona Gora, 65-417 Zielona Gora, Poland

Piotr Prowans
Clinic of Plastic, Endocrine and General Surgery, Pomeranian Medical University in Szczecin, 72-009 Police, Poland

Diji Kuriakose and Zhicheng Xiao
Development and Stem Cells Program, Monash Biomedicine Discovery Institute and Department of Anatomy and Developmental Biology, Monash University, Melbourne, VIC 3800, Australia

Jacob Story, Willie Davis and Ike C. dela Peña
Department of Pharmaceutical and Administrative Sciences, Loma Linda University School of Pharmacy, Loma Linda, CA 92350, USA

Talia Knecht
Department of Pharmaceutical and Administrative Sciences, Loma Linda University School of Pharmacy, Loma Linda, CA 92350, USA
Department of Psychology, University of California, San Diego, CA 92093, USA

Jeffrey Liu
Department of Pharmaceutical and Administrative Sciences, Loma Linda University School of Pharmacy, Loma Linda, CA 92350, USA
Department of Neuroscience, University of California, Riverside, CA 92521, USA

Cesar V. Borlongan
Department of Neurosurgery and Brain Repair, Center of Excellence for Aging and Brain Repair, University of South Florida College of Medicine, Tampa, FL 33612, USA

Grzegorz Meder
Department of Interventional Radiology, Jan Biziel University Hospital No. 2, Ujejskiego 75 Street, 85-168 Bydgoszcz, Poland

Piotr Płeszka and Violetta Palacz-Duda
Stroke Intervention Centre, Department of Neurosurgery and Neurology, Jan Biziel University Hospital No. 2, Ujejskiego 75 Street, 85-168 Bydgoszcz, Poland

Milena Świtońska
Stroke Intervention Centre, Department of Neurosurgery and Neurology, Jan Biziel University Hospital No. 2, Ujejskiego 75 Street, 85-168 Bydgoszcz, Poland
Department of Neurosurgery and Neurology, Faculty of Health Sciences, Nicolaus Copernicus University in Toruń, Ludwik Rydygier Collegium Medicum, Ujejskiego 75 Street, 85-168 Bydgoszcz, Poland

Paweł Sokal
Department of Neurosurgery and Neurology, Faculty of Health Sciences, Nicolaus Copernicus University in Toruń, Ludwik Rydygier Collegium Medicum, Ujejskiego 75 Street, 85-168 Bydgoszcz, Poland

Dorota Dzianott-Pabijan
Neurological Rehabilitation Ward Kuyavian-Pomeranian Pulmonology Centre, Meysnera 9 Street, 85-472 Bydgoszcz, Poland

Adam Wiśniewski
Department of Neurology, Faculty of Medicine, Nicolaus Copernicus University in Toruń, Collegium Medicum in Bydgoszcz, 85-094 Bydgoszcz, Poland

Karolina Filipska and Robert Ślusarz
Department of Neurological and Neurosurgical Nursing, Faculty of Health Sciences, Nicolaus Copernicus University in Toruń, Collegium Medicum in Bydgoszcz, 85-821 Bydgoszcz, Poland

Joanna Sikora
Experimental Biotechnology Research and Teaching Team, Department of Transplantology and General Surgery, Nicolaus Copernicus University in Toruń, Collegium Medicum in Bydgoszcz, 85-094 Bydgoszcz, Poland

Grzegorz Kozera
Medical Simulation Centre, Medical University of Gdańsk, Faculty of Medicine, 80-210 Gdańsk, Poland
Medical Simulation Centre, Medical University of Gdańsk, Faculty of Medicine, Dębowa 17 Street, 80-208 Gdańsk, Poland

Minho Han, Jin Kyo Choi, Junghye Choi and Jimin Ha
Department of Neurology, Yonsei University College of Medicine, Seoul 03722, Korea

Adam Lemanowicz and Zbigniew Serafin
Department of Radiology, Collegium Medicum in Bydgoszcz, Nicolaus Copernicus University in Toruń, Skłodowskiej 9 Street, 85-094 Bydgoszcz, Poland

Eunjeong Park
Cardiovascular Research Institute, Yonsei University College of Medicine, Seoul 03722, Korea

Tae-Jin Song
Department of Neurology, Seoul Hospital, Ewha Womans University College of Medicine, Seoul 07804, Korea

Chrissoula Liantinioti, Lina Palaiodimou, Aikaterini Theodorou, Maria Chondrogianni, Christina Zompola, Sokratis Triantafyllou, Andromachi Roussopoulou, Anastasios Bonakis, Konstantinos Voumvourakis and Georgios Tsivgoulis
Second Department of Neurology, "Attikon" University Hospital, School of Medicine, National and Kapodistrian University of Athens, 12462 Athens, Greece

Konstantinos Tympas, John Parissis, Ignatios Ikonomidis and Gerasimos Filippatos
Second Department of Cardiology, "Attikon" University Hospital, Medical School, National and Kapodistrian University of Athens, 12462 Athens, Greece

Odysseas Kargiotis
Stroke Unit, Metropolitan Hospital, 18547 Piraeus, Greece

Aspasia Serdari and Konstantinos Vadikolias
Department of Neurology, University Hospital of Alexandroupolis, Democritus University of Thrace, School of Medicine, 68100 Alexandroupolis, Greece

Leonidas Stefanis
Second Department of Neurology, "Attikon" University Hospital, School of Medicine, National and Kapodistrian University of Athens, 12462 Athens, Greece
First Department of Neurology, Eginition Hospital, National and Kapodistrian University of Athens, School of Medicine, 11528 Athens, Greece

Young Dae Kim, Ji Hoe Heo, JoonNyung Heo, Minyoung Kim, Jin Kyo Choi and Hyo Suk Nam
Department of Neurology, Yonsei University College of Medicine, Seoul 03722, Korea

Sung-Il Sohn and Jeong-Ho Hong
Department of Neurology, Brain Research Institute, Keimyung University School of Medicine, Daegu 41931, Korea

Joonsang Yoo and Hyungjong Park
Department of Neurology, Yonsei University College of Medicine, Seoul 03722, Korea
Department of Neurology, Brain Research Institute, Keimyung University School of Medicine, Daegu 41931, Korea

Byung Moon Kim and Dong Joon Kim
Department of Radiology, Yonsei University College of Medicine, Seoul 03722, Korea

Oh Young Bang, Woo-Keun Seo and Jong-Won Chung
Department of Neurology, Samsung Medical Center, Sungkyunkwan University School of Medicine, Seoul 06351, Korea

Hyeon Chang Kim
Department of Preventive Medicine, Yonsei University College of Medicine, Seoul 03722, Korea

Euna Han
College of Pharmacy, Yonsei Institute for Pharmaceutical Research, Yonsei University, Incheon 21983, Korea

Kyung-Yul Lee
Department of Neurology, Gangnam Severance Hospital, Severance Institute for Vascular and Metabolic Research, Yonsei University College of Medicine, Seoul 06273, Korea

Hye Sun Lee
Department of Research Affairs, Biostatistics Collaboration Unit, Yonsei University College of Medicine, Seoul 06273, Korea

Dong Hoon Shin
Department of Neurology, Gachon University Gil Medical Center, Incheon 21565, Korea

Hye-Yeon Choi
Department of Neurology, Kyung Hee University Hospital at Gangdong, Kyung Hee University School of Medicine, Seoul 05278, Korea

Chulho Kim
Department of Neurology, Chuncheon Sacred Heart Hospital, Chuncheon 24253, Korea
Chuncheon Translational Research Center, Hallym University College of Medicine, Chuncheon 24252, Korea

Gyu Sik Kim
Department of Neurology, National Health Insurance Service Ilsan Hospital, Ilsan 10444, Korea

Seo Hyun Kim
Department of Neurology, Yonsei University Wonju College of Medicine, Wonju 26426, Korea

Sang Won Han and Joong Hyun Park
Department of Neurology, Sanggye Paik Hospital, Inje University College of Medicine, Seoul 01757, Korea

Jinkwon Kim
Department of Neurology, Gangnam Severance Hospital, Severance Institute for Vascular and Metabolic Research, Yonsei University College of Medicine, Seoul 06273, Korea
Department of Neurology, CHA Bundang Medical Center, CHA University, Seongnam 13496, Korea
Department of Neurology, Yongin Severance Hospital, Yonsei University College of Medicine, Yongin-si 16995, Korea

Yo Han Jung
Department of Neurology, Changwon Fatima Hospital, Changwon 51394, Korea

Han-Jin Cho
Department of Neurology, Pusan National University School of Medicine, Busan 49241, Korea

Seong Hwan Ahn
Department of Neurology, Chosun University School of Medicine, Gwangju 61453, Korea

Sung Ik Lee
Department of Neurology, Sanbon Hospital, Wonkwang University School of Medicine, Sanbon 15865, Korea

Kwon-Duk Seo
Department of Neurology, National Health Insurance Service Ilsan Hospital, Ilsan 10444, Korea
Department of Neurology, Sanbon Hospital, Wonkwang University School of Medicine, Sanbon 15865, Korea

Jang-Hyun Baek
Department of Neurology, Kangbuk Samsung Hospital, Sungkyunkwan University School of Medicine, Seoul 03181, Korea
Department of Neurology, Severance Stroke Center, Severance Hospital, Yonsei University College of Medicine, Seoul 03722, Korea

Ji Hoe Heo, Hyo Suk Nam and Young Dae Kim
Department of Neurology, Severance Stroke Center, Severance Hospital, Yonsei University College of Medicine, Seoul 03722, Korea

Byung Moon Kim and Dong Joon Kim
Interventional Neuroradiology, Severance Stroke Center, Severance Hospital, Department of Radiology, Yonsei University College of Medicine, Seoul 03722, Korea

Jin Woo Kim
Department of Radiology, Gangnam Severance Hospital, Yonsei University College of Medicine, Seoul 06273, Korea

Ioannis Tsogkas, Amélie Carolina Hesse, Daniel Behme, Katharina Schregel and Michael Knauth
Department of Neuroradiology, University Medical Center Goettingen, 37075 Goettingen, Germany

Marios-Nikos Psychogios and Alex Brehm
Department of Neuroradiology, University Medical Center Goettingen, 37075 Goettingen, Germany
Department of Neuroradiology, Clinic for Radiology & Nuclear Medicine, University Hospital Basel, 4031 Basel, Switzerland

Ilko L. Maier, Marlena Schnieder, Mathias Bähr and Jan Liman
Department of Neurology, University Medical Center Goettingen, 37075 Goettingen, Germany

Ismini Papageorgiou
Department of Neuroradiology, Südharz Klinikum, 99734 Nordhausen, Germany

David S. Liebeskind
Neurovascular Imaging Research Core and Stroke Center, Department of Neurology, University of California Los Angeles, Los Angeles, CA 90095, USA

Mayank Goyal
Calgary Stroke Program, Department of Clinical Neurosciences, University of Calgary, Calgary, AB 2500, Canada

Eunhee Park, Ae-Ryoung Kim and Tae-Du Jung
Department of Rehabilitation Medicine, School of Medicine, Kyungpook National University, Daegu 41944, Korea
Department of Rehabilitation Medicine, Kyungpook National University Hospital, Daegu 41944, Korea

Dae-Won Gwak and Seung-Hwan Jung
Department of Rehabilitation Medicine, School of Medicine, Kyungpook National University, Daegu 41944, Korea

Yu-Sun Min
Department of Rehabilitation Medicine, School of Medicine, Kyungpook National University, Daegu 41944, Korea
Department of Rehabilitation Medicine, Kyungpook National University Hospital, Daegu 41944, Korea
Department of Biomedical Engineering, Seoul National University College of Medicine, Seoul 03080, Korea

Jang Woo Park and Hyunsil Cha
Department of Medical & Biological Engineering, Kyungpook National University, Daegu 41944, Korea

Yongmin Chang
Department of Medical & Biological Engineering, Kyungpook National University, Daegu 41944, Korea
Department of Radiology, Kyungpook National University Hospital, Daegu 41944, Korea

Department of Molecular Medicine, School of Medicine, Kyungpook National University, Daegu 41944, Korea

Jens Eyding
Department of Neurology, Klinikum Dortmund gGmbH, Beurhausstr 40, 44137 Dortmund, Germany
Department of Neurology, University Hospital Knappschaftskrankenhaus, Ruhr University Bochum, 44892 Bochum, Germany

Christian Fung
Department of Neurosurgery, University hospital, University of Freiburg, 79106 Freiburg, Germany

Wolf-Dirk Niesen
Department of Neurology, University hospital, University of Freiburg, 79106 Freiburg, Germany

Christos Krogias
Department of Neurology, St. Josef-Hospital, Ruhr University Bochum, 44791 Bochum, Germany

Giovanni Merlino and Simone Lorenzut
Stroke Unit, Department of Neuroscience, Udine University Hospital, Piazzale S. Maria della Misericordia 15, 33100 Udine, Italy

Carmelo Smeralda, Andrea Surcinelli and Mariarosaria Valente
Clinical Neurology, Udine University Hospital, 33100 Udine, Italy
Department of Medical Area (DAME), University of Udine, 33100 Udine, Italy

Gian Luigi Gigli
Clinical Neurology, Udine University Hospital, 33100 Udine, Italy
Department of Mathematics, Informatics and Physics (DMIF), University of Udine, 33100 Udine, Italy

Minho Han, Young Dae Kim, Jin Kyo Choi, Ji Hoe Heo and Hyo Suk Nam
Department of Neurology, Yonsei University College of Medicine, Seoul 03722, Korea

Joonsang Yoo
Department of Neurology, Keimyung University School of Medicine, Daegu 42601, Korea

Hyungjong Park
Department of Neurology, Yonsei University College of Medicine, Seoul 03722, Korea
Department of Neurology, Keimyung University School of Medicine, Daegu 42601, Korea

Joanna Boinska, Katarzyna Ziołkowska and Danuta Rość
Department of Pathophysiology, Collegium Medicum in Bydgoszcz, Nicolaus Copernicus University in Toruń, Skłodowskiej 9 Street, 85-094 Bydgoszcz, Poland

Sang-Hwa Lee
Department of Neurology, Chuncheon Sacred Heart Hospital, Chuncheon 24253, Korea

Jae-Sung Lim, Mi Sun Oh, Kyung-Ho Yu and Byung-Chul Lee
Department of Neurology, Hallym University Sacred Heart Hospital, Anyang 14068, Korea

Yerim Kim and Ju-Hun Lee
Department of Neurology, Kangdong Sacred Heart Hospital, Seoul 05355, Korea

Min Uk Jang
Department of Neurology, Dongtan Sacred Heart Hospital, Hwaseong 18450, Korea

San Jung
Department of Neurology, Kangnam Sacred Heart Hospital, Seoul 07440, Korea

Index

Printed in the USA
CPSIA information can be obtained
at www.ICGtesting.com
JSHW052128021123
51365JS00005B/27